Protocols for High-Risk Pregnancies

An Evidence-Based Approach

Protocols for High-Risk Pregnancies

An Evidence-Based Approach

EDITED BY

John T. Queenan MD

Professor and Chairman, Emeritus
Department of Obstetrics & Gynecology
Georgetown University School of Medicine
Washington, DC, USA

Catherine Y. Spong MD

Bethesda, MD, USA

Charles J. Lockwood MD, MHCM

Dean, Morsani College of Medicine
Senior Vice President, USF Health
Professor of Obstetrics and Gynecology and Public Health
University of South Florida
Tampa, FL

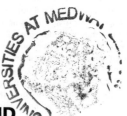

SIXTH EDITION

WILEY Blackwell

This edition first published 2015, © 1982, 1987, 1996, 2005, 2010, 2015 by John Wiley & Sons, Ltd

Registered office: John Wiley & Sons, Ltd, The Atrium, Southern Gate, Chichester, West Sussex, PO19 8SQ, UK

Editorial offices: 9600 Garsington Road, Oxford, OX4 2DQ, UK

The Atrium, Southern Gate, Chichester, West Sussex, PO19 8SQ, UK

111 River Street, Hoboken, NJ 07030-5774, USA

For details of our global editorial offices, for customer services and for information about how to apply for permission to reuse the copyright material in this book please see our website at www.wiley.com/wiley-blackwell

The right of the author to be identified as the author of this work has been asserted in accordance with the UK Copyright, Designs and Patents Act 1988.

Designations used by companies to distinguish their products are often claimed as trademarks. All brand names and product names used in this book are trade names, service marks, trademarks or registered trademarks of their respective owners. The publisher is not associated with any product or vendor mentioned in this book. It is sold on the understanding that the publisher is not engaged in rendering professional services. If professional advice or other expert assistance is required, the services of a competent professional should be sought.

The contents of this work are intended to further general scientific research, understanding, and discussion only and are not intended and should not be relied upon as recommending or promoting a specific method, diagnosis, or treatment by health science practitioners for any particular patient. The publisher and the author make no representations or warranties with respect to the accuracy or completeness of the contents of this work and specifically disclaim all warranties, including without limitation any implied warranties of fitness for a particular purpose. In view of ongoing research, equipment modifications, changes in governmental regulations, and the constant flow of information relating to the use of medicines, equipment, and devices, the reader is urged to review and evaluate the information provided in the package insert or instructions for each medicine, equipment, or device for, among other things, any changes in the instructions or indication of usage and for added warnings and precautions. Readers should consult with a specialist where appropriate. The fact that an organization or Website is referred to in this work as a citation and/or a potential source of further information does not mean that the author or the publisher endorses the information the organization or Website may provide or recommendations it may make. Further, readers should be aware that Internet Websites listed in this work may have changed or disappeared between when this work was written and when it is read. No warranty may be created or extended by any promotional statements for this work. Neither the publisher nor the author shall be liable for any damages arising herefrom.

Library of Congress Cataloging-in-Publication Data

Protocols for high-risk pregnancies : an evidence-based approach / edited by John T. Queenan, Catherine Y. Spong, Charles J. Lockwood. – Sixth edition.

p. ; cm.

Includes bibliographical references and index.

ISBN 978-1-119-00087-7 (cloth)

I. Queenan, John T., editor. II. Spong, Catherine Y., editor. III. Lockwood, Charles J., editor.

[DNLM: 1. Pregnancy Complications. 2. Pregnancy, High-Risk. 3. Evidence-Based Medicine. WQ 240]

RG571

618.3–dc23

2015003151

A catalogue record for this book is available from the British Library.

Wiley also publishes its books in a variety of electronic formats. Some content that appears in print may not be available in electronic books.

Cover image: ©iStock.com/stereohype

Set in 9.5/13pt Meridien by Laserwords Private Limited, Chennai, India

Printed and bound in Malaysia by Vivar Printing Sdn Bhd

1   2015

Contents

List of Contributors

Richard M.K. Adanu
Population Family and Reproductive Health
Department, University of Ghana School of
Public Health, Accra, Ghana, Africa

Brenna L. Hughes (Anderson)
Department of Obstetrics and Gynecology,
Warren Alpert Medical School of Brown
University/Women & Infants Hospital,
Providence, RI, USA

Raul Artal
Department of Obstetrics, Gynecology and
Women's Health, Saint Louis University,
St. Louis, MO, USA

Vincenzo Berghella
Department of Obstetrics and Gynecology,
Division of Maternal-Fetal Medicine, Thomas
Jefferson University, Philadelphia, PA, USA

Richard L. Berkowitz
Department of Obstetrics and Gynecology,
Division of Maternal Fetal Medicine, Columbia
University Medical Center, New York, NY, USA

Robert L. Brent
Alfred I. duPont Hospital for Children, Thomas
Jefferson University, Wilmington, DE, USA

Joshua A. Copel
Departments of Obstetrics, Gynecology and
Reproductive Sciences, and Pediatrics, Yale
School of Medicine, New Haven, CT, USA

F. Garry Cunningham
Department of Obstetrics and Gynecology,
University of Texas Southwestern Medical
Center, Dallas, TX, USA

Mary E. D'Alton
Department of Obstetrics and Gynecology,
Columbia University College of Physicians and
Surgeons, New York Presbyterian Hospital,
New York, NY, USA

Mara J. Dinsmoor
Department of Obstetrics and Gynecology,
NorthShore University Health System,
Evanston, IL, USA
Department of Obstetrics and Gynecology,
Pritzker School of Medicine, University of
Chicago, Chicago, IL, USA

Patrick Duff
Department of Obstetrics and Gynecology,
University of Florida College of Medicine,
Gainesville, FL, USA

Roger K. Freeman
Long Beach Memorial Medical Center,
University of California Irvine, Long Beach,
CA, USA

Steven G. Gabbe
Department of Obstetrics and Gynecology,
The Ohio State University College of Medicine,
Columbus, OH, USA

Henry L. Galan
Department of Obstetrics and Gynecology,
University of Colorado School of Medicine,
Aurora, CO, USA

Sreedhar Ghaddipati
Department of Obstetrics and Gynecology,
Division of Maternal Fetal Medicine,
Columbia University Medical Center,
New York, NY, USA

Robert Gherman
Division of Maternal Fetal Medicine, Frannklin
Square Medical Center, Baltimore, MD, USA

Alessandro Ghidini
Perinatal Diagnostic Center, Inova Alexandra
Hospital, Alexandria, VA, USA

Jane Hitti
Department of Obstetrics and Gynecology,
University of Washington, Seattle, WA, USA

G. Justus Hofmeyr
Department of Obstetrics and Gynecology,
Frere Maternity Hospital/University of the
Witwatersrand/University of Fort Hare/
Eastern Cape Department of Health, Bhisho,
South Africa

Fred M. Howard
Department of Obstetrics and Gynecology,
University of Rochester School of Medicine
and Dentistry, Rochester, NY, USA

Andra H. James
Division of Maternal-Fetal Medicine,
Department of Obstetrics & Gynecology,
Duke University, Durham, NC, USA

Jeffrey R. Johnson
Women and Children's Hospital, Buffalo,
NY, USA

Mark B. Landon
Department of Obstetrics and Gynecology,
The Ohio State University College of Medicine,
Columbus, OH, USA

Charles J. Lockwood
Dean, Morsani College of Medicine
Senior Vice President, USF Health
Professor of Obstetrics and Gynecology and
Public Health
University of South Florida, Tampa, FL

Men-Jean Lee
Department of Obstetrics & Gynecology, Icahn
School of Medicine at Mount Sinai, New York,
NY, USA

George A. Macones
Department of Obstetrics & Gynecology,
Washington University School of Medicine,
St Louis, MO, USA

Maureen P. Malee
University of Illinois McKinley Health Center,
Urbana, IL, USA

Fergal D. Malone
Department of Obstetrics and Gynecology, Royal
College of Surgeons in Ireland, Dublin, Ireland
The Rotunda Hospital, Dublin, Ireland

David S. McKenna
Maternal-Fetal Medicine, Miami Valley Hospital,
Dayton Ohio, USA

Brian Mercer
Department of Obstetrics & Gynecology, Case
Western University-MetroHealth Medical
Center, Cleveland, OH, USA

Kenneth J. Moise Jr
Department of Obstetrics, Gynecology and
Reproductive Sciences, UT Health School of
Medicine, Houston, TX, USA

Thomas R. Moore
Department of Reproductive Medicine, Division
of Perinatal Medicine, University of California at
San Diego, San Diego, CA, USA

Michael P. Nageotte
Miller Children's and Women's Hospital,
Long Beach, CA, USA
Department of Obstetrics and Gynecology,
University of California, Irvine, CA, USA

Gayle Olson
Department of Obstetrics & Gynecology,
University of Texas Medical Branch, Galveston,
TX, USA

John Owen
Department of Obstetrics and Gynecology,
Division of Maternal-Fetal Medicine,
University of Alabama at Birmingham,
Birmingham, AL, USA

Yinka Oyelese
Atlantic Health System, Morristown, NJ, USA

Marc R. Parrish
Department of Obstetrics and Gynecology,
University of Kansas Medical Center, Kansas
City, KS, USA

Alan Peaceman
Division of Maternal-Fetal Medicine,
Northwestern University Feinberg School
of Medicine, Chicago, IL, USA

John T. Queenan, Jr.
Department of Obstetrics and Gynecology,
University of Rochester Medical Center,
Rochester, NY, USA

Susan Ramin
Department of Obstetrics and Gynecology,
Baylor College of Medicine, Texas Children's
Hospital Pavilion For Women, Houston, TX, USA

Robert Resnik
Department of Reproductive Medicine, UCSD
School of Medicine, La Jolla, CA, USA

Dwight J. Rouse
Maternal-Fetal Medicine Division, Women &
Infants Hospital of Rhode Island, Providence,
RI, USA
Department of Obstetrics and Gynecology,
Warren Alpert School of Medicine at Brown
University, Providence, RI, USA

George Saade
Department of Obstetrics & Gynecology,
Division of Maternal Fetal Medicine,
University of Texas Medical Branch, Galveston,
TX, USA

Michael Schatz
Department of Allergy, Kaiser-Permanente
Medical Center, San Diego, CA, USA

James R. Scott
Department of Obstetrics and Gynecology,
University of Utah Medical Center, Salt Lake
City, UT, USA

Jeanne S. Sheffield
Division of Maternal-Fetal Medicine, University
of Texas Southwestern Medical Center, Dallas,
TX, USA

Baha M. Sibai
Department of Obstetrics and Gynaecology and
Reproductive Sciences, The University of Texas
Medical School at Houston, Houston, TX, USA

Robert M. Silver
Department of Obstetrics & Gynecology,
Division of Maternal-Fetal Medicine, University
of Utah Health Sciences Center, Salt Lake City,
UT, USA

Lynn L. Simpson
Department of Obstetrics and Gynecology,
Columbia University Medical Center, New York,
NY, USA

Catherine Y. Spong
Bethesda, MD, USA

Stephen F. Thung
Department of Obstetrics and Gynecology,
The Ohio State University College of Medicine,
Columbus, OH, USA

Jorge E. Tolosa
Department of Obstetrics and Gynecology,
Division of Maternal-Fetal Medicine, Oregon
Health & Science University, Portland, OR, USA
Departamento de Obstetricia y Ginecología,
Facultad de Medicina, NACER Salud Sexual y
Reproductiva, Universidad de Antioquia,
Colombia

Katharine D. Wenstrom
Division of Maternal-Fetal Medicine, Women &
Infants' Hospital of Rhode Island and Brown
Alpert Medical School, Providence, RI, USA

Deborah A. Wing
Department of Obstetrics and Gynecology,
Division of Maternal-Fetal Medicine, University
of California, Irvine, CA, USA

Kimberly Yonkers
Department of Psychiatry, Yale University
School of Medicine, New Haven, CT, USA
Department of Obstetrics, Gynecology and
Reproductive Sciences, Yale University School
of Medicine, New Haven, CT, USA
School of Epidemiology and Public Health,
Yale University School of Medicine, New Haven,
CT, USA

Preface

Today's pressures of healthcare reform, rapidly changing technology, "information overload," and medically sophisticated patients make it essential to have correct, concise, and relevant information at hand. The nature and training of physicians instills a constant drive to always try to do the right thing. Therefore, it is necessary to have appropriate, current, and practical information available as protocols to make good decisions. Why use protocols? Having a protocol or guideline organizes essential clinical material in a systematic, logical order and avoids omissions in patient care. It is to this end that we have created the sixth edition of *Protocols for High-Risk Pregnancies*.

Evaluating all pregnancies for risk factors is an effective way of identifying patients who need special care. Some patients have factors present at the outset of pregnancies such as diabetes or history of prematurity that place them at increased risk. Others start with uneventful pregnancies but subsequently develop complications such as fetal growth restriction, preeclampsia, or premature rupture of the membranes. These conditions may develop quickly and, therefore, it is important to have a protocol for management. Of course, care must be taken to be sure that the term "high risk" does not cause alarm or anxiety for your patient.

Since the fifth edition was published, advances in medicine and technology have dictated changes in management. Thus, in the sixth edition, all protocols have been reviewed and new protocols added to cover advances in Doppler and sonography, as well as changes in approach to prematurity, depression, diagnosis and treatment of venous thromboembolism, and fetal growth restriction, among others. We have included protocols in areas of critical importance to the developing world such as malaria, tuberculosis, and chronic iron deficiency anemia.

For each protocol, we have invited physicians who are outstanding authorities on the topics. They start with a brief introduction and pathophysiology and write the protocol as if they were working up their patients and following them through the various stages of management.

We required that each protocol is evidence-based to the maximum extent possible. In areas where no clear evidence exists, we have asked the experts to exercise their best judgment and make necessary recommendations. All protocols represent the individual thoughts and opinions of the experts.

We thank John C. Hobbins who was the codeveloper and coeditor for the first five editions. We are indebted to our Editorial Coordinator, Michele Prince, whose skills made this edition exceptional in every aspect. At Wiley-Blackwell we have enjoyed excellent expertise from Martin Sugden, Rob Blundell, Priyanka Gibbons, and their outstanding editorial and production staffs.

This edition, as the others, was created to be practical, cost effective, and clearly presented: a format that is easy to carry with you on rounds and consultations. We have designed this book to help you in your practice. Make it your own!

John T. Queenan, MD
Professor and Chairman, Emeritus
Department of Obstetrics & Gynecology
Georgetown University School of Medicine
Washington, DC, USA

Catherine Y. Spong, MD
Bethesda, MD, USA

Charles J. Lockwood, MD
Department of Obstetrics and Gynecology and Reproductive Sciences,
University of South Florida, Morsani College of Medicine,
Tampa, FL, USA

PART I
Concerns in Pregnancy

PROTOCOL 1

Tobacco, Alcohol, and the Environment

Jorge E. Tolosa[1,2] & George Saade[3]

[1]Department of Obstetrics and Gynecology, Division of Maternal-Fetal Medicine, Oregon Health & Science University, Portland, OR, USA
[2]Departamento de Obstetricia y Ginecología, Facultad de Medicina, NACER Salud Sexual y Reproductiva, Universidad de Antioquia, Colombia
[3]Department of Obstetrics & Gynecology, Division of Maternal Fetal Medicine, University of Texas Medical Branch, Galveston, TX, USA

Tobacco
Clinical significance

Globally, 22% of the world's adult population aged 15 years and over are estimated to be current tobacco smokers, including 36% of men and 8% of women. The World Health Organization European and Americas regions have the highest prevalence of current tobacco smoking among adult women. There is a stark difference in smoking rates between women of low income countries (whose tobacco smoking rates are low to very low) and women of middle and high-income countries (whose tobacco smoking rates are high to very high). Global tobacco use continues to shift to low and middle-income countries, with a recent increase in the rates of tobacco smoking among women, which is expected to rise to 20% by 2025. About 250 million women worldwide are daily smokers. Women 18–19 years old show the highest prevalence (17.1%); 26% smoked half a pack or more of cigarettes a day. An estimated 19.8 million women in the United States smoke. The annual average rate of past month cigarette use in 2012 and 2013 among women aged 15 to 44 who were pregnant was 15.4 percent. Rates of current cigarette use in 2012–2013 among pregnant women aged 15 to 44 were 19.9 percent in the first trimester, 13.4 percent in the second trimester, and 12.8 percent in the third trimester. The women most likely to smoke are among the most vulnerable—those disadvantaged by low income, low education, and mental health disorders, further exacerbating the adverse health effects from smoking on mothers and their offspring. Women in these groups are also less likely to quit smoking when they become pregnant and are more likely to relapse after delivery.

Tobacco exposure in pregnancy is associated with an increased rate of adverse outcomes including low birth weight, resulting from preterm birth

Protocols for High-Risk Pregnancies: An Evidence-Based Approach, Sixth Edition.
Edited by John T. Queenan, Catherine Y. Spong and Charles J. Lockwood.
© 2015 John Wiley & Sons, Ltd. Published 2015 by John Wiley & Sons, Ltd.

and/or fetal growth restriction. In 2003 in the United States, nonsmokers had a rate of 7.7% of low-birth-weight babies compared with 12.4% born to smokers. Tobacco dependence is a chronic addictive condition that requires repeated intervention for cessation. Although a light smoker is defined as a cigarette smoker of fewer than 10 per day, smoking is unsafe at all levels, as is exposure to any form of tobacco in pregnancy. Tobacco cessation in pregnancy results in reduction in preterm birth, fetal growth restriction, low birth weight and perinatal death, as well as in improved neonatal outcomes. It is the most important preventable cause of low birth weight.

Pathophysiology

Tobacco smoke contains thousands of compounds that may have adverse effects. The major compounds suspected of causing harm to the developing fetus are nicotine and carbon monoxide. Nicotine crosses the placenta and can be detected in the fetal circulation at levels that exceed maternal concentrations by 15%, while amniotic fluid concentrations of nicotine are 88% higher than maternal plasma. The actions of nicotine include vasoconstriction and decreased uterine artery blood flow. Carbon monoxide also crosses the placenta rapidly and is detectable in the fetal circulation at levels that are 15% higher than maternal. It has a higher affinity for hemoglobin than oxygen to form the compound carboxyhemoglobin that shifts the oxygen dissociation curve to the left. Consequently, the availability of oxygen to fetal tissues is decreased. Levels of cyanide in the circulation are higher in smokers, a substance that is toxic to rapidly dividing cells. In addition, smokers frequently have other clinical characteristics that may account for some adverse pregnancy outcomes, such as poor nutrition, and alcohol or drug abuse.

Screening for tobacco exposure and increasing tobacco cessation

Smoking cessation interventions for pregnant women result in fewer low-birth-weight newborns and perinatal deaths, fewer physical, behavioral and cognitive problems during infancy and childhood, and important health benefits for the mothers. Women who discontinue smoking even as late as 30 weeks of gestation have infants with higher birth weight than those who continue smoking. In contrast, "cutting down" seems to improve fetal growth only slightly.

Smoking cessation interventions should be included as part of prenatal care. Women are more likely to quit smoking during pregnancy than at any other time in their lives. An office-based cessation counseling session of 5–15 minutes, when delivered by a trained provider with the provision of pregnancy-specific educational materials, increases rates of cessation among pregnant smokers. Trials have shown that a five-step intervention program (the 5 As) is effective:

1 *Ask* pregnant women about smoking status using a multiple-choice question method to improve disclosure.

2 *Advise* women who smoke to quit smoking, with unequivocal, personalized and positive messages about the benefits for her, the baby and family. Review the risks associated with continued smoking. Congratulate women who have quit and reinforce the decision by reviewing the benefits resulting from not smoking.

3 *Assess* the woman's willingness to make an attempt to quit smoking within the next 30 days. If the woman wants to try to quit, the provider should move to the next step, Assist. For women who are unwilling to attempt cessation, the advice, assessment and assistance should be offered at each future visit.

4 *Assist*
   • Provide self-help smoking cessation materials that contain messages to build motivation and confidence in support of a cessation attempt.
   • Suggest and encourage the use of problem-solving methods and skills for cessation for issues that the woman believes might adversely influence her attempt to quit. Avoid "trigger situations."
   • Arrange social support in the smoker's environment by helping her identify and solicit help from family, friends, co-workers and others who are most likely to be supportive of her quitting smoking.
   • Provide social support as part of the treatment. This means that the counselor is encouraging, communicates care and concern, and encourages the patient to talk about the process of quitting.

5 *Arrange* follow up. Smoking status should be monitored throughout pregnancy, providing opportunities to congratulate and support success, reinforce steps taken toward quitting, and advise those still considering a cessation attempt.

Pharmaceutical cessation aids such as nicotine replacement therapy (NRT), varenicline, or bupropion SR have efficacy as first-line agents in the general non-pregnant population. *The use of these medications is not yet routinely recommended in pregnancy*, as there is inconclusive data of their effectiveness and safety. NRT is available in transdermal patch, nasal spray, chewing gum, or lozenge. If used, it should be with extreme caution and women should be warned of uncertain side effects in pregnancy. Bupropion SR is an atypical antidepressant that has been approved by the FDA for use in smoking cessation. It is contraindicated in patients with bulimia, anorexia nervosa, use of MAO inhibitors within the previous 14 days, or a known or history of seizures. It carries a black box warning due to an association of antidepressant medications with suicidality in children, adolescents, and young adults under the age of

24 years. Varenicline is approved for smoking cessation in the general population. Serious neuropsychiatric symptoms have been associated with its use including agitation, depression, and suicidality. The FDA issued a public health advisory in 2008 cautioning its use in populations with a history of psychiatric illness. To date, contingency management, or the use of tangible reinforcement to promote desired behaviors, is the most promising technique to achieve smoking cessation and has been shown to be an effective motivational tool for overcoming other addictions, including alcohol and substance abuse. Four small randomized trials and a recent systematic review of the published literature of contingency management in pregnancy demonstrate an increase in smoking quit rates and potential beneficial effects in reducing adverse pregnancy outcomes. However, the generalizability of these studies in the U.S. and globally is limited especially for women of lower socio-economic status. Adequately powered randomized controlled trials are needed in the US and globally to determine the effectiveness and cost-effectiveness of this intervention.

An increasing proportion of smokers are now using e-cigarettes, either for nicotine delivery or as an attempt to stop smoking. There are limited data on e-cigarettes in pregnancy. In addition to nicotine, some of the e-cigarettes may contain other chemicals such as preservatives. Pregnant women should be discouraged from using e-cigarettes.

ACOG and other organizations including the Centers for Disease Control and Prevention have a number of resources to assist providers in counseling and managing smokers in pregnancy (CDC's Smoking Cessation for Pregnancy and Beyond: A Virtual Clinic: www .smokingcessationandpregnancy.org, ACOG's Smoking Cessation During Pregnancy: A Clinician's guide to helping pregnant women quit smoking: https://www.acog.org/~/media/Departments/Tobacco%20Alcohol%20 and%20Substance%20Abuse/SCDP.pdf, and Clean Air for Healthy Children: www.cleanairforhealthychildren.org).

Complications

Pregnancies among women who smoke have been associated with increased risks for miscarriage, ectopic pregnancy, fetal growth restriction, placenta previa, abruptio placentae, preterm birth, premature rupture of the membranes and low birth weight. Overall, the perinatal mortality rate among smokers is 150% greater than that in nonsmokers.

The progeny of smoking mothers face additional risks during childhood. There is a strong association between maternal smoking and sudden infant death syndrome, and a clear dose–response relationship has been demonstrated. Prenatal and postnatal tobacco smoke exposure also has been associated with increased risk of persisting reduced lung function, respiratory infections, and childhood asthma. Recent studies suggest that infants born to women who smoke during pregnancy may be at increased risk for childhood obesity. In addition, there is evidence suggesting a neurotoxic effect of prenatal tobacco exposure on newborn behavior, i.e., being more excitable and hypertonic. The behavioral and cognitive deficits associated with in utero exposure to tobacco seem to continue into late childhood and adolescence with increased risk for attention-deficit hyperactivity disorder and conduct disorder.

Follow up and prevention

It is essential to identify the pregnant woman who is a smoker, ideally before pregnancy, when the risks associated with smoking in pregnancy should be discussed and the benefits of smoking cessation emphasized. Cotinine, a metabolite of nicotine, is an accurate assay for nicotine exposure when measured in urine and can be part of a cost-effective cessation program. Studies indicate higher success rates when participants are aware that compliance is measured with biochemical tests. Postnatal relapse rates are high, averaging 50–60% in the first year after delivery. Counseling should be continued at each postpartum visit including unequivocal, personalized and positive messages about the benefits to the patient, her baby and family resulting from smoking cessation. If indicated, pharmacotherapy could be recommended to the lactating woman, after giving consideration to the risk for the nursing infant of passage of small amounts of the medications through breast milk, compared to the increased risks associated with smoking for children such as sudden infant death syndrome, respiratory infections, asthma, and middle ear disease.

Alcohol

Clinical significance

In the mother, chronic alcohol abuse is associated with pneumonia, hypertension, hepatitis and cirrhosis, among other serious medical complications. For the fetus, it is a known teratogen. *Alcohol exposure in pregnancy is the leading known cause of mental retardation and the leading preventable cause of birth defects in Western societies.* As many as 1 in 100 births are affected in the United States. Fetal alcohol syndrome is characterized by fetal growth restriction, central nervous system abnormalities and facial dysmorphology, with an average IQ of 70. Functionally, the spectrum of disease even when fetal alcohol syndrome is not fully expressed includes hyperactivity, inattention, memory deficits, inability to solve problems, and mood disorders.

It has been estimated that the risk of fetal alcohol syndrome is 20% if the pregnant woman consumes four drinks per day, increasing to 50% with eight drinks per day. No safe level of exposure to alcohol has been identified, thus alcohol consumption during pregnancy should be avoided.

Public health warnings about the importance of avoiding alcohol in pregnancy were initiated 30 years ago. Despite this, the 2007 National Survey on Drug Use and Health found that among pregnant women between 15 and 44 years of age, 11.6% used alcohol in the previous 30 days and 0.7% were classified as heavy drinkers (five or more drinks on one occasion, on 5 or more days in the last 30 days) and 6.6% reported binge drinking in the first trimester.

Screening for alcohol abuse in pregnancy

Identifying women who drink during pregnancy is difficult. While a recent report reveals that 97% of women are asked about alcohol use as part of their prenatal care, only 25% of practitioners use standard screening tools.

There is no validated biological marker for alcohol available for use in the clinical setting. Healthcare providers have to rely on self-reported use, resulting in significant underreporting. Of available screening tools, the T-ACE is validated for pregnant women.

Tolerance (T): The first question is "How may drinks can you hold?" A positive answer, scored as a 2, is at least a 6-pack of beer, a bottle of wine or 6 mixed drinks. This suggests a tolerance of alcohol and very likely a history of at least moderate to heavy alcohol consumption.

Annoyed (A): "Have people annoyed you by criticizing your drinking?"

Cut down (C): "Have you felt you ought to cut down on your drinking?"

Eye opener (E): "Have you ever had a drink first thing in the morning to steady your nerves or get rid of a hangover?"

These last three questions, if answered positively, are worth 1 point each. A score on the entire scale of 2 or higher is considered positive for excessive or risk drinking. Follow up of a positive screen should include questions about volume and frequency. A report of more than seven standard drinks per week, less if any single drinking episode involves more than three standard drinks, should be considered at risk. A standard drink is defined as 12 ounces of beer, 5 ounces of wine, or 1.5 ounces of liquor in a mixed drink. The T-ACE has been reported to identify 90% or more of women engaging in risk drinking during pregnancy.

Treatment of risk drinking in pregnancy

Advice by the healthcare provider is valid, effective and feasible in the clinical office setting. Brief behavioral counseling interventions with follow up in the clinical setting have been demonstrated to produce significant reductions in alcohol consumption lasting at least 12 months. Practitioners need to be aware of the possibility of concurrent psychiatric and/or social problems. Consultation with mental health professionals and social workers is indicated and can be powerful adjuvants to assist women to discontinue use of alcohol.

Brief interventions for pregnancy risk drinking generally involve systematic counseling sessions, approximately 5 minutes in length, which are tailored to the severity of the identified alcohol problem. In the first intervention, the provider should state her/his concern, give advice, and help to set a goal. Educational written materials should be provided. Routine follow up is essential and should involve encouragement, information and re-evaluation of goals at each prenatal visit. Women who are actually alcohol-dependent may require additional assistance to reduce or eliminate consumption during pregnancy. For these women, referral for more intensive intervention and alcohol treatment needs to be recommended. No randomized clinical trials for pregnant women enrolled in alcohol treatment in pregnancy have been conducted to test the use of pharmacological or psychosocial interventions as reported by the Cochrane collaboration.

Environmental hazards

In 1970, the Occupational Safety and Health Act was implemented with a surge of interest in the reproductive effects of working and the workplace. While an adult worker with an occupational exposure is best served by referral to an occupational medicine specialist, workplace exposures of pregnant women tend to be avoided by occupational physicians and the responsibility for these issues thus falls to the obstetrician. In their *Guidelines for Perinatal Care*, the American Academy of Pediatrics and the American College of Obstetricians and Gynecologists include environmental and occupational exposures among the components of the preconceptional and antepartum maternal assessment and counseling. Help is available in the form of Teratogen Information Services, accessed through local health departments, and via the databases, such as REPROTOX (http://reprotox.org/) and TERIS (http://depts.washington.edu/~terisweb/teris/), which were set up to provide information to physicians and the Teratogen Information Services on potential teratogens from any source, including the workplace.

Physical agents
Heat
The metabolic rate increases during pregnancy, and the fetus's temperature is approximately 1°C above the mother's. Because pregnant women have to eliminate the physiological excess heat, they may be less tolerant of high

environmental temperatures. Exposure to heat and hot environments can occur in many occupations and industries. Few studies specifically address the hazards of occupational heat stress in pregnancy. Data from animal studies and fever during pregnancy indicate that core temperature elevations to 38.9°C or more may increase the rate of spontaneous abortion or birth defects, most notably neural tube defects. Women with early pregnancy hyperthermic episodes should be counseled about possible effects and offered alpha-fetoprotein screening and directed sonogram studies.

Chemical exposures
Hairstylists
Hair colorants and dyes contain aromatic amines that may be absorbed through the skin. These agents are mutagenic but are not teratogenic in rats and cause embryotoxicity in mice only at high doses that are also maternally toxic. Permanent wave solutions may cause maternal dermatitis but are not known to be teratogenic in animals.

There is no direct evidence that hair dyes and permanent wave solutions are teratogenic in human pregnancy, but very limited data are available. One study found a higher rate of spontaneous abortion among cosmetologists. Exposure to these agents should be minimized by the use of gloves and, if possible, reduction of chronic exposures in the first trimester.

Painters and artists
Organic and inorganic pigments may be used in paints. The raw materials for organic pigments may contain aromatic hydrocarbons, such as benzene, toluene, naphthalene, anthracene, and xylene. Inorganic pigments may contain lead, chromium, cadmium, cobalt, nickel, mercury, and manganese. Workers in battery plants and those involved in the removal of old paint are also exposed to lead salts.

Reproductive concerns about inorganic pigments are focused primarily on lead, which is readily transferred across the placenta. Inorganic lead salts have been associated with increased spontaneous abortion, infant cognitive impairment, and stillbirth rates in humans, and central nervous system abnormalities and clefting in rodents. Women at risk of lead exposure should be monitored for blood lead levels before becoming pregnant. If blood lead concentration is greater than 10 micrograms/mL, the patient should be removed from exposure and chelation considered before pregnancy. Chronically exposed workers will have significant bone lead stores and should remain in a lead-free environment until safe lead levels are reached before attempting pregnancy. There is no consensus on how to manage elevated blood lead levels during pregnancy as chelation will at least temporarily elevate blood lead levels by releasing bone stores. Further, the chelating agent, calcium edetate, may be developmentally toxic, probably by decreasing zinc stores.

Solvent workers

Some organic hydrocarbons may cause a fetal dysmorphogenesis syndrome comparable to fetal alcohol syndrome if ingested in large amounts. This has best been evaluated for gasoline, in a group of individuals who habitually "sniffed" the fuel for its euphoric effects. An excess of mental retardation, hypotonia, and microcephaly was found in the offspring. The effects of lower levels of gasoline are not known. Similar effects were reported with toluene sniffing.

   Ethylene glycol is another solvent used in a large number of industrial processes (paint, ink, plastics manufacture). No human studies exist, but in rodents many studies report abnormal development and skeletal and central nervous system abnormalities. If a woman has a considerable exposure level as determined by blood and urine levels or abnormal liver function tests, increased monitoring of fetal development is recommended.

Pesticide workers

Pesticides are often encountered in agricultural workers and landscape artists. Two common agents are carbaryl and pentachlorophenol. A suspected workplace exposure may be quantitated by urine levels. Human studies for these agents are not available but animal studies suggest that high doses, particularly those that produce maternal toxicity, may impair reproductive success and be responsible for skeletal and body wall defects. These outcomes may be related to maternal toxicity and may not be a specific developmental effect.

Exposure to inhalational anesthetics

The studies that have suggested an association between occupational exposure to inhalational anesthetics and adverse reproductive outcomes have been heavily criticized. The available scientific evidence, while weak, does lead to concern over occupational exposure to inhalational anesthetics in the trace concentrations encountered in adequately scavenged operating rooms. Recommending limitation of exposure may be reasonable in environments where scavenging equipment is not available, such as some dentists' offices.

Other occupational hazards
Air travel

The environment in passenger cabins of commercial airlines is maintained at the equivalent of 5000–8000 feet. While living at high altitude has significant effects on maternal and fetal physiology, air travel has not been associated with harmful fetal effects because of the short duration of most flights. Adequate hydration is essential as the humidity is also reduced to less than 25% in most cabins. Intermittent ambulation and changing posture is recommended in order to prevent deep vein thrombosis. Reports indicate that flight attendants experience twice the incidence of first trimester spontaneous abortions as other women, but not other employed women. Most airlines restrict the working air travel of flight attendants after 20 weeks of gestation, and restrict commercial airline pilots from flying once pregnancy is diagnosed. Counseling for women with medical or obstetric complications should be individualized. It should be noted that air travel could contribute to background radiation. The magnitude of in-flight exposure to radiation depends on altitude and the solar cycle. A round trip between New York and Seattle can result in exposure to 6 mrem (0.06 mSv), well below the safe upper limit accepted by most experts. Because the effect may be cumulative, frequent flyers need to keep track of their exposure. Patients and physician can consult the FAA's radiation estimation software (http://jag.cami.jccbi.gov./cariprofile.asp) to calculate the exposure and the National Oceanic and Atmospheric Administration (http://www.sec.noaa.gov) to check for solar flares.

Suggested reading

Tobacco

Fiore MC, Jaén CR, Baker TB, *et al.* Treating Tobacco Use *and Dependence: 2008 Update.* Clinical Practice Guideline. Rockville, MD: US Department of Health and Human Services, Public Health Service, May 2008.Hamilton, BE., Martin, JA., Ventura, SJ. (2013). Births: Final data for 2011. National vital statistics reports 61(5). Hyattsville, MD: National Center for Health Statistics. Retrieved July 2, 2013, from http://www.cdc.gov/nchs/data/nvsr/nvsr62/nvsr62_01.pdf.

Chamberlain C, O'Mara-Eves A, Oliver S, Caird JR, Perlen SM, Eades SJ, Thomas J. Psychosocial interventions for supporting women to stop smoking in pregnancy. Cochrane Database of Systematic Reviews 2013, Issue 10. Art. No.: CD001055. DOI: 10.1002/14651858.CD001055.pub4.

Smoking cessation during pregnancy. Committee Opinion No. 471. American College of Obstetricians and Gynecologists. *Obstet Gynecol* 2010;116:1241–4. (Reaffirmed 2013).

U.S. Department of Health and Human Services. The Health Consequences of Smoking: 50 Years of Progress. A Report of the Surgeon General. Atlanta, GA: U.S. Department of Health and Human Services, Centers for Disease Control and Prevention, National Center for Chronic Disease Prevention and Health Promotion, Office on Smoking and Health, 2014. Printed with corrections, January 2014.

Likis FE, Andrews JC, Fonnesbeck CJ, Hartmann KE, Jerome RN, Potter SA, Surawicz TS, McPheeters ML. Smoking Cessation Interventions in Pregnancy and Postpartum Care. Evidence Report/Technology Assessment No.214. (Prepared by the Vanderbilt Evidence-based Practice Center under Contract No. 290-2007-10065-I.) AHRQ Publication no. 14-E001-EF. Rockville, MD. Agency for Healthcare Research and Quality; February 2014. www.effectivehealthcare.ahrq.gov/reports/final.cfm.

World Health Organization. *WHO Recommendations for the Prevention and Management of Tobacco Use and Second-Hand Smoke Exposure in Pregnancy*. Geneva: World Health Organization; 2013.

U.S. Department of Health and Human Services Substance Abuse and Mental Health Services Administration Center for Behavioral Health Statistics and Quality. National Survey on Drug Use and Health, 2013. Inter-University Consortium for Political and Social Research (ICPSR) [distributor].

Alcohol

At-Risk Drinking and Illicit Drug Use: Ethical Issues in Obstetric and Gynecologic Practice. ACOG Committee Opinion No.422. American College of Obstetricians and Gynecologists. *Obstet Gynecol* 2008;112:1449–1460.

Chang G. Screening and brief intervention in prenatal care settings. *Alcohol Res Health* 2004;28(2):80–84.

Lui S, Terplan M, Smith EJ. Psychosocial interventions for women enrolled in alcohol treatment during pregnancy. *Cochrane Database Syst Rev* 2008;(3).

Sokol RJ, Martier S, Ager J. The T-ACE questions: practical prenatal detection of risk-drinking. *Am J Obstet Gynecol* 1989;160:863–70.

Substance Abuse and Mental Health Services Administration. *Results from the 2007 National Survey on Drug Use and Health*. (www.oas.samhsa.gov/nsduh/reports.htm).

Environmental agents

Barish RJ. In-flight radiation exposure during pregnancy. *Obstet Gynecol* 2004;103: 1326–30.

Chamberlain G. Women at work in pregnancy. In: Chamberlain G (ed.) *Pregnant Women at Work*. New York: Macmillan, 1984.

Frazier LM, Hage ML (eds) *Reproductive Hazards of the Workplace. New York*; Chichester: John Wiley & Sons, 1998.

Mittlemark RA, Dorey FJ, Kirschbaum TH. Effect of maternal exercise on pregnancy outcome. In: Mittlemark RA, Drinkwater BL (eds) *Exercise in Pregnancy*, 2nd edn. Baltimore: Williams & Wilkins, 1991.

Paul M (ed.) *Occupational and Environmental Reproductive Hazards: A Guide for Clinicians*. Baltimore: Williams & Wilkins, 1993.

Scialli AR. The workplace. In: Scialli AR (ed.) *A Clinical Guide to Reproductive and Developmental Toxicology*. Boca Raton: CRC Press, 1992.

PROTOCOL 2

Ionizing Radiation

Robert L. Brent

Alfred I. duPont Hospital for Children, Thomas Jefferson University, Wilmington, DE, USA

In 2013, an extensive update of radiation risks was published by the National Council on Radiation Protection and Measurements (NCRP 174, 2013). The new material dealing with the preconception and postconception risks of ionizing will be summarized in this protocol.

Ionizing radiation associated with medical procedures is typically the radiation exposure that causes the greatest concern and anxiety to pregnant women. However, if imaging examinations are medically indicated and performed with proper equipment and careful technique, then the potential immediate benefit to the health of the patient and the embryo or fetus will outweigh the radiation risks. Most diagnostic medical imaging procedures in radiography, computed tomography (CT), conventional fluoroscopy, and nuclear medicine subject the embryo or fetus to absorbed doses of less than 0.1 Gy (10 rad). Doses delivered to the embryo or fetus during fluoroscopically guided interventional procedures and during the course of radiation therapy may be higher.

Preconception ionizing radiation risks

There is no convincing direct evidence of heritable disease in the offspring of humans attributable to ionizing radiation, yet radiation clearly induces mutations in microbes and somatic cells of rodents and humans, and transgenerational effects in irradiated drosophila and mice are established. It would be imprudent to ignore the possibility of human germ-cell mutation. However, the data indicated that the risk is not measurable in humans.

The inheritance of mutations is a process that, in theory, has both a background component that is intrinsic in an individual and an induced component that results from environmental exposures such as ionizing radiation. A very small but undefined fraction of hereditary human disease is attributable to the environmental agents with mutagenic potential.

Protocols for High-Risk Pregnancies: An Evidence-Based Approach, Sixth Edition.
Edited by John T. Queenan, Catherine Y. Spong and Charles J. Lockwood.

In the absence of adequate human data, modeling and extrapolation have guided radiation protection.

Genetic risk is generally estimated using three components:

- doubling dose for radiation-induced germ-cell mutations in mice;
- background rate of sporadic genetic disease in humans; and
- population-genetics theory and experience.

One additional consideration is that some deleterious mutations (spontaneous or as a result of preconception radiation exposure) would not be expressed as effects in an offspring because they are lethal to the developing ova (eggs) or sperm or to the developing embryo because of defective ova or sperm, a consideration that has been described as biological filtration.

There is little to no convincing or consistent evidence among the offspring of childhood cancer survivors, atomic-bomb survivors, environmentally exposed populations, or occupationally exposed workers for an excess of cytogenetic syndromes, single-gene disorders, malformations, stillbirths, neonatal deaths, cancer, or cytogenetic markers that would indicate an increase of heritable genetic mutations in the exposed parents.

James V. Neel, M.D., Ph.D., a geneticist, spent a major part of his scientific life studying the genetic effects of the atomic bomb in the children of the exposed parents (Neel 1990, Annual Review in Genetics 24: 327–362). Studies of eight indicators in the children of the atomic bomb survivors and suitable controls suggested that the genetic doubling dose for the spectrum of acute gonadal radiation (experienced by survivors of the atomic bombings) is in the neighborhood of 2.0 Gy. For extrapolation to the effects of chronic radiation Neel used a dose rate factor of 2, resulting in a doubling dose estimate of 4.0 Gy. Using the specific locus test of Russell (Russell 1956, 1965, 1976) Russell *et al.* 1958; Schull *et al.* 1981, Neel concluded that his estimate of the doubling dose was acceptable. It would be impossible to demonstrate this risk in a human population exposed to less than 0.1 Gy (10 rad). You would need tens of thousands of exposed humans in the study. Preconception gonadal (sperm, ova) exposure to diagnostic radiological tests are unlikely to have a measurable genetic risk.

Exposure during pregnancy

What are the reproductive and developmental risks of in utero exposures to ionizing radiation exposure?

1 Birth defects, mental retardation and other neurobehavioral effects, growth retardation and embryonic death are deterministic effects (threshold effects). This indicates that these effects have a NOAEL (no adverse effect level). Almost all diagnostic radiological procedures

provide exposures that are below the NOAEL for these developmental effects. Diagnostic radiological studies rarely exceed 0.1 Gy (10 rad), while the threshold for congenital malformations or miscarriage is more than 20 rad (0.2 Gy) (Table 2.1).

2 For the embryo to be deleteriously affected by ionizing radiation when the mother is exposed to a diagnostic study, the embryo has to be exposed above the NOAEL in order to increase the risk of deterministic effects. This rarely happens when pregnant women have X-ray studies of the head, neck, chest or extremities.

3 During the pre-implantation and pre-organogenesis stages of embryonic development, the embryo is least likely to be malformed by the effects of ionizing radiation because many of the cells of the very young embryo are omnipotential and can replace adjacent cells that have been deleteriously affected. This early period of development has been designated as the "all or none" period.

4 Protraction and fractionation of exposures of ionizing radiation to the embryo decrease the magnitude of the deleterious effects of deterministic effects.

5 The increased risk of cancer following high exposures to ionizing radiation exposure to adult populations has been demonstrated in the atomic bomb survivor population. Radiation-induced carcinogenesis is assumed to be a stochastic effect (non-threshold effect), so that there is theoretically a risk at low exposures. While there is no question that high exposures of ionizing radiation can increase the risk of cancer, the magnitude of the risk of cancer from embryonic exposures following diagnostic radiological procedures is very controversial. Recent publications and analyses indicate that the risk is lower for the irradiated embryo than for the irradiated child which surprised many scientists interested in this subject (Preston *et al.* 2008).

Evaluating the risks

The responsibility of evaluating risks of environmental toxicants to the pregnant patient and her embryo frequently is the responsibility of the obstetrician. When evaluating the risks of ionizing radiation, the physician is faced with several different clinical situations, as outlined below.

1 The pregnant patient presents with clinical symptoms that need to be evaluated. What is the appropriate utilization of diagnostic radiological procedures that may expose the embryo or fetus to ionizing radiation?

A pregnant or possibly pregnant woman complaining of gastrointestinal bleeding, abdominal or back pain, or an abdominal or pelvic mass that cannot be attributed to pregnancy deserves the appropriate studies

Table 2.1 Radiation exposure and risk at different gestational phases

Stage, Gestation weeks	Effect
First and second weeks post first day of the last menstrual period (LMP). (Prior to conception)	First two weeks post first day of the last menstrual period. This is a preconception radiation exposure. Mother has not yet ovulated
Third and fourth week of gestation (First two weeks post conception)	Minimum human acute lethal dose (from animal studies) approximately 0.15–0.20 Gy. Most sensitive period for the induction of embryonic death
Fourth to eighth week of gestation (Second to sixth week post conception)	Minimum lethal dose (from animal studies) at 18 days post conception is 0.25 Gy (25 rad).
	After 50 days post conception, more than 0.50 Gy (50 rad) predisposes embryo to the induction of major malformations and growth retardation.
	Minimum dose for growth retardation at 18–36 days is 0.20–0.50 Gy (20 rad-50 rad and at 36–110 days is 0.25–0.5 Gy (25–50 rad). But the induced growth retardation during this period is not as severe as during mid-gestation from similar exposures
Eighth to fifteenth week of gestation	Most vulnerable period for irreversible whole body growth retardation, microcephaly and severe mental retardation. Threshold for severe metal retardation is 0.35–0.50 Gy (35–50 rad) (Schull and Otake 1999). Miler indicated that the threshold was more than 50 rad (1999). Decrease in I.Q. may occur at lower exposures but is difficult to document. There is no increased risk for mental retardation with exposures less than 0.10 Gy
Sixteenth week to term of gestation	Higher exposures can produce growth retardation and decreased brain size and intellect, although the effects are not as severe as what occurs from similar exposures during mid-gestation. There is no risk for major anatomical malformations. The threshold dose for lethality (from animal studies) from 15 weeks to term is more than 1.5 Gy (150 rad).
	Minimum dose for severe mental retardation at 15 weeks to term is more than1.50 Gy, but decrease in I.Q. can occur at lower exposures.

There is no evidence that radiation exposure in the diagnostic ranges (less than 0.10 Gy, less than 10 rad) is associated with measurably increased incidence of congenital malformation, stillbirth, miscarriage, growth, and mental retardation.

to diagnose and treat her clinical problems, including radiological studies. Furthermore, these studies should not be relegated to one portion of the menstrual cycle if she has not yet missed her period. The studies should be performed at the time they are clinically indicated whether or not the woman is in the first or second half of the menstrual cycle.

2 The patient has completed a diagnostic procedure that has exposed her uterus to ionizing radiation. Her pregnancy test was negative. She now believes she was pregnant at the time of the procedure. What is your response to this situation?

Explain that you would have proceeded with the necessary X-ray diagnostic test whether she was pregnant or not, since diagnostic studies that are indicated in the mother have to take priority over the possible risk to her embryo, because almost 100% of diagnostic studies do not increase the risks to the embryo (Table 2.1). Secondly, she must have been very early in her pregnancy, since her pregnancy test was negative. At this time, obtain the calculated dose to the embryo and determine her stage of pregnancy. If the dose is below 0.1 Gy (10 rad) (0.1 Sv), you can inform the mother that her risks for birth defects and miscarriage have not been increased. In fact, the threshold for these effects is 20 rad (0.2 Gy) at the most sensitive stage of embryonic development (Tables 2.1 and 2.2). Of

Table 2.2 Risk of less than 0.1 Gy (less than 10 rad).

Risk	Zero rad exposure	Additional risk of less than 0.1 Gy (less than 10 rad) exposure
Risk of very early pregnancy loss, before the first missed period	350,000/10^6 pregnancies	0
Risk of spontaneous abortion in known pregnant women	150,000/10^6 pregnancies	0
Risk of major congenital malformations	30,000/10^6	0
Risk of severe mental retardation	5,000/10^6	0
Risk of childhood leukemia/year	40/10^6 /year	less than 2/10^6/year
Risk of early-onset or late-onset genetic disease	100,000/10^6	Very low risk is in next generation and there is not measurable increase with small populations
Prematurity	40,000/10^6 pregnancies	0
Growth retardation	30,000/10^6 pregnancies	0
Stillbirth	20–2000/10^6 pregnancies	0
Infertility	7% of couples	0

course, you are obligated to tell her that every healthy woman is at risk for the background incidence of birth defects and miscarriage, which is 3% for birth defects and 15% for miscarriage.

3 A woman delivers a baby with serious birth defects. On her first post-partum visit, she recalls that she had a diagnostic x-ray study early in her pregnancy. What is your response when she asks you whether the baby's malformation could be caused by the radiation exposure?

In most instances, the nature of the clinical malformations will rule out radiation teratogenesis. At this time, a clinical teratologist or radiation embryologist could be of assistance. On the other hand, if the exposure is below 0.1 Gy (10 rad), it would not be scientifically supportable to indicate that the radiation exposure was the cause of the malformation. As mentioned before, the threshold for malformations is 0.20 Gy (20 rad) exposure. The nature of the malformation would enter into this analysis.

In order to appropriately and more completely respond to these questions, the obstetrician should rely on the extensive amount of information that has accumulated on the effects of radiation to the embryo. There is no environmental hazard that has been more extensively studied or on which more information is available (Tables 2.1 and 2.2).

Radiation risks to the embryo

There is no question that an acute exposure to ionizing radiation above 0.5 Gy represents a significant risk to the embryo, regardless of the stage of gestation. The threshold dose for low LET ionizing radiation that results in an increase in malformations is approximately 0.02–0.1 Gy (Table 2.1). Although congenital malformations are unlikely to be produced by radiation during the first 14 days of human development, there would be a substantial risk of embryonic loss if the dose is high. From approximately the 18th day to the 40th day postconception, the embryo would be at risk for an increased frequency of anatomical malformations if the embryonic exposure is greater than 20–25 rad (0.2–0.25 Gy). Up until about the 15th week, the embryo maintains an increased susceptibility to central nervous system (CNS) effects, major CNS malformations early in gestation and mental retardation in mid-gestation. Of course, with very high doses, more than 1 Gy, mental retardation can be produced in the latter part of gestation. While it is true that the embryo is sensitive to the deleterious effects of these mid-range exposures of ionizing radiation, the measurable effects fall off rapidly as the exposure approaches the usual exposures that the embryo receives from diagnostic radiological procedures less than 0.1 Gy (10 rad). The threshold of 20 rad at the most sensitive stage of development (20–25 days postconception) is raised by protraction of the radiation exposure, for example, following several clinical diagnostic radiological procedures occurring over a period of days.

That is why the recommendation of most official organizations, including the National Council on Radiation Protection and Measurements (NCRP), indicates that exposures in the diagnostic range will not increase the risk of birth defects or miscarriage. The risks of radiation exposure to the human embryo when the exposure exceeds the no-effect dose (20 rad) are:

- Embryonic loss
- Growth retardation
- Congenital malformations
- Carcinogenesis (the magnitude of the risk is controversial)
- Microcephaly and mental retardation.

Because all of the above effects are threshold phenomena, except for carcinogenesis, radiation exposure below 0.1 Gy (10 rad) literally presents no measurable risk to the embryo. Even if one accepts the controversial concept that the embryo is more vulnerable to the carcinogenic effects of radiation than the child, the risk at these low exposures is much smaller that the spontaneous risks. Furthermore, other studies indicate that Stewart's estimate of the risk involved is exaggerated.

Table 2.2 compares the spontaneous risks facing an embryo at conception and the risks from a low exposure of ionizing radiation.

Therefore, the hazards of exposures in the range of diagnostic roentgenology less than 0.1 Gy (10 rad) present an extremely low risk to the embryo, when compared with the spontaneous mishaps that can befall human embryos (Table 2.2). Approximately 30–40% of human embryos abort spontaneously (many abort before the first missed menstrual period). Human infants have a 2.75% major malformation rate at term, which rises to approximately 4–6% once all malformations become manifest. When the data and risks are explained to the patient, the family with a wanted pregnancy invariably continues with the pregnancy.

The difficulty that frequently arises is that the risks from diagnostic radiation are evaluated outside the context of the significant normal risks of pregnancy. Furthermore, many physicians approach the evaluation of diagnostic radiation exposure with either of two extremes: a cavalier attitude or panic. The usual procedures in clinical medicine are ignored, and an opinion based on meager information is given to the patient. Frequently, it reflects the physician's bias about radiation effects or his or her ignorance of the field of radiation biology. We have patient records in our files of scores of patients who were not properly evaluated but were advised to have an abortion following radiation exposure.

Evaluating the patient

After thorough evaluation in most instances, the dose to the embryo is estimated to be less than 0.1 Gy (10 rad) and frequently is less than 1 rad (0.01 Gy). Our experience has taught us that there are many variables involved in radiation exposure to a pregnant or potentially pregnant woman. Therefore, there is no routine or predetermined advice that can be given in this situation. However, if physicians take a systematic approach to the evaluation of the possible effects of radiation exposure, they can help the patient make an informed decision about continuing the pregnancy. This systematic evaluation can begin only when the following information has been obtained:

- Stage of pregnancy at the time of exposure
- Menstrual history
- Previous pregnancy history
- Family history of congenital malformations and miscarriages
- Other potentially harmful environmental factors during the pregnancy
- Ages of the mother and father
- Type of radiation study, dates and number of studies performed
- Calculation of the embryonic exposure by a medical physicist or competent radiologist when necessary
- Status of the pregnancy: wanted or unwanted.

An interpretation should be made of the information, with both patient and counselor arriving at a decision. The physician should place a summary of the information in the medical record. It should state that the patient has been informed that every pregnancy has a significant risk of problems and that the decision to continue the pregnancy does not mean that the counselor is guaranteeing the outcome of the pregnancy. The use of amniocentesis and ultrasound to evaluate the fetus is an individual decision that would have to be made in each pregnancy but is rarely indicated.

The carcinogenic effects of radiation

The carcinogenic risk of in-utero radiation is an important topic that cannot be addressed completely in this protocol. Alice Stewart published the results of her case–control studies indicating that diagnostic radiation from pelvimetry increased the risk of childhood leukemia by 50% (Table 2.2). That would change the risk of childhood leukemia from four cases per 100,000 to six cases per 100,000 in the population of exposed fetuses. This has been a very controversial subject. A recent publication by Preston *et al.* (2008) presented data from the in utero population of the A-bomb survivors, which indicated that the embryo was less vulnerable to the

Table 2.3 Parameter estimates and 95% confidence intervals for solid cancer excess risks for atomic-bomb survivors in the in utero and childhood cohorts

Risk Estimates (per unit weighted organ dose)*,†	Cohort Age at Exposure	Male	Female	Sex-Averaged
ERR Gy^{-1}	*In utero*	0.3 (0.0–2.0)	0.5 (0.0–2.4)	0.4 (0.0–2.0)
	Early childhood	1.3 (0.6–2.2)	2.2 (1.3–3.4)	1.7 (1.1–2.5)
EAR (104 PY Gy)$^{-1}$ at 50 y of age	*In utero*	4.3 (0.001–36)	9.2 (0.002–65)	6.8 (0.002–48)
	Early childhood	36 (16–63)	76 (49–100)	56 (36–79)

*Weighted organ doses are the estimated absorbed dose from gamma rays plus 10 times the estimated absorbed dose from neutrons. In this report, the weighted organ dose is presented in gray; it has also been reported in the literature in sievert.
†For the in utero cohort, weighted uterine dose; for the early childhood cohort, weighted colon dose.
The *excess relative risk* (ERR) is the ratio of the excess risk of a specified disease to the probability of the same effect in the unexposed population.
The *excess absolute rate* (EAR) is the excess rate of a specified disease in a specified population among exposed persons per unit dose. In radiation-exposed populations, the EAR is designated as the number of excess cases of a specific disease in radiation-exposed persons per 10,000 persons-years per gray [$(10^4$PY Gy$)^{-1}$].
The *excess absolute risk* (of solid tumors) is much greater for irradiated children than for exposed embryos.
Source: Preston *et al.* 2008. Adapted with permission of Oxford University Press.

oncogenic effects of ionizing radiation than the child (Table 2.3). Patients can be told that the fetal risks are extremely small, so small that we cannot measure the risks because that would require a large exposed population.

The risk of cancer in offspring that have been exposed to diagnostic x-ray procedures while in utero has been debated for 55 years. High doses at high dose rates to the embryo or fetus (e.g., more than 0.5 Gy) increase the risk of cancer. This has been demonstrated in human epidemiology studies as well as in mammalian animal studies. Most pregnant women exposed to diagnostic x-ray procedures or the diagnostic use of radionuclides receive doses to the embryo or fetus less than 0.1 Gy (10 rad). The risk of cancer in offspring exposed in utero at a low dose such as less than 0.1 Gy (10 rad) is controversial and has not been definitively determined.

Research at the University of Rochester in 1951 demonstrated that the rat embryo was less vulnerable to the carcinogenic risks of ionizing radiation than the postnatal animal. The use of chemical carcinogens such as urethane also indicated that the postnatal animal was more vulnerable than the embryo to the carcinogenic risks of some chemical carcinogens.

In the 1950s, Stewart and others published numerous case–control studies that indicated that the embryo was the most vulnerable organism to the carcinogenic effects of low exposures of ionizing radiation (pelvimetry). There are 17 cohort studies of pregnant women exposed to diagnostic radiological studies, none of which were positive, however many of the studies contained too few subjects to negate the impact of the many case control studies. In 2008, Preston *et al.* published the results of the in utero exposed population to the atomic bomb, which indicated that the embryo was less vulnerable to the carcinogenic effect of ionizing radiation (Table 2.3).

The Preston *et al.* (2008) study is important because it demonstrates that radiation exposure in utero is associated with increased risks of adult-onset solid tumors, which was not new information.

> The difference in ERRs and EARs between the two cohorts suggests that lifetime cancer risks at 57 y of age following in utero exposure are lower than risks for early childhood exposure

However, the investigators state, "additional follow-up of this cohort is necessary before definitive conclusions can be made about the nature of the risks for those exposed in utero" (Preston *et al.* 2008). Mortality follow-up for the in utero cohort, however, was available from 1950 and indicated no deaths from childhood leukemia (Delongchamp *et al.* 1997). Another limitation is the small numbers of cancers in each dose category in the in utero cohort. Nevertheless, this investigation is the only cohort study with long-term, continuous, active follow-up of a population with in utero radiation exposure and high-quality estimated doses for each subject.

At this time (2014), diagnostic imaging procedures utilizing ionizing radiation that are clinically indicated for the pregnant patient should be performed because the clinical benefits outweigh the potential carcinogenic risks. However, when it has been determined that the procedure is necessary, it should be tailored to effectively manage the dose to the embryo or fetus (i.e., use only the least amount of radiation necessary to achieve the clinical purpose).

The background risk for lethal cancers is 23% (23,000 per 100,000 individuals) due to the background spontaneous incidence of cancer. That is thousands of times greater than the estimated cancer risks of low dose radiation to the developing embryo, with the possibility that there might not be an increase risk.

Diagnostic or therapeutic abdominal radiation in women of reproductive age

In women of reproductive age, it is important for the patient and physician to be aware of the pregnancy status of the patient before performing any type of x-ray procedure in which the ovaries or uterus will be exposed. If the embryonic exposure will be 0.1 Gy (10 rad) or less, the radiation risks to the embryo are very small when compared with the spontaneous risks (Table 2.2). Even if the exposure is less than 0.1 Gy (10 rad), this exposure is far from the threshold or no-effect dose of 20 rad. The patient will accept this information if it is offered as part of the *preparation* for the x-ray studies at a time when both the physician and patient are aware that a pregnancy exists or may exist. The pregnancy status of the patient should be determined and noted.

Because the risks of less than 0.1 Gy (10-rad) fetal irradiation are so small, the immediate medical care of the mother should take priority over the risks of diagnostic radiation exposure to the embryo. X-ray studies that are essential for optimal medical care of the mother and evaluation of medical problems that need to be diagnosed or treated should not be postponed. Elective procedures such as employment examinations or follow-up examinations, once a diagnosis has been made, need not be performed on a pregnant woman even though the risk to the embryo is not measurable. If other procedures (e.g., MRI or ultrasound) can provide adequate information without exposing the embryo to ionizing radiation, then of course they should be used. Naturally, there is a period when the patient is pregnant but the pregnancy test is negative and the menstrual history is of little use. However, the risks of less than 0.1 Gy (10 rad) or less are extremely small during this period of pregnancy (all or none period, first two weeks postconception). The patient will benefit from knowing that the diagnostic study was indicated and should be performed in spite of the fact that she may be pregnant.

Scheduling the examination

In those instances in which elective X-ray studies need to be scheduled, it is difficult to know whether to schedule them during the first half of the menstrual cycle just before ovulation or during the second half of the menstrual cycle, when most women will not be pregnant. The genetic risk of diagnostic exposures to the oocyte or the embryopathic effects on the preimplanted embryo is extremely small, and there are no data available to compare the relative risk of less than 0.1 Gy (10 rad) to the oocyte or the preimplanted embryo. If the diagnostic study is performed in the first 14 days of the menstrual cycle, should the patient be advised to defer conception for several months, based on the assumption that the deleterious effect of radiation to the ovaries decreases with increasing time between radiation exposure and a subsequent ovulation? Physicians are in a quandary because they may be warning the patient about a very-low-risk phenomenon. On the other hand, avoiding conception for several months is not an insurmountable hardship. This potential genetic hazard is quite speculative for man, as indicated by the report by the BEIR V and NCRP 174 committee report dealing with preconception radiation.

> "It is not known whether the interval between irradiation of the gonads and conception has a marked effect on the frequency of genetic changes in human offspring, as has been demonstrated in the female mouse. Nevertheless, patients receiving high doses to the gonads (>25 rad) may be advised to wait for several months after such exposures before conceiving additional offspring."

Because the patients exposed during diagnostic radiological procedures absorb considerably less than 25 rad, the recommendations made here may be unnecessary, but it involves no hardship to the patient or physician. Because both the NCRP and ICRP have previously recommended that elective radiological examinations of the abdomen and pelvis be performed during the first part of the menstrual cycle (10-day rule, 14-day cycle) to protect the zygote from possible but largely conjectural hazards, the recommendation to avoid fertilization of recently irradiated ova perhaps merits equal attention.

Importance of determining pregnancy status of patient

If exposures less than 0.1 Gy (10 rad) do not measurably affect the exposed embryos, and it is recommended that diagnostic procedures should be performed at any time during the menstrual cycle, if necessary, for the medical care of the patient, why expend energy to determine the pregnancy status of the patient?

There are several reasons why the physician and patient should share the burden of determining the pregnancy status before performing an x-ray or nuclear medicine procedure that exposes the uterus:

1 If the physician is forced to include the possibility of pregnancy in the differential diagnosis, a small percentage of diagnostic studies may no longer be considered necessary. Early symptoms of pregnancy may mimic certain types of gastrointestinal or genitourinary disease.

2 If the physician and patient are both aware that pregnancy is a possibility and the procedure is still performed, it is much less likely that the patient will be upset if she subsequently proves to be pregnant.

3 The careful evaluation of the reproductive status of women undergoing diagnostic procedures will prevent many unnecessary lawsuits. Even more important, the patient will have more confidence if the decision

to continue the pregnancy is made before the medical x-ray procedure is performed, because the necessity of performing the procedure
would have been determined with the knowledge that the patient
was pregnant.

In every consultation dealing with the exposure of the embryo to diagnostic studies involving ionizing radiation (X-ray, CT scans, use of radionuclides) in which her reproductive risks or developmental risks for her fetus
have not been increased by the radiation exposure, the patient should be
informed that every healthy woman with a negative personal and genetic
family reproductive history has background reproductive risks which are
3% for birth defects and 15% for miscarriage. We cannot change these
background risks, which every women faces.

Suggested reading

Brent RL. Biological factors related to male mediated reproductive and developmental
toxicity. In: Olshan, AF and Mattison, DR (Eds). *Male-Mediated Developmental Toxicity*.
Plenum Press, New York, pp. 209–242, 1994.

Brent, R.L. Saving lives and changing family histories: Appropriate counseling of pregnant women and men and women of reproductive age, concerning the risk of radiation
exposures during and before pregnancy. *Am J Obstet Gynecol* 2009;200(1):4–24.

Brent RL, Frush DP, Harms RW, *et al.* Preconception and prenatal radiation exposure:
Health effects and protective guidance. NCRP Report No. 174. Recommendations of
the National Council on Radiation Protection and Measurements, 342 pp., May 24,
2013.

Neel JV. The comparative radiation genetics of human and mice. *Annu Rev Genet*
1990;24:327–362.

Preston DL, Cullings H, Suyama A, *et al.* Solid cancer incidence in atomic bomb survivors
exposed in utero or as young children. *J Natl Cancer inst* 2008;100:428–436.

Russell LB. Numerical sex-chromosome anomalies in mammals: Their spontaneous
occurrence and use in mutagenesis studies. Hollaender A, *Chemical Mutagens. Principles
and Methods for their Detection*, 1976;4:55–91, New York: Plenum.

Russell WL. Comparison of x-ray-induced mutation rates in Drosophila and mice. *Am
Nat* 1956;90:69–80.

Russell WL. Effect of the interval between irradiation and conception on mutation
frequency in female mice. *Proc Natl Acad Sci USA* 1965;54:1552–1557.

Russell WL, Russell LB, Kelly EM. Radiation dose rate and mutation frequency. *Science*
1958;128:1546–1550.

PROTOCOL 3

Depression

Kimberly Yonkers[1,2,3]

[1] Department of Psychiatry, Yale University School of Medicine, New Haven, CT, USA
[2] Department of Obstetrics, Gynecology and Reproductive Sciences, Yale University School of Medicine, New Haven, CT, USA
[3] School of Epidemiology and Public Health, Yale University School of Medicine, New Haven, CT, USA

Clinical significance

Approximately 20% of women suffer from a depressive disorder at some point in their lives. The risk of being depressed is greatest for women during their reproductive years and thus clinicians may encounter a pregnant woman with pre-existing depression or a woman who becomes depressed during her pregnancy. Some research finds an association between maternal depression and particular perinatal complications, including preterm birth and/or delivery of a low-birth-weight baby, although there are dissenting results. These findings, along with the potentially devastating toll that a major depressive episode (MDE) has on a mother, underscore the need to treat depressed pregnant women. However, when the needed treatment is pharmacotherapy, there are additional concerns because antidepressants, and the anxiolytics that are often used concurrently, are linked with adverse perinatal and fetal outcomes. Researchers note a risk of fetal malformations although this appears to be a small risk that has largely centered on atrial and ventricular septal defects and only with some antidepressants. Other worrisome associations include delivery of an infant who is preterm or small for gestational age, as well as a very small increased likelihood of persistent pulmonary hypertension. The evidence for a number of these outcomes among women treated with antidepressants in pregnancy is mixed, with the strongest support for preterm birth. However, even the smallest risk can lead to apprehension on the part of patients and uneasiness for their prescribing physicians.

Protocols for High-Risk Pregnancies: An Evidence-Based Approach, Sixth Edition.
Edited by John T. Queenan, Catherine Y. Spong and Charles J. Lockwood.
© 2015 John Wiley & Sons, Ltd. Published 2015 by John Wiley & Sons, Ltd.

Pathophysiology

As with many psychiatric disorders, the pathophysiology of a depressive disorder is unknown, although evidence suggests that underlying risk is determined by biology (e.g., genetic factors), stress, and trauma. Co-occurring general medical conditions and exposure to selected medications and other substances can also lead to development of depressive symptoms or an MDE. Brain imaging studies show that individuals with depression have changes in neurocircuitry and volume reductions in critical brain areas such as anterior cingulate cortex, amygdala, and hippocampus. These regions are also affected by elevations in glucocorticoids and there are longstanding theories that implicate dysregulation of the hypothalamic–pituitary–adrenal axis in depression. For example, the introduction of stress leads to secretion of cortisol. The integrity of the feedback systems between cortisol, adrenocorticotrophic hormone, and corticotrophin releasing hormone is compromised in many individuals with depression leading to overexpression of these hormones. Ongoing exposure to these hormones can lead to anatomic and dynamic (signaling) changes in the aforementioned brain regions.

Diagnosis

There are several mood disorders that fall under the category of "depression" and they are outlined in the Diagnostic and Statistical Manual version 5 (Association 2013). The prototypic depressive disorder is an MDE. There are nine candidate symptoms of an MDE including depressed mood, diminished interest, significant weight change, insomnia or hypersomnia, psychomotor retardation or agitation, fatigue, feelings of guilt or worthlessness, decreased concentration and recurrent thoughts of death or suicide. A woman should have at least five of these symptoms, including either depressed mood and/or diminished interest, most of the time for 2 weeks. If a woman has a history of manic/hypomanic episodes as well as MDEs, she suffers from bipolar disorder but is presenting in the depressed phase. Mania is characterized by elevated/expansive/irritable mood, increased energy, grandiosity, decreased need for sleep, pressured speech, and increased participation in goal-related or risky activities. If she has never had manic or hypomanic episodes, and she meets the above criteria, then her diagnosis is unipolar major depressive disorder.

Management

The management of a pregnant woman with an MDE will vary depending upon whether she has unipolar or bipolar illness. In either case, she may benefit from psychotherapy although she should be monitored to ensure that this treatment is sufficient for response. If she requires pharmacotherapy, she should be apprised of the risks and benefits and this should be documented in her medical chart. Along with her obstetrician, it may be prudent to have her evaluated and followed concurrently by a psychiatrist. If she experiences thoughts of self-harm or suicide, she should be evaluated by a psychiatrist or clinical psychologist as soon as possible.

Women with MDE, who suffer from bipolar disorder, will require treatment with a mood stabilizer and an antidepressant. Valproate and carbamazepine are effective mood stabilizers but also established teratogens and should not be used early in pregnancy. Lamotrigine is FDA approved for treatment of individuals with bipolar disorder and may be useful although it must be titrated up slowly. Lithium has been associated with cardiac defects and should be avoided early in pregnancy, although the risk is now considered to be smaller than it was after publication of results from the lithium registry. It is currently thought that the risk of the heart malformation, Ebstein's anomaly is 1–2 per thousand for lithium-exposed babies. However, the risk of other types of cardiac malformations has been reported to be nearly 8-fold higher for lithium-exposed offspring as compared to those nonexposed in the first trimester. First- and second-generation antipsychotics have good mood stabilizing properties and appear to have lower teratogenic risk than anticonvulsants and lithium. If mood improves, there is no need to add an antidepressant.

Women with unipolar MDE who are not sufficiently treated with psychotherapy or women with bipolar disorder who did not respond to a mood stabilizer alone will need treatment with an antidepressant agent. The reproductive safety profile for the older tricyclic antidepressants is no better than for the newer, serotonin or serotonin-norepinephrine reuptake inhibitors. However, older agents have more side effects. It is reasonable to start with either a selective serotonin reuptake inhibitor or bupropion. If a woman is struggling to avoid nicotine cigarettes, use of bupropion may help treat her nicotine addiction and her depression. Given data associating paroxetine use in pregnancy with malformations of the heart, many experts recommend that this agent not be prescribed to pregnant women in the first trimester. However, if a woman presents well into her first trimester of pregnancy, there may be little benefit to switching to a different agent since exposure has already occurred. In any case, women should be counseled to minimize use of other harmful licit and illicit substances such as cigarettes, alcohol or recreational drugs. Use of substances is more common in women with depression as compared to without depression and patients may not realize that cigarettes, alcohol or other drugs are as harmful, if not more problematic than antidepressant agents.

Follow up

It is ideal to see a woman a week after initiation of pharmacotherapy for MDE to determine side effects to the medication and assess further deterioration in psychiatric status. Subsequently, she can be seen again after 2 weeks and then monthly. Some degree of mood improvement may be noticeable within a few weeks. However, it may take 6–8 weeks to see full response to treatment. The patient should be assessed for suicidal thoughts at each visit. While some clinicians have concerns that asking about suicidal thoughts will "suggest" this action to patients, this is not the case. Appropriate emergency medical care can be arranged if the patient endorses suicidal thoughts. If the obstetrician is unable to provide follow-up care at these intervals, the patient may be referred to a psychiatrist who can communicate with the obstetrician with regard to the patient's progress. Once response has been obtained, the patient's mood can be re-evaluated at routine obstetrical visits.

Conclusion

The risk period for an episode of MDE coincides with the period of women's fertility. While some women benefit from psychotherapy and can avoid pharmacotherapy in pregnancy, this is not always the case. Women who have underlying bipolar disorder and those with severe recurrent major depressive disorder will likely require medication management. Antipsychotic agents have a lower risk profile than anticonvulsant mood stabilizers, which should be avoided early in pregnancy. Antidepressants are not major teratogens but clinicians need to apprise patients of potential risks and benefits of treatment, including perinatal complications such as preterm birth or transient neonatal distress.

Suggested reading

American Psychiatric Association. *Diagnostic and Statistical Manual of Mental Disorders*, Fifth Edition. Washington, DC, American Psychiatric Association, 2013.

Chambers C, Hernandez-Diaz H, Marter LV, Werler M, Louik C, Jones K, Mitchell A. Selective serotonin-reuptake inhibitors and risk of persistent pulmonary hypertension of the newborn. *New Eng J Med* 2006;354:579–587.

Kallen B, Reis M. Neonatal complications after maternal concomitant use of SSRI and other central nervous system active drugs during the second or third trimester of pregnancy. *Journal Of Clinical Psychopharmacology* 2012;32(5):608–614.

McKenna K, Koren G, Tetelbaum M, Wilton L, Shakir S, Diav-Citrin O, Levinson A, Zipursky RB, Einarson A. Pregnancy outcome of women using atypical antipsychotic drugs: a prospective comparative study. *J Clin Psych* 2005;66(4):444–449; quiz 546.

Moore JA. An assessment of lithium using the IEHR evaluative process for assessing human developmental and reproductive toxicity of agents. *Reprod Tox* 1995;9(2):175–210.

Ross LE, Grigoriadis S, Mamisashvili L, Vonderporten EH, Roerecke M, Rehm J, Dennis CL, Koren G, Steiner M, Mousmanis P, Cheung A. Selected pregnancy and delivery outcomes after exposure to antidepressant medication: a systematic review and meta-analysis. *JAMA Psychiatry* 2013;70(4):436–443.

Yonkers K, Blackwell K, Glover J, Forray A. Antidepressant use in pregnant and postpartum women. *Ann Rev Clin Psyc* 2014;10:369–392.

Yonkers KA, Norwitz ER, Smith MV, Lockwood CJ, Gotman N, Luchansky E, Lin H, Belanger K. Depression and serotonin reuptake inhibitor treatment as risk factors for preterm birth. *Epidemiology* 2012;23(5):677–685.

PART II

Antenatal Testing

PROTOCOL 4

Prenatal Detection of Fetal Chromosome Abnormality

Fergal D. Malone[1,2]
[1] Department of Obstetrics and Gynecology, Royal College of Surgeons in Ireland, Dublin, Ireland
[2] The Rotunda Hospital, Dublin, Ireland

Overview

Fetal aneuploidy refers to an abnormal number of chromosomes, other than the usual diploid complement of 46 chromosomes. Presence of a single additional chromosome, known as trisomy, is an important cause of congenital malformations. The most common autosomal trisomies are Down syndrome (trisomy 21), Edward syndrome (trisomy 18), and Patau syndrome (trisomy 13). In addition, microdeletions and microduplications of portions of chromosomes are increasingly being recognized as being associated with pediatric abnormalities, such as del22q11 (DiGeorge syndrome) and del7q11.23 (Williams syndrome). Recently, chromosomal microarray analysis has demonstrated submicroscopic abnormalities which cannot be seen with conventional karyotyping, and there is increasing evidence that such "copy number variants" are associated with significant genetic diseases.

Pathophysiology

The phenotype of trisomy 21 occurs when there is a triplication of genes at a particular part of chromosome number 21, known as band 21q22. Nondisjunction of the pair of chromosomes number 21 during egg or sperm meiosis accounts for 95% of cases of trisomy 21. In the vast majority of cases the extra chromosome is maternal in origin, and there is a strong correlation between maternal age and the chances of fetal trisomy 21. In less than 5% of cases, the additional chromosome 21 material is a result of an unbalanced translocation, usually affecting chromosomes 14 and 21,

Protocols for High-Risk Pregnancies: An Evidence-Based Approach, Sixth Edition.
Edited by John T. Queenan, Catherine Y. Spong and Charles J. Lockwood.
© 2015 John Wiley & Sons, Ltd. Published 2015 by John Wiley & Sons, Ltd.

but occasionally also involving chromosomes 15 or 22. About 50% of such cases occur as *de novo* translocations and 50% are inherited from one parent who is a carrier of a balanced translocation. Rarer cases of trisomy 21 are mosaic, in which some cell lines carry three copies of chromosome number 21 while others are normal. Trisomies 18 and 13 are also due to meiotic nondisjunction in approximately 85% of cases, while 10% of cases are mosaic and 5% are due to a translocation.

Diagnosis and screening protocols

Prenatal screening and diagnosis of autosomal trisomies should be offered to all pregnant women, regardless of maternal age. Prenatal diagnosis requires an invasive procedure, with chorionic villus sampling (CVS) and amniocentesis being the most commonly performed procedures to provide a certain diagnosis. In contrast, prenatal screening provides a patient-specific risk of chromosomal abnormality, with the most common current approaches being combined first trimester serum and sonographic screening, second trimester serum and sonographic screening, and noninvasive prenatal testing (NIPT).

Invasive prenatal diagnosis

When a diagnosis of fetal chromosomal status is required in the first trimester of pregnancy, the procedure of choice is CVS. This is typically performed between 10 and 14 weeks of gestation using a 20-gauge spinal needle sonographically guided through the maternal abdominal and uterine walls into the placenta, or using a plastic canula or biopsy forceps sonographically guided through the vagina and cervix into the placenta. Both transabdominal and transcervical CVS are associated with an overall pregnancy loss rate of 1%, but it is unclear how much of this loss is related to the procedure and how much reflects the background natural pregnancy loss rate at such an early gestational age. CVS performed prior to 9 weeks of gestation may be associated with a slightly higher rate of fetal limb reduction defect, although such early CVS procedures are rarely performed in contemporary practice.

Amniocentesis is the procedure of choice when prenatal diagnosis of fetal chromosome status is required from 15 weeks of gestation. Sonographically directed placement of a 22-gauge spinal needle into the amniotic cavity is a very safe procedure, with older studies suggesting a procedure-related loss rate of 1 in 200–500, while more contemporary data suggest loss rates lower than 1 in 1000. While conventional cell culture for karyotype may provide a diagnosis more quickly with CVS compared with amniocentesis, this is no longer of practical importance as additional tests to provide rapid diagnosis of aneuploidy within 1–2 days is usually also performed by means of polymerase chain reaction (PCR) or florescence in situ hybridization (FISH).

First trimester combined screening

The ability to provide an accurate, patient-specific, risk assessment for fetal trisomy 21 during the first trimester is an established part of routine clinical practice. This allows patients the option of CVS to confirm or exclude fetal aneuploidy, and the possibility of pregnancy termination, earlier in gestation. Such patient-specific risk estimation is currently performed using a combination of maternal age, sonographic measurement of nuchal translucency (NT), and assay of the maternal serum markers pregnancy-associated plasma protein A (PAPP-A) and either the free beta-subunit (fß) or the intact molecule of human chorionic gonadotropin (hCG).

Nuchal translucency sonography

Nuchal translucency (NT) refers to the normal space that is visible between the spine and overlying skin at the back of the fetal neck during the first trimester sonography (Figs. 4.1 and 4.2). The larger this space, the higher the risk for trisomy 21, while the smaller the space the lower the risk for trisomy 21. Measurement of this NT space has been shown to be a powerful sonographic marker for trisomy 21, when obtained between 10 weeks 3 days and 13 weeks 6 days of gestation. Table 4.1 describes the components of a standardized NT sonographic protocol.

NT sonography can be technically challenging to master initially, and requires considerable effort to maintain quality over time. Given the

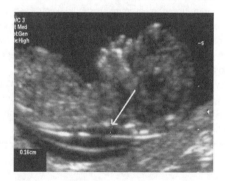

Figure 4.1   Nuchal translucency (NT) ultrasound measurement at 13 weeks in a chromosomally normal fetus, measuring 1.6 mm. Various features of good NT ultrasound technique are evident in this image: adequate image magnification, mid-sagittal plane, neutral neck position, inner to inner caliper placement perpendicular to the fetal body axis (as indicated by white arrow), and separate visualization of the overlying fetal skin and amnion.   Source: Malone *et al.*, Obstet Gynecol 2003;102:1066. Reproduced with permission of Lippincott Williams & Wilkins.

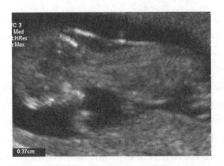

Figure 4.2   Increased nuchal translucency measurement of 3.7 mm at 12 weeks in a fetus with Down syndrome.   Source: Malone *et al.*, Obstet Gynecol 2003;102:1066. Reproduced with permission of Lippincott Williams & Wilkins.

Table 4.1   Sonographic technique to optimize nuchal translucency (NT) sonography

1 Nuchal translucency ultrasound should only be performed by sonographers or sonologists trained and experienced in the technique
2 Transabdominal or transvaginal approach should be left to the sonographer's discretion, based on maternal body habitus, gestational age and fetal position
3 Gestation should be limited between 10 weeks 3 days and 13 weeks 6 days, which are equivalent to approximate fetal crown : rump lengths of 36–79 mm (some centers use 45–84 mm for eligibility for NT imaging)
4 Fetus should be examined in a mid-sagittal plane
5 Fetal neck should be in a neutral position
6 Fetal image should occupy at least 75% of the viewable screen
7 Fetal movement should be awaited to distinguish between amnion and overlying fetal skin
8 Calipers should be placed on the inner borders of the nuchal fold
9 Calipers should be placed perpendicular to the long axis of the fetal body
10 At least three nuchal translucency measurements should be obtained, with either the maximum or the mean value (depending on the requirements of each laboratory's risk assessment protocol) of those used in risk assessment and patient counseling
11 At least 20 minutes may need to be dedicated to the nuchal translucency measurement before abandoning the effort as failed
12 Nuchal translucency measurements for each sonographer should be monitored as part of an ongoing quality assurance program to ensure optimal screening performance (such as is available with the NTQR Program from the Perinatal Quality Foundation in the US, or the Fetal Medicine Foundation in Europe)

importance of maintaining such accuracy, it is now accepted that sono-graphers and physicians who provide this form of screening should be enrolled in an ongoing quality assurance program. Examples of such QA programs include the NT Quality Review managed by the Perinatal Quality Foundation in the US (www.ntqr.org) and the Fetal Medicine Foundation in Europe (www.fetalmedicine.org).

In order to use an NT measurement to calculate a patient's risk for trisomy 21, a special software program is required to convert the raw millimeter measurement into a multiple of the median (MoM) value. Use of MoM values takes into account the normal gestational age variation in NT size, and allows integration of maternal age and serum results into the final risk assessment.

PAPP-A and fßhCG

Maternal serum levels of PAPP-A are approximately 50% lower in trisomy 21 pregnancies compared with normal pregnancies at 10–13 weeks of gestation. By contrast, maternal serum levels of fßhCG are approximately twice as high in trisomy 21 pregnancies compared with normal pregnancies at this gestational age. Depending on which laboratory is used, either total hCG or fßhCG can be used for such first trimester screening. The combination of maternal age, NT sonography, PAPP-A, and fßhCG will detect 85% of cases of trisomy 21, for a 5% false-positive rate, between 10 and 13 weeks of gestation. The test is best performed earlier in the first trimester, as it has been shown to have trisomy 21 detection rates of 87% at 11 weeks, compared with 82% at 13 weeks of gestation, for a 5% false-positive rate.

Secondary sonographic markers

While measurement of the NT space combined with serum markers is the mainstay of general population screening, it is also apparent that there are other useful sonographic features of aneuploidy in the first trimester. Cystic hygroma is found in about 1 of every 300 first trimester pregnancies, and refers to a markedly enlarged NT space, often extending along the entire length of the fetus, with septations clearly visible. Cystic hygroma is the most powerful predictor of fetal aneuploidy yet described, being associated with a 50% risk for fetal aneuploidy. Of the 50% of such pregnancies that are proven to have a normal fetal karyotype, almost half will be complicated by major structural fetal malformations, such as cardiac defects and skeletal anomalies. Less than 25% of all cases of first trimester septated cystic hygroma will result in a normal liveborn infant. Therefore, this finding should prompt immediate referral for CVS, and pregnancies found to be euploid should be evaluated carefully for other malformations, by means of a detailed fetal anomaly scan and fetal echocardiography at 18–22 weeks of gestation.

It has also been suggested that the fetus with trisomy 21 may have underdeveloped nasal bones when imaged in a perfect mid-sagittal plane at 10–13 weeks of gestation (Fig. 4.3). It has been suggested that failure to visualize this echogenic line, suggesting absence of the fetal nasal bones, may be an independent marker for fetal trisomy 21. Similarly, it has been suggested that the fetus with trisomy 21 may have an abnormal Doppler

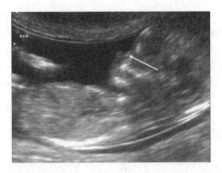

Figure 4.3   Nasal bone image of a euploid fetus at 13 weeks. Various features of good nasal bone technique are evident in this image: a good mid-sagittal plane, clear fetal profile, downward-facing spine, slight neck flexion, and two echogenic lines, representing the overlying fetal skin and the nasal bone. The white arrow represents the fetal nose bone, which loses its echogenicity distally. Source: Malone *et al.*, Obstet Gynecol 2003;102:1066. Reproduced with permission from Lippincott Williams & Wilkins.

blood flow pattern in the ductus venosus during the first trimester. Normally, this vessel shows a triphasic flow pattern, with forward flow reaching peaks during ventricular systole and early ventricular diastole. There should normally be forward flow even during the nadir coinciding with the atrial contraction (Fig. 4.4). Reversal of blood flow during the atrial contraction phase is considered abnormal, and has been suggested as

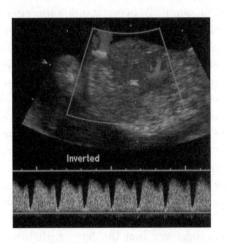

Figure 4.4   Ductus venous flow velocity waveform in a normal 13-week fetus. The Doppler is placed in the ductus venosus between the umbilical venous sinus and the inferior vena cava. Note that there is triphasic pulsatile flow with constant forward flow. The troughs of flow during the atrial contraction also demonstrate forward flow. Source: Malone *et al.*, Obstet Gynecol 2003;102:1066 with permission from Lippincott Williams & Wilkins.

an additional marker for trisomy 21 during the first trimester. Additionally, the fetus with trisomy 21 may be more likely to have abnormal blood flow waveforms across the tricuspid valve, with tricuspid regurgitation being described in the first trimester in such pregnancies.

However, it should be noted that studies suggesting a role for sonographic evaluation of nasal bones, ductus venosus, and tricuspid regurgitation in the first trimester have been derived from select high-risk populations, and likely significantly overestimate the performance in general population screening. At this time, first trimester evaluation of these secondary markers is not recommended for general population screening, but instead is used in select tertiary referral centers as a second-line screening tool to evaluate a patient who has a high-risk first trimester screening result but who is uncertain about whether to proceed with invasive testing. If these secondary tests appear abnormal then this might be used as an additional indicator to proceed with CVS.

Second trimester screening

The mainstay of risk assessment for fetal trisomy 21 had previously been second trimester serum and sonographic screening. Second trimester serum screening in particular has fallen greatly in popularity due to the superiority of first trimester combined screening, although there may still be a role for such serum markers in the minority of patients who may not present for care sufficiently early to avail of first trimester approaches. Techniques used to evaluate risk for trisomy 21 during the second trimester include sonographic detection of major structural fetal malformations, sonographic detection of minor markers, and maternal serum assay of alphafetoprotein (AFP), hCG, unconjugated estriol (uE3) and inhibin-A.

Sonographic detection of major malformations

The genetic sonogram is a term used to describe second trimester sonographic assessment of the fetus for signs of aneuploidy. The detection of certain major structural malformations that are known to be associated with aneuploidy should prompt an immediate consideration of genetic amniocentesis. Table 4.2 summarizes the major structural malformations that are associated with the most common trisomies. Given the increasing popularity of first trimester screening, many advanced obstetric ultrasound practitioners have attempted to bring the genetic sonogram forward in gestation so that an anomaly scan may also be performed toward the end of the first trimester. Little data however are available to validate the accuracy of the genetic sonogram in the first trimester for general population screening, and therefore the optimal time remains at about 18–22 weeks of gestation. When a major structural malformation is found, such as an atrioventricular canal defect or a double-bubble suggestive of duodenal atresia, the risk of trisomy 21 in that pregnancy can be increased

Table 4.2   Sonographic findings associated with trisomies 21, 18, and 13

Trisomy 21	Trisomy 18	Trisomy 13
Major structural malformations		
Cardiac defects:	Cardiac defects:	Holoprosencephaly
• AV canal defect	• Double outlet right ventricle	Orofacial clefting
• Ventricular septal defect	• Ventricular septal defect	Cyclopia
• Tetralogy of Fallot	• AV canal defect	Proboscis
Duodenal atresia	Meningomyelocele	Omphalocele
Cystic hygroma	Agenesis corpus callosum	Cardiac defects:
Hydrops	Omphalocele	• Ventricular septal defect
	Diaphragmatic hernia	• Hypoplastic left heart
	Esophageal atresia	Polydactyly
	Clubbed or rocker bottom feet	Clubbed or rocker bottom feet
	Renal abnormalities	Echogenic kidneys
	Orofacial clefting	Cystic hygroma
	Cystic hygroma	Hydrops
	Hydrops	
Minor sonographic markers		
Nuchal thickening	Nuchal thickening	Nuchal thickening
Mild ventriculomegaly	Mild ventriculomegaly	Mild ventriculomegaly
Short humerus or femur	Short humerus or femur	Echogenic bowel
Echogenic bowel	Echogenic bowel	Enlarged cisterna magna
Renal pyelectasis	Enlarged cisterna magna	Echogenic intracardiac focus
Echogenic intracardiac focus	Choroid plexus cysts	Single umbilical artery
Hypoplastic nasal bones	Micrognathia	Overlapping fingers
Brachycephaly	Strawberry-shaped head	Growth restriction
Clinodactyly	Clenched or overlapping fingers	
Sandal gap toe	Single umbilical artery	
Widened iliac angle	Growth restriction	
Growth restriction		

by approximately 20-fold to 30-fold. For almost all patients, such an increase in their background risk for aneuploidy will be sufficiently high to justify immediate genetic amniocentesis.

Sonographic detection of minor markers

Second trimester sonography can also detect a range of minor markers for aneuploidy. The latter are not considered structural abnormalities of the fetus *per se* but, when noted, may be associated with an increased probability that the fetus is aneuploid. Table 4.2 also summarizes the minor sonographic markers that, when visualized, may increase the probability of an aneuploid fetus. The minor markers that may be of most value are nuchal fold measurement, nasal bone sonography, echogenic bowel, and short femur or humerus. It is likely that other minor markers, such as echogenic intracardiac focus, minimal pyelectasis, and choroid plexus cysts, have minimal value when found in isolation in an otherwise low-risk patient. It should be noted that most data supporting the role of second trimester sonography for minor markers for aneuploidy are derived from high-risk populations, such as patients of advanced maternal age or with abnormal maternal serum screening results. The detection of isolated minor markers in lower-risk patients from the general population will likely have minimal impact on an already low background risk of aneuploidy.

To objectively counsel patients following the prenatal diagnosis of a minor sonographic marker, likelihood ratios can be used to create a more precise risk assessment for the patient that their fetus might be affected with trisomy 21. Table 4.3 summarizes the likelihood ratios that can be used to modify a patient's risk for trisomy 21, depending on which minor marker is detected. If no markers are present, the patient's *a priori* risk can be multiplied by 0.4, effectively reducing their chances of carrying a fetus with trisomy 21 by 60%. The likelihood ratio values listed for each marker assume that the marker is an isolated finding. By contrast, when more than one minor marker is noted in the same fetus different likelihood ratios must be used, with the risk for trisomy 21 being increased by a factor of 10 when two minor markers are detected and by a factor of 115 when three or more minor markers are found. It should also be noted that the 95% confidence interval values for each marker's likelihood ratios are rather wide. These values should therefore be used only as a general guide for counseling patients, and care should be exercised to avoid implying too much precision in the final risk estimates. Accuracy of risk estimates, however, can be maximized by using the best available *a priori* risk value for a

Table 4.3 Likelihood ratios for trisomy 21 when an isolated minor sonographic marker is detected

Minor marker	Likelihood ratio	95% confidence intervals
Nuchal fold .5 mm	11	6–22
Echogenic bowel	6.7	3–17
Short humerus	5.1	217
Short femur	1.5	0.8–3
Echogenic intracardiac focus	1.8	1–3
Pyelectasis	1.5	0.6–4
Any two minor markers	10	6.6–14
Any three or more minor markers	115	58–229
No markers	0.4	0.3–0.5

The patient's *a priori* risk is multiplied by the appropriate positive likelihood ratio to yield an individualized post-test risk for fetal trisomy 21.

Source: Data from Nyberg *et al.*, *J Ultrasound Med* 2001, 20:1053.

particular patient, such as the results of maternal serum marker screening, rather than maternal age, when available.

AFP, hCG, uE3, and inhibin-A

Maternal serum levels of AFP and uE3 are both approximately 25% lower in pregnancies complicated by trisomy 21, compared with euploid pregnancies. By contrast, levels of hCG and inhibin-A are approximately twice as high in pregnancies complicated by trisomy 21. Maternal serum levels of AFP, uE3, and hCG all tend to be decreased in pregnancies complicated by trisomy 18. The combination of AFP, uE3, hCG and inhibin-A, commonly known as the quad screen, can detect over 80% of cases of trisomy 21, for a 5% false-positive rate. Performance of serum screening tests can be maximized by accurate ascertainment of gestational age, and, wherever possible, sonographic dating should be used instead of menstrual dating. It is optimal to provide serum screening between 15 and 16 weeks of gestation, thereby allowing the results to be available at the time of second trimester sonographic evaluation, although as discussed earlier, the main role of such second trimester serum markers is for screening for those few patients who present for initial antenatal care after 14 weeks of gestation.

Combined first and second trimester screening

Given that some of the markers used for second trimester serum screening are independent of those used in the first trimester, some centers have combined multiple makers across both trimesters to optimize screening performance. There are three approaches to combining different screening modalities across different gestational ages, namely: integrated screening, stepwise screening and contingent screening. However, the complexity of these screening arrangements, especially in the era of NIPT, will likely make such combined first and second trimester screening tests increasingly irrelevant.

Integrated screening refers to a two-step screening protocol, with results not being released until all screening steps are completed. Sonographic measurement of NT, together with serum assay for PAPP-A, are obtained between 10 and 13 weeks of gestation, followed by a second serum assay for AFP, hCG, uE3 and inhibin-A obtained between 15 and 16 weeks of gestation. A single risk assessment is then calculated at 16 weeks. This "fully integrated" test has a trisomy 21 detection rate of 95%, for a 5% false-positive rate. A variant of this approach, referred to as the "serum integrated" test, involves blood tests only, including PAPP-A in the first trimester, followed by AFP, hCG, uE3 and inhibin-A in the second trimester. This latter test, which does not require an NT ultrasound assessment, has a trisomy 21 detection rate of 86%, for a 5% false-positive rate. The main criticism of this approach is that patients have no opportunity to avail of CVS for first trimester diagnosis.

In contrast to integrated screening, stepwise screening refers to multiple different trisomy 21 screening tests being performed, with risk estimates being provided to patients upon completion of each step. A key concept in performing stepwise screening is to ensure that each subsequent screening test that is performed should use the trisomy 21 risk from the preceding test as the new *a priori* risk for later screening. If sequential screening tests are performed independently for trisomy 21, without any modification being made for earlier screening results, the positive predictive value of the later tests will inevitably deteriorate, and it is likely that the overall false-positive rate will increase. The advantage of stepwise screening over integrated screening is that it allows patients in the first trimester to avail of an immediate CVS, should their risk estimate justify this test.

Contingent screening is a modification of stepwise screening in which patients are counseled in different clinical directions depending on first trimester screening results. With this form of screening, patients have a standard combined first trimester screening test using NT, PAPP-A, and fßhCG. Those with very high-risk screening results, for example 1 in 30 or higher, have immediate invasive diagnostic testing with CVS, while those with very low-risk results, for example 1 in 1500 or lower, are reassured and have no further screening or diagnostic testing. The remaining patients who have intermediate first trimester screening results (for example, between 1 in 30 and 1 in 1500 risk) return at 15–16 weeks for quad serum markers. These markers are then combined with the first trimester markers in an integrated test, with those having a final risk of 1 in 270 or higher then undergoing amniocentesis. The advantage of such contingent screening is that 75% of patients complete aneuploidy screening in the first trimester, with either a diagnostic test or such low-risk results that there is little value in further screening. Only 25% of patients need to return in the second trimester for further evaluation. Detection rates of at least 90% for a 5% false-positive rate should be achievable with this form of screening.

Noninvasive prenatal testing

The newest approach to screening for fetal aneuploidy, NIPT, relies on the detection of fetal cell-free DNA (cfDNA) in the maternal circulation. Fetal cfDNA crosses the placenta into the maternal circulation and accounts for approximately 10% of the total maternal circulating cfDNA after 9 weeks of gestation. Unlike fetal cells in the maternal circulation which can persist for years, fetal cfDNA is cleared within hours after delivery. The two different approaches to quantifying cfDNA in the maternal circulation are massively parallel shotgun sequencing (MPSS), or targeted sequencing using single nucleotide polymorphisms (SNPs). The performance of the test depends on the proportion of fetal cfDNA, with no result being provided when this fetal fraction is less than 4%. Early gestational age and increasing maternal body mass index may compromise this fetal fraction and increase the chances of a failed test.

Initial studies from high-risk populations suggest a trisomy 21 detection rate of greater than 99% with a false-positive rate of less than 0.1%, and similarly high performance for trisomy 18. The detection rate for trisomy 13 appears to be somewhat lower, varying from 80% to 99%, and with false-positive rates varying from 0.1% to 0.3%, depending on the particular commercial platform used. It is important to realize that NIPT is a screening, rather than a diagnostic, test with false-positive and false-negative results being possible, in particular at low fetal fractions. The presence of mosaicism or an earlier vanishing twin may also compromise the performance of NIPT. This form of screening is now available from a number of commercial laboratories, with each test having slightly different performance characteristics in terms of earliest gestational age, use in twin gestations, use in pregnancies conceived with assisted reproductive technology techniques including donor egg, ability to detect triploidy, and ability to detect microdeletion syndromes.

Currently, NIPT is considered a reasonable screening test to offer to patients considered to be at increased risk for fetal aneuploidy, for example women older than 35 years, those with a prior fetal aneuploidy, or those with fetal sonographic abnormalities. It involves a maternal blood sample, obtained at 9 weeks of gestation or later, with a turnaround time typically of 5–10 days. As NIPT becomes more prevalent, there will inevitably be a significant reduction in the number of invasive diagnostic procedures.

Conclusion

A wide range of screening tests for fetal aneuploidy, in particular trisomy 21, is now available in both the first and second trimesters. Given the simplicity of NIPT, national screening algorithms will become more straightforward, with more complex screening tests using different modalities across different gestational ages likely becoming redundant. Because of the huge array of available tests, and because of the potential for inefficient combinations of screening approaches or confusion among patients and providers, it would be ideal if all pregnant patients could be provided with formal pretest counseling to select the most appropriate risk assessment algorithm for their particular circumstances. Frequent updates to clinical guidelines will be required from professional bodies in order to empower providers to remain aware of the rapid changes in this area.

Suggested reading

Bianchi DW, Crombleholme TM, D'Alton ME, Malone FD. *Fetology: Diagnosis and Management of the Fetal Patient*, 2nd edn.. New York, London: McGraw Hill, 2010.

Bianchi DW, Platt LD, Goldberg JD, Abuhamad AZ, Sehnert AJ, Rava RP. Genome-wide fetal aneuploidy detection by maternal plasma DNA sequencing. MatErnal Blood IS Source to Accurately diagnose fetal aneuploidy (MELISSA) Study Group. *Obstet Gynecol* 2012;119:890–901.

Invasive Prenatal Testing for Aneuploidy. ACOG Practice Bulletin No. 88. American College of Obstetricians and Gynecologists. *Obstet Gynecol* 2007;110:1459–67. (Reaffirmed 2013).

Malone FD, Canick JA, Ball RH, *et al.* A comparison of first trimester screening, second trimester screening, and the combination of both for evaluation of risk for Down syndrome. *N Engl J Med* 2005;353:2001–11.

Noninvasive prenatal testing for fetal aneuploidy. Committee Opinion No. 545. American College of Obstetricians and Gynecologists. *Obstet Gynecol* 2012;120:1532–34.

Nyberg DA, Souter VL. Chromosomal abnormalities. In: Nyberg DA, McGahan JP, Pretorius DH, Pilu G (eds) *Diagnostic Imaging of Fetal Anomalies*. Philadelphia; London: Lippincott Williams & Wilkins, 2003; pp. 861–906.

Palomaki GE, Kloza EM, Lambert-Messerlian GM, Haddow JE, Neveus LM, Ehrich M, *et al.* DNA sequencing of maternal plasma to detect Down syndrome: an international clinical validation study. *Genet Med* 2011;13:913–20.

PROTOCOL 5

Fetal Echocardiography

Joshua A. Copel

Departments of Obstetrics, Gynecology and Reproductive Sciences, and Pediatrics, Yale School of Medicine, New Haven, CT, USA

Overview

Congenital heart disease occurs in approximately 8 of 1000 live births. Of these, approximately half are relatively minor ventricular septal defects or valve stenoses that are of little hemodynamic significance. Some of these can be identified prenatally with sensitive color Doppler flow mapping with little clinical impact, while many others are undetectable prenatally. The remainder are significant lesions that may benefit from prenatal detection, parental counseling, and obstetric–pediatric planning for delivery and neonatal care.

Pathophysiology

Most types of congenital heart disease are thought to be inherited in multifactorial fashion, with both genetic and environmental contributions. The indications used for fetal echocardiography, a prenatal ultrasound technique that can detect most significant congenital heart disease, reflect that. Many patients referred for fetal echocardiography have had prior affected children or other affected family members, and the recurrence risk for these families is about 2–3% if there has been a prior affected child, and 3–5% if one of the parents has congenital heart disease.

The pathophysiology of congenital cardiac anomalies varies with the type of anatomic abnormality that is present. The underlying mechanisms include failures of cell migration leading to failure of a structure to form, or diminished flow, inhibiting the normal growth of a downstream structure (e.g., poor flow across the foramen ovale and mitral valve predisposing to a coarctation of the aorta).

Protocols for High-Risk Pregnancies: An Evidence-Based Approach, Sixth Edition.
Edited by John T. Queenan, Catherine Y. Spong and Charles J. Lockwood.
© 2015 John Wiley & Sons, Ltd. Published 2015 by John Wiley & Sons, Ltd.

Structural heart disease

Diagnosis and workup

In patients without risk factors for congenital heart disease, full fetal echocardiography, which is generally more time-consuming and expensive than general obstetric sonography, is not indicated unless cardiac anomalies are suspected. Many risk factors for congenital heart disease have been described (Table 5.1).

The four-chamber view of the heart has been suggested as an easy way of screening for congenital heart disease, although its sensitivity to significant

Table 5.1 Indications for fetal echocardiography

Familial risk factors
- History of congenital heart disease (CHD)
  - Previous sibling with CHD
  - Paternal CHD
  - Second-degree relative to fetus with CHD
- Mendelian syndromes that include congenital heart disease (e.g., Noonan, Tuberous sclerosis)

Maternal risk factors
- Congenital heart disease
- Cardiac teratogen exposure
  - Lithium carbonate
  - Phenytoin
  - Valproic acid
  - Trimethadione
  - Carbamazepine
  - Isotretinoin
  - Paroxetine
- Maternal metabolic disorders
  - Diabetes mellitus
  - Phenylketonuria
- In vitro fertilization

Fetal risk factors
- Suspected cardiac anomaly
- Extracardiac anomalies
  - Chromosomal
  - Anatomic
- Fetal cardiac arrhythmia
  - Irregular rhythm
  - Tachycardia (greater than 200 bpm) in absence of chorioamnionitis
  - Fixed bradycardia
- Nonimmune hydrops fetalis
- Lack of reassuring four-chamber view during basic obstetric scan
- Monochorionic twins
- Increased nuchal translucency space at 11–14 weeks of gestation

cardiac anomalies has varied in the literature. Approximately one-third of cases of major heart disease are detected on screening prenatal ultrasound, according to a review of the world's literature. Our own experience suggests that it has a very high positive predictive value, with about half of patients referred for abnormal four-chamber views actually having cardiac anomalies. Current recommendations from US medical societies, including the American College of Obstetricians and Gynecologists, and the American Institute of Ultrasound in Medicine, all call for including outflow tract views in the standard (or so-called "Level 1") obstetric scan.

Full fetal echocardiography includes obtaining all of the views in the fetus routinely obtained in postnatal echocardiography (Table 5.2) using both real-time grayscale and color Doppler imaging. Additionally, spectral Doppler, cardiac biometry and M-mode data can be obtained as indicated. Fetal echocardiographers use these latter techniques variably. The two-dimensional examination should be sufficient to exclude significant heart disease in the vast majority of affected individuals. The more sophisticated studies are especially useful in cases of suspected structural or functional abnormalities.

Table 5.2   Standard fetal echocardiographic views and what to see

---

Four chamber
   Situs: check fetal position and stomach
   Axis of heart to the left
   Intact interventricular septum
   Atria approximately equal sizes
   Ventricles approximately equal sizes
   Free movement of mitral and tricuspid valves
   Heart occupies about one-third of chest area
   Foramen ovale flap (atrial septum primum) visible in left atrium

Long-axis left ventricle
   Intact interventricular septum
   Continuity of the ascending aorta with mitral valve posteriorly
   Interventricular septum anteriorly

Short axis of great vessels
   Vessel exiting the anterior (right) ventricle bifurcates, confirming it is the pulmonary artery

Aortic arch
   Vessel exiting the posterior (left) ventricle arches and has three head vessels, confirming it is the aorta

Pulmonary artery-ductus arteriosus
   Continuity of the ductus arteriosus with the descending aorta

Venous connections
   Superior and inferior vena cavae enter right atrium
   Pulmonary veins entering left atrium from both right and left lungs

---

Management

When a cardiac anomaly is found, a full detailed fetal scan to detect any other extracardiac anomalies is mandatory. Many fetal syndromes include cardiac anomalies, and accurate counseling requires complete enumeration of associated anomalies. Fetal karyotype testing should be offered to the parents, as chromosome abnormalities are seen in a large segment of fetuses with congenital heart disease. Additional testing for a microdeletion of chromosome 22q11 can be helpful in fetuses with conotruncal malformations (e.g., tetralogy of Fallot, truncus arteriosus). As for all fetal anomalies, microarray testing for microdeletions and microduplications has also become routine.

Overall survival once a cardiac lesion is found depends on the nature of the cardiac problem, the presence of extracardiac anomalies, the karyotype and the presence of fetal hydrops. Fetal hydrops in association with structural heart disease is virtually universally fatal. Aneuploid fetuses may have dismal prognoses even in the absence of heart disease; for example, fetal trisomy 18 may make repairing even a straightforward ventricular septal defect inadvisable.

Lesions that can be repaired into a biventricular heart carry a better long-term prognosis than those that result in a univentricular heart. In general, infants who are known to have congenital heart disease prenatally do better than those whose cardiac defects are only found after birth.

Fetal arrhythmias

Diagnosis and management

The largest group of fetal arrhythmias are intermittent and due to atrial, junctional or ventricular extrasystoles. They carry a small risk of coexistent structural abnormality. A greater risk exists of an unrecognized tachyarrhythmia, or the development of a tachyarrhythmia later in gestation. Atrial extrasystoles predispose the fetus to development of re-entrant atrial tachycardia, which can lead to fetal hydrops. We recommend weekly auscultation of the fetal heart, along with avoidance of caffeine or other sympathomimetics, until resolution of the arrhythmia.

Fetal tachycardias represent a management challenge, because determination of the precise electrophysiological cause of the arrhythmia is essential to any rational management strategy, but fetal electrocardiography is not yet clinically practical in the presence of intact membranes. The differential diagnoses of fetal tachycardias include re-entrant atrial tachycardia, atrial flutter, and ventricular tachycardia. The treatment of these disorders differs significantly, and appropriate medications for one may be contraindicated for another. The correct diagnosis, which should be based on combinations of M-mode, Doppler and color Doppler–M-mode imaging, is essential to appropriate therapy.

   If there is a fetal bradycardia, the first step is to determine if there is a regular or an irregular atrial rate. If the atrial rate is regular and slow, that is, below 100 beats per minute, there may be sinus bradycardia, which should prompt a complete evaluation of fetal well-being. The most common clinically important fetal bradycardia results from complete heart block, which will demonstrate a normal regular atrial rate with a slower ventricular rate whose beats do not occur in conjunction with atrial beats. In structurally normal hearts this is usually caused by maternal antibodies associated with lupus erythematosus and Sjogren syndrome, termed SSA/Ro and SSB/La. A smaller group of patients, without maternal antibodies, may present with congenital complete heart block in a setting of complex congenital heart disease involving the central fibrous body of the heart (e.g., left atrial isomerism, corrected transposition of the great arteries). In these patients, the prognosis is directly related to the complexity of the heart disease and the association with congestive heart failure. A more benign cause of fetal bradycardia, which may be mistaken for 2:1 heart block, is blocked atrial bigeminy. In such cases the atrial rate is not regular, but rather demonstrates paired beating in which a premature atrial beat follows closely after a normal atrial beat with no ventricular response to the premature beat. This arrhythmia has no significance beyond that of isolated atrial extrasystoles.

Follow up

The fetus with congenital heart disease should be carefully followed by ultrasound up to delivery. Structural lesions may evolve prenatally even as they do postnatally. It is particularly important to evaluate areas of potential obstruction, and the relationships of the great arteries to the ventricles. Fetuses with significant arrhythmias (including re-entrant tachycardias, atrial flutter, and complete heart block) should also be followed at a center with experience in the prenatal medical management of fetal arrhythmias, by a team that includes perinatologists, pediatric cardiologists and adult electrophysiologists. Delivery need not be by cesarean except in the presence of selected fetal arrhythmias that do not permit adequate fetal heart rate monitoring. For fetuses with lesions that are expected to render the neonate dependent on ductus arteriosus patency for systemic or pulmonary perfusion, prostaglandin E1 should be available in the nursery at the time of delivery to keep the ductus open.

Suggested readings

American Institute of Ultrasound in Medicine. AIUM Practice Guideline for the Performance of Obstetric Ultrasound Examinations. http://aium.org/resources/guidelines/obstetric.pdf (accessed 5/14/14).

Bahtiyar MO, Dulay AT, Weeks BP, Friedman AH, Copel JA. Prenatal course of isolated muscular ventricular septal defects diagnosed only by color Doppler sonography: single-institution experience. *J Ultrasound Med* 2008;27:715–720.

Copel JA, Liang RI, Demasio K, Ozeren S, Kleinman CS. The clinical significance of the irregular fetal heart rhythm. *Am J Obstet Gynecol* 2000;182:813–817.

Copel JA, Tan AS, Kleinman CS. Does a prenatal diagnosis of congenital heart disease alter short-term outcome? *Ultrasound Obstet Gynecol* 1997;10:237–241.

Donofrio MT, Moon-Grady AJ, Hornberger LK, et al. Diagnosis and treatment of fetal cardiac disease: a scientific statement. *Amer Heart Assoc Circ* 2014 doi: 10.1161/01.cir.0000437597.44550.5d

Kleinman CS, Copel JA. Electrophysiological principles and fetal antiarrhythmic therapy. *Ultrasound Obstet Gynecol* 1991;4:286–297.

Miller A, Riehle-Colarusso T, Alverson MS, *et al.* Congenital heart defects and major structural noncardiac anomalies, Atlanta, Georgia, 1968 to 2005. *J Pediatr* 2011;159:70–78.

Pierpont ME, Basson CT, Benson D, *et al.* Genetic basis for congenital heart defects: current knowledge. *Circulation* 2007;115:3015–3038 (doi: 10.1161/CIRCULATIONAHA.106.183056)

Silverman NH, Kleinman CS, Rudolph AM, *et al.* Fetal atrioventricular valve insufficiency associated with nonimmune hydrops: a two-dimensional echocardiographic and pulsed Doppler study. *Circulation* 1985;72:825–832.

Todros T, Faggiano F, Chiappa E, Gaglioti P, Mitola B, Sciarrone A. Accuracy of routine ultrasonography in screening heart disease prenatally. Gruppo piemontese for prenatal screening of congenital heart disease. *Prenatal Diag* 1997;17:901–906.

PROTOCOL 6

Clinical Use of Doppler

Henry L. Galan

Department of Obstetrics and Gynecology, University of Colorado School of Medicine, Aurora, CO, USA

Overview

Doppler ultrasound depends upon the ability of an ultrasound beam to be changed in frequency when encountering moving objects such as red blood cells (RBC). The change in frequency (Doppler shift) between the emitted beam and the reflected beam is proportional to the velocity of the RBC and dependent on the angle between the ultrasound beam and the vessel. Pulsed-wave Doppler velocimetry provides a flow velocity waveform from which information can be obtained to determine three basic characteristics of blood flow that are useful in obstetrics: velocity, resistance indices, and volume blood flow. Doppler velocimetry is applied in a broad number of clinical circumstances in high-risk pregnancies including diagnostic fetal echocardiography, intrauterine growth restriction (IUGR), fetal anemia, adverse pregnancy outcome assessment, twin-twin transfusion syndrome (TTTS), and preterm labor (tocolysis with indomethacin). Pulsed-wave Doppler velocimetry is also used to evaluate the ductus venosus (DV) in first trimester risk assessment for Down syndrome, but is not discussed in this protocol.

Pathophysiology

Normal fetal circulation

The umbilical vein is a conduit vessel bringing oxygen and nutrient-rich blood from the placenta to the fetus. The umbilical vein enters the umbilicus, courses anteriorly along the abdominal wall prior to entering the liver, and becomes the hepatic portion of the umbilical vein. The umbilical vein eventually becomes the portal vein, but first gives off the left inferior and superior portal vein, the DV, and finally the right portal vein. Approxi-

Protocols for High-Risk Pregnancies: An Evidence-Based Approach, Sixth Edition.
Edited by John T. Queenan, Catherine Y. Spong and Charles J. Lockwood.
© 2015 John Wiley & Sons, Ltd. Published 2015 by John Wiley & Sons, Ltd.

mately 50% of umbilical vein blood is directed into the DV and then to an area under the diaphragm that is referred to as the subdiaphragmatic vestibulum. The subdiaphragmatic vestibulum also receives blood from the inferior vena cava and blood exiting the liver via the right, middle and left hepatic veins. The process of preferential streaming begins in the subdiaphragmatic vestibulum with blood from the DV and the left and middle hepatic veins preferentially shunted across the foramen ovale into the left atrium and left ventricle so that the heart and the head receive the most oxygenated and nutrient-rich blood. In contrast, blood coming from the inferior vena cava and the right hepatic vein are preferentially streamed into the right atrium and right ventricle and then out the pulmonary artery and then shunted to the descending aorta via the ductus arteriosus. Blood leaving the fetus does so via two umbilical arteries arising from the hypogastric arteries which course around the lateral aspects of the bladder in an anterior and cephalad direction, exiting the umbilicus, returning back to the placenta.

There are three primary shunts in the fetus that require closure after delivery in order for normal postnatal circulation and subsequent adult circulation to take place. As mentioned above, the DV shunts blood from the umbilical vein toward the heart. The ductus arteriosus shunts approximately 90% of the blood in main pulmonary artery to the descending aorta leaving only 10% of pulmonary artery blood to reach the fetal lungs. The third shunt is the foramen ovale, which is maintained in a patent state in utero to allow the process of preferential streaming to occur from the right atrium to the left atrium. Failure of any one of these shunts to close properly may result in adverse cardiopulmonary transition in the newborn.

Intrauterine growth restriction
Fetuses that fail to reach genetically determined growth potential due to uteroplacental dysfunction may develop abnormal resistance to blood flow in the placenta. This abnormal resistance is due to numerous placental vascular abnormalities (poor villous capillarization, reduced number and branching of stem arteries, luminal reduction and wall hypertrophy), which can be detected with Doppler velocimetry in the umbilical artery located upstream from the placenta. Progression of placental disease with concomitant worsening of blood flow resistance may lead to additional Doppler velocimetry changes in the precordial venous system or in the heart. Once the fetus decompensates to that level of Doppler abnormality, acidemia is nearly always present.

Fetal anemia
In Rh disease, a fetal RBC antigen enters the maternal bloodstream and stimulates antibody production against that RBC antigen. An amnestic response may occur in a subsequent pregnancy if the same RBC antigen is

presented to the mother's immune system and this may lead to a series of events that include fetal anemia, extramedullary hematopoiesis, hydrops fetalis and fetal death. Historically, the degree of fetal anemia and need for fetal RBC transfusion involved an amniocentesis to determine the amniotic fluid $\Delta OD450$ to assess the degree of RBC-derived hemoglobin breakdown products and to estimate anemia. If moderate to severe anemia is suspected, the fetus should undergo a fetal blood sampling and transfusion. Isoimmunization with the Kell antibody also results in fetal anemia, but does so through bone marrow suppression rather than hemolysis. Thus, the $\Delta OD450$ will not be abnormal. Fetal anemia can also result from infections such as parvovirus.

Preterm labor

Although the pathophysiology of preterm labor is still largely unknown, tocolytic use is widespread. Use of agents that inhibit prostaglandin synthesis can result in premature closure of the ductus arteriosus and oligohydramnios. Doppler velocimetry is useful in assessment of ductus arteriosus closure by determining the peak systolic velocity as well as whether there is continuous flow throughout diastole.

Cardiac abnormalities

Fetuses with known cardiac abnormalities including congenital or structural heart disease, arrhythmias and congestive failure may have intracardiac and outflow tract flow velocity abnormalities that can be detected with Doppler velocimetry. Depending on the nature of the abnormality, this can affect other flow velocity waveforms including the DV, hepatic veins, inferior vena cava and the umbilical vein.

Diagnosis

Doppler techniques and measurements

As mentioned in the overview, pulse-wave Doppler velocimetry can be used to obtain the following information from a flow velocity waveform:

1 Velocity of the blood – requires an angle of insonation of zero degrees between the transducer and the vessel of interest (Fig. 6.1). Angle correction function available on most ultrasound machines can be used but the actual angle between the vessel and the ultrasound beam should be less than 30°. For middle cerebral artery peak systolic velocity (MCA PSV), the sample volume should be placed in the proximal 1/3 of the MCA as it branches from the circle of Willis.

2 Resistance indices (S/D ratio, resistance index, pulsatility index) – these are angle independent measurements such that the value obtained for

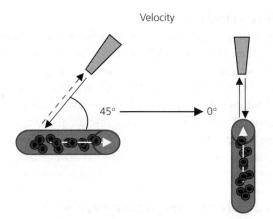

Figure 6.1 Schematic representing zero angle of insonation between the Doppler transducer and the vessel of interest.

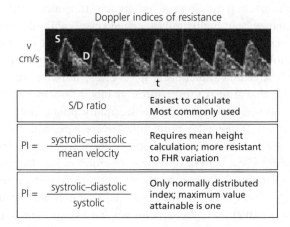

Figure 6.2 Flow velocity waveform of the umbilical artery and definitions for the different Doppler indices of resistance.

any one of these indices is not dependent upon the angle between the transducer and the vessel being interrogated (Fig. 6.2).

3 Volume blood flow (milliliters per minute) – this is determined by obtaining the velocity of the blood and multiplying it by the cross-sectional area of the vessel (obtained by two-dimensional ultrasound) times 60 seconds:

Volume flow (mL/min) = velocity (cm/ sec)

$\times$ cross − sectional area (cm^2) $\times$ 60 seconds

Cardiac flow velocities

Normal values and blood flow velocity patterns have been previously reported for cardiac Doppler velocities. More specifically, blood flow velocity values and patterns have been described for the pulmonary and aortic outflow tracts, ductus arteriosus, DV and arteriosus, pulmonary veins, tricuspid and mitral valve, and the inferior vena cava. Any fetal structural cardiac abnormality or precordial or postcordial vascular abnormality can affect the blood flow velocity and waveform of the aforementioned vessels and valves. Further discussion of fetal echocardiography is found in Protocol 5.

Prediction of adverse pregnancy events

There has been considerable effort over the past two decades with the application of maternal Doppler studies of the uterine arteries in the prediction of adverse pregnancy outcomes including preeclampsia, IUGR, fetal demise and preterm birth. The most distal branches of the uterine artery (spiral arteries) undergo a remarkable transition during the first half of pregnancy from highly muscularized vessels with high resistance to remodeled vessels with low resistance. This is in response to differentiation of cytotrophoblast to non-invasive and invasive cytotrophoblast with the latter literally invading and altering spiral artery muscular architecture. It is this change that leads to the enormous blood flow eventually seen in pregnancy (600–800 mL/min). There are many publications on the use of uterine artery Doppler for predicting adverse pregnancy outcomes in both low-risk and high-risk populations. In the low-risk population, there does not seem to be a benefit of wide application of this Doppler test as a screening tool for adverse pregnancy events. There may be a role in uterine artery Doppler testing in high-risk pregnancy as it may identify a subgroup of patients at a particular higher risk for adverse events, which may lead to useful additional monitoring during pregnancy or preventative strategies. In addition, the high negative predictive value for adverse pregnancy events can provide reassurance. However, before this test can be applied to the general or even the high-risk pregnancy population, further evidence is needed to elucidate a clear predictive capability, the optimum gestational age for screening, standardization for study technique and abnormal test criteria, and an effective prevention therapy or strategy; this position has been supported by the Society for Maternal-Fetal Medicine.

Intrauterine growth restriction

Blood flow velocity waveforms obtained by pulsed-wave Doppler velocimetry change in any given vessel across gestation. In the umbilical artery of a normal pregnancy, there is a progressive increase in diastolic flow velocity across gestation, which reflects a decrease in the resistance within the placenta. One characteristic of IUGR due to uteroplacental insufficiency is an increase in blood flow resistance within the placenta, which can be detected by Doppler velocimetry upstream in the umbilical arteries. Approximately 40% of cardiac output is directed toward the placenta via the umbilical artery. Thus, as placental disease progresses and blood flow resistance increases, the heart is subject to increased workload (afterload). However, prior to significant cardiac dysfunction becoming apparent, abnormalities arise in the "prechordial" venous circulation (inferior vena cava, DV, and hepatic veins) in up to 70% of preterm, severely IUGR fetuses. Use of Doppler velocimetry in the management of IUGR is further discussed in Protocol 40.

Rh sensitization

As previously mentioned, fetal anemia resulting from maternal alloimmunization (except anti-Kell) was historically detected by amniocentesis and assessment of the ΔOD450 and then confirmed by fetal blood sampling. Assessment of the middle cerebral artery (MCA) peak systolic velocity (PSV) has essentially replaced the ΔOD450 as the gold standard test for fetal anemia. The MCA PSV has greater sensitivity for moderate to severe anemia than does the ΔOD450. Moreover, the ΔOD450 is not useful in Kell sensitization because fetal anemia in this condition is caused by bone marrow suppression rather than hemolysis and thus does not lead to RBC breakdown products in the amniotic fluid normally detected by the ΔOD450.

One of the resultant pathophysiological features present in Rh disease is a reduction in the viscosity of the fetal blood, which is secondary to a lower hematocrit. This results in an increase in the velocity of blood flow, which can be detected by pulsed-wave Doppler velocimetry. One of the vessels branching off the circle of Willis is the MCA, which lends itself to interrogation by Doppler because of its location and because the paired middle cerebral arteries carry 80% of the cerebral blood flow. The MCA is first identified with the use of color flow Doppler. With an angle of insonation of 0° (or less than 30° with angle correction), pulse-wave Doppler velocimetry is used to obtain the flow velocity waveform. From the flow velocity waveform, one can determine the PSV across serial peaks of the systolic component of the flow velocity waveform profile and obtain a mean systolic peak velocity of the MCA flow waveform. Nomograms are available for PSV in the MCA across gestation. Web-based MCA PSV multiples of the median (MoM) calculators for a given gestational age are also available at perinatology.com. When the MCA PSV surpasses the threshold of 1.55 MoM, there is a high risk of moderate-to-severe anemia in the fetus. The cut-off 1.55 MoM has a sensitivity of 100% and a negative predictive value of 100% for moderate to severe anemia. Subsequent studies have shown similar favorable performance characteristics of this screening test. Once this value is surpassed, the fetus can undergo a blood sampling to determine the actual fetal hematocrit and determine if a transfusion is necessary. Using Doppler to assess the MCA PSV and identifying anemia in the fetus in this fashion avoids the standard invasive procedural risks of amniocentesis (needed for the ΔOD450) including exacerbation of the Rh sensitization. The MCA PSV measurement has also been used to guide management in the cases of anemia due to infections such as parvovirus.

Management

Congenital heart disease and arrhythmia

A number of clinical scenarios may warrant fetal echocardiography, which is discussed in more detail in Protocol 5. The ideal time to obtain a fetal echocardiogram is between 18 and 22 weeks of gestation; however, there are several specialized perinatal centers performing this in the first trimester. Counseling and management of the patient with a congenital heart defect involves a variety of steps including a karyotypic analysis of the fetus, defining the type and severity of cardiac legion, consideration of the patient's moral and religious disposition, and the presence of extracardiac abnormalities. In many instances, one of the most important things to determine in a fetus with congenital heart disease is whether the cardiac lesion will be ductal dependent and require newborn prostaglandin administration to maintain patency of the ductus arteriosus. This is an important step in the management of the pregnant patient, as it will determine whether the patient needs to be delivered a hospital with a nursery capable of administering IV prostaglandin.

Fetal arrhythmias are typically first detected by routine Doppler auscultation during a prenatal clinic visit or by external electronic fetal monitoring. Further identification of the specific type of arrhythmia requires the use of M-mode cardiography and full assessment of the cardiac structure and flow velocities. Some patients with autoimmune conditions will be SSA/SSB antibody positive and require serial fetal echo for evaluation of P-R intervals as one indicator of risk for developing complete heart block.

Management of a patient with congenital heart disease should be a collaborative effort with a team consisting of a perinatologist, genetic counselor, pediatric cardiologist, neonatologist, pediatric cardiothoracic surgeon, and the primary obstetrical provider.

Intrauterine growth restriction

Once the fetus has been diagnosed by ultrasound to be growth restricted, a full assessment of the fetus should be performed to exclude fetal anomalies, possible karyotypic abnormalities, and congenital infection. The dating criteria for the pregnancy should be reviewed and estimated date of confinement confirmed. Early-onset, structural abnormalities, or symmetric IUGR should result in consideration of excluding karyotype abnormalities and congenital infection. Treatment options are limited in IUGR and include avoidance of strenuous activities and work, increase fluid intake, and elimination of adverse social habits such as tobacco, alcohol or recreational drug use. Strict bed rest should not be recommended and if more rest is desired by the practitioner or patient, this should simply be "modified" rest at home with movement within the household and ability to prepare meals and perform light duties at home. In pregnant patients with a history of IUGR in a previous pregnancy, a baby aspirin (81 mg) has been shown to have some benefit in reducing the risk of recurrence and should be started in the first half of pregnancy, preferably prior to 16 weeks of gestation.

Surveillance of the growth-restricted fetus includes the use of fetal activity count, serial assessment of fetal growth with ultrasound (every 2–3 weeks), nonstress test and/or biophysical profile and Doppler velocimetry. Early-onset IUGR fetuses who deteriorate in utero from an acid–base standpoint, often demonstrate sequential Doppler changes in different vessels, while these changes occur far less frequently in late-onset IUGR. Use of Doppler in the management of the IUGR fetus is further discussed in Protocol 42.

Fetal anemia

The management of fetal anemia requires careful consideration of the etiologic factors. The majority of cases will be due to RBC alloimmunization of the mother or parvovirus B19 infection. Rh sensitization begins with identification of an isoimmunized patient from routine blood type and Rh, and antibody screening tests. When the antibody screen shows the presence of an antibody that places the fetus(es) at risk for fetal anemia, the patient needs to undergo serial screening with antibody titers. An alternative to serial antibody titers that is now more commercially available is the use of cf fDNA to see if the fetus carries the RBC antigen in question. If the antigen is absent in the fetus, no further testing is needed. If the antigen is present, the patient should be followed with antibody titers. Once a critical threshold has been reached by a specific titer of a given RBC antigen antibody, the patient must undergo evaluation for fetal anemia. Most hospital laboratories use either a 1:16 or 1:32 threshold cut-off and it is essential that each practitioner know the threshold for their particular hospital or laboratory. Once the critical threshold has been reached, the patient needs to undergo either (1) an amniocentesis for assessment of $\Delta OD450$ in the amniotic fluid or (2) middle cerebral artery PSV assessment using pulse-wave Doppler velocimetry. If the latter is available, it should receive priority over the amniocentesis simply because it avoids the risk associated with the amniocentesis and has very good performance characteristics as a screening test for moderate to severe anemia. If an amniocentesis is performed and the ΔOD450 is in the high zone 2 or zone 3 of the Liley or Queenan curve, then that fetus must undergo fetal blood sampling for documentation of the anemia and transfusion (see Protocol 43). Alternatively, if the MCA PSV is used to assess fetal anemia, a 1.55 multiple of the median (MoM) value should be used as a threshold above which fetal blood sampling and transfusion is needed. After one blood transfusion, the MCA PSV loses some accuracy and a different threshold for subsequent transfusion should be used (1.32 MoM has been suggested). The MCA PSV becomes increasingly less reliable for timing of subsequent transfusions and empiric intervals between transfusions are usually used: 7–10 days after the first transfusion, then 2 weeks until fetal marrow suppression achieved by Kliehauer-Betke stain and then 3 weeks thereafter. Administration of phenobarbitol (30 mg PO TID) to enhance hepatic maturation should be considered at 34 weeks gestation or one week prior to delivery. Delivery of the anemic fetus receiving blood transfusion can generally be accomplished at between 36 and 37 weeks. If fetal blood sampling will be performed at a very preterm gestation, administration of betamethasone or dexamethasone should be considered prior to the procedure.

Preterm labor

Use of anti-prostaglandin medications such as indocin for tocolysis results in inhibition of prostaglandin synthase activity and reduction in prostaglandin synthesis, which may constrict the ductus arteriosus. The effect on the ductus arteriosus is gestational-age dependent and generally, indomethacin is not used beyond 32 weeks of gestation. A ductus arteriosus effect is not typically seen within the first 48 hours of treatment. Assessment of the velocity within the ductus arteriosus should be performed beyond that time if the patient continues on a prostaglandin synthase inhibitor. Constriction is typically reversible with discontinuation of anti-prostaglandin drugs.

Summary

Color and pulse-wave Doppler velocimetry are useful ultrasound tools for the evaluation and management of fetuses with Rh disease, growth restriction, congenital heart disease and fetal arrhythmias. While Doppler ultrasound has been used in other fetal conditions, no study has demonstrated any clear clinical benefit for its use outside those stated above. Widespread use of the DV FVW in the diagnosis of Down syndrome in the first trimester has not yet occurred. Although this is a noninvasive tool to assess for Down syndrome, the emergence of maternal cell-free fetal DNA screening is far more accurate with extremely high sensitivity for the detection of this chromosomal abnormality. While uterine artery Doppler evaluation of the high-risk pregnancy might identify a subgroup of women who are at higher risk for adverse pregnancy outcome, the use of Doppler should not be considered a standard medical practice in the general population until further studies demonstrate benefit.

Suggested reading

Fetal Growth Restriction. Practice Bulletin. No 134. American College of Obstetricians and Gynecologists. *Obstet Gynecol* 2013;121:1122–33.

Hecher K, Snijders R, Campbell S, Nicolaides K. Fetal venous, intracardiac, and arterial blood flow measurements in intrauterine growth retardation: Relationship with fetal blood gases. *Am J Obstet Gynecol* 1995;173:10–15.

Rizzo G, Arduini D. Fetal cardiac function in intrauterine growth retardation. *Am J Obstet Gynecol* 1991;165:876–82.

Reed KL, Anderson CF, Shenker L. Changes in intracardiac Doppler blood flow velocities in fetuses with absent umbilical artery diastolic flow. *Am J Obsetet Gynecol* 1987;157:774.

Society for Maternal-Fetal Medicine Publications Committee, Berkley E, Chauhan SP, Abuhamad A. Doppler assessment of the fetus with intrauterine growth restriction. *Am J Obstet Gynecol* 2012;206(4):300–308.

Biggio JR Jr., Bed rest in pregnancy: time to put the issue to rest. *Obstet Gynecol* 2013; 121(6):1158–1160.

Mavrides E, Moscoso G, Carvalho JS *et al.* The anatomy of the umbilical, portal and hepatic venous systems in the human fetus at 14-19 weeks of gestation. *Ultrasound Obstet Gynecol* 2001;18(6):598–604.

Mari G, Deter RL, Carpenter RL, *et al.* Collaborative group for doppler assessment of the blood velocity in anemic fetuses. noninvasive diagnosis by Doppler ultrasonography of fetal anemia due to maternal red-cell alloimmunization. *N Eng J Med* 2000; 342:9–14.

Galan HL, Jozwik M, Rigano S, Regnault TRH, Hobbins JC, Battaglia FC, Ferrazzi E. Umbilical vein blood flow in the ovine fetus: comparison of Doppler and steady-state techniques. *Am J Obstet Gynecol* 1999;181:1149–1153.

Ferrazzi E, Bellotti M, Bozzo M, Rigano S, Pardi G, Battaglia F, Galan HL. The temporal sequence of changes in fetal velocimetry indices for growth restricted fetuses. *Ultrasound Obstet Gynecol* 2002;19:140–146.

Hecher K, Bilardo CM, Stigter RH, *et al.* Monitoring of fetuses with intrauterine growth restriction: a longitudinal study. *Ultrasound Obstet Gynecol* 2001;18:564–570.

Baschat AA, Genbruch U, Harman CR. The sequence of changes in Doppler and -biophysical parameters as severe fetal growth restriction worsens. *Ultrasound Obstet Gynecol* 2001;18:571–577.

Moise KJ, Huhta JC, Sharif DS, *et al.* Indomethacin in the treatment of premature labor: effects on the fetal ductus arteriosus. *N Engl J Med* 1998;319:327.

Ciscione AC, Hayes EJ. Uterine artery Doppler flow studies in obstetric practice. *Am J Obstet Gynecol* 2009;201(2):121–126.

Scheier M, Hernandez-Andrade E, Fonseca EB, Nicolaides KH. Prediction of severe fetal anemia in red blood cell alloimmunization after previous intrauterine transfusion. *Am J Obstet Gynecol* 2006;195:1550–1556.

Opinion, MG. Middle cerebral artery peak systolic velocity for diagnosis of fetal -anemia: the untold story. *Ultrasound Obstet Gynecol* 2005;25:323–330.

Moise KJ. The usefulness of middle cerebral artery Doppler assessment in the treatment of the fetus at risk for anemia. *Am J Obstet Gynecol* 2008;198:161.e1–161.e4.

PROTOCOL 7

Antepartum Testing

Michael P. Nageotte[1,2]

[1] Miller Children's and Women's Hospital, Long Beach, CA, USA
[2] Department of Obstetrics and Gynecology, University of California, Irvine, CA, USA

Antepartum fetal testing is utilized to assess fetal well-being, especially in the complicated pregnancy. Several tests are utilized including the non-stress test (NST), the biophysical profile (BPP), the modified BPP, and the contraction stress test (CST).

Nonstress test

The NST is currently the most common means of evaluation of fetal oxygenation status during the antepartum period. Less intensive than the CST in many regards, the NST evolved as an excellent means of fetal assessment following observations that the occurrence of two or more accelerations of the fetal heart during a CST most often predicted a negative CST while the absence of these accelerations of baseline fetal heart rate was associated with a positive test and poor perinatal outcome. The basic premise of the NST is that the fetal heart will accelerate its rate with fetal movement if the fetus is not acidotic or depressed neurologically.

A reactive NST is defined by the presence of two or more accelerations of the fetal heart rate of at least 15 beats per minute lasting for at least 15 seconds within 20 minutes. Other definitions of reactivity have been proposed with a requirement of two or more accelerations in as little as 10 minutes before the test is considered reactive. If such accelerations are not elicited either spontaneously or with repeated vibroacoustic stimulation within 40 minutes of monitoring, the NST is interpreted as nonreactive. Options for further management include admission to the hospital for delivery or extended monitoring or more commonly some form of backup test (e.g., a CST or BPP) is performed immediately. If the variable decelerations are repetitive or prolonged (lasting greater than 1 minute), the test is read as equivocal and a backup test is indicated at that time. The NST has a false-negative rate of approximately 0.3% but this is influenced by indica-

Protocols for High-Risk Pregnancies: An Evidence-Based Approach, Sixth Edition.
Edited by John T. Queenan, Catherine Y. Spong and Charles J. Lockwood.
© 2015 John Wiley & Sons, Ltd. Published 2015 by John Wiley & Sons, Ltd.

tion for test and testing interval. Of note, most nonreactive NSTs have a normal backup test, which allows continuation of the pregnancy in most instances. The current recommendation is that the NST should be performed at least twice weekly.

Biophysical profile

The fetal BPP is a frequently utilized method of antepartum fetal surveillance. The BPP score is a composite of four acute or short-term variables (fetal tone, movement, breathing and nonstress test) and one chronic or long-term variable (amniotic fluid index). All four short-term variables of the BPP are regulated by the fetal central nervous system (CNS). The fetal CNS is highly sensitive to decreases in the level of oxygenation and these biophysical variables are directly influenced by changes in the state of oxygenation of the fetus.

In the presence of progressive hypoxemia, clinical studies have confirmed that reactivity is the first biophysical variable to disappear. This is followed by the loss of fetal breathing and subsequently the loss of fetal movement. Fetal tone is the last variable to be lost in the presence of ongoing in utero hypoxemia.

Fetal urine production is the predominant source of amniotic fluid volume and is directly dependent upon renal perfusion. In response to sustained fetal hypoxemia, there is a long-term adaptive response mediated by chemoreceptors located in the aortic arch and carotid arteries. This results in chemoreceptor-mediated centralization of fetal blood flow by differential channeling of blood to vital organs in the fetus (brain, heart, adrenals), at the expense of nonessential organs (lung, kidney) by means of peripheral vasoconstriction. In cases of prolonged or repetitive episodes of fetal hypoxemia, there is a persistent decrease in blood flow to the lungs and kidneys resulting in a reduction in the amniotic fluid production leading to oligohydramnios. Amniotic fluid volume, therefore, is a reflection of chronic fetal condition. On an average, it takes approximately 13 days for a fetus to progress from a normal to an abnormal amniotic fluid volume.

The NST is first performed followed by the sonographic evaluation of fetal biophysical activities including fetal tone, movement, and breathing. Amniotic fluid volume is measured by holding the transducer perpendicular to the floor. The largest vertical pocket is selected in each quadrant. The composite of all four quadrants' deepest vertical pockets is the amniotic fluid index (AFI). A total of 30 minutes are assigned for obtaining ultrasound variables. A normal variable is assigned a score of 2 and an abnormal variable a score of zero (see Table 7.1).

A composite score of 8 or 10 is considered normal and correlates with the absence of fetal acidemia. A score of 6 is equivocal, and the test should be

Table 7.1 Fetal biophysical profile

Biophysical variable	Normal (score = 2)	Abnormal (score = 0)
Nonstress test	Reactive: More than two accelerations of greater than 15 bpm for more than 15 seconds in 20 minutes	Nonreactive: Less than two accelerations of greater than 15 bpm for more than 15 seconds in 20 minutes
Fetal breathing movements	More than one episode of more than 30 seconds in 30 minutes	Absence or less than 30 seconds in 30 minutes
Gross body movements	More than three discrete body/limb movements in 30 minutes	Fewer than two discrete body/limb movements in 30 minutes
Fetal tone	More than one active extension/flexion of limb, trunk, or hand	Slow or absent fetal extension/flexion
Amniotic fluid volume	More than one pocket of fluid greater than 2 cm in two perpendicular planes	No pocket greater than 1 cm in two perpendicular planes

Source: Adapted from Manning *et al.*, 1980. Reproduced with permission of Elsevier.

repeated in 24 hours, except in cases of oligohydramnios with intact membranes. In this particular instance, either delivery or close fetal surveillance is indicated depending on the gestational age. BPP scores of 4, 2 or 0 indicate fetal compromise and delivery should be strongly considered. The BPP score correlates linearly with fetal pH. A normal BPP score virtually rules out the possibility of fetal acidemia being present at the time of testing. A normal BPP result is highly reassuring with a stillbirth (false negative) rate of 0.8 per 1000 within one week of the test. The positive predictive value of an abnormal BPP for evidence of fetal compromise (nonreassuring fetal heart rate tracing in labor, acidemia, etc.) is approximately 50%, and a negative predictive value of 99.9% with a normal BPP. A BPP score of 6 has a positive predictive value of 25% while a score of 0 correlates with a compromised fetus in close to 100% of cases. Vibroacoustic stimulation (VAS) can be used as an adjunct in the assessment of BPP score without changing the predictive value of the test. Further, this may reduce unnecessary obstetric interventions. The BPP can either be used as a primary test for fetal well-being in high-risk conditions or, more commonly, a back-up test for a nonreactive NST.

Modified biophysical profile

Modified BPP is a commonly employed primary mode of fetal surveillance in many institutions. It takes into consideration the two most important predictors of fetal well-being – fetal heart rate reactivity and the amniotic fluid volume. The NST is an excellent predictor of acute fetal status when reactive. The amniotic fluid assessment is a means to evaluate the chronic uteroplacental function. The NST is performed in the usual manner and interpreted as previously defined. An amniotic fluid index is obtained as in the BPP and a value of greater than 5 is considered to represent a normal amount of amniotic fluid. The combination of the NST and ultrasonographic evaluation of amniotic fluid volume appears to be as reliable as BPP in acutely assessing fetal well-being with a very low incidence of false negativity. Indeed, the rate of stillbirth within 1 week of a normal modified BPP is the same as a normal BPP (0.8 per 1000). Consequently, the modified BPP is reliable, easy to perform and can be utilized as a primary means of surveillance. The testing frequency should be at least once per week. In a setting of an AFI of less than 8 but greater than 5, a repeat evaluation of the amniotic fluid is recommended within 3–4 days.

Contraction stress test

The CST was historically the first method of fetal assessment using the noninvasive technique of fetal heart rate monitoring during the antepartum period. The test is based upon the fact that normal uterine contractions will restrict fetal oxygen delivery in a transient manner resulting from stasis of blood flow secondary to compression of maternal blood vessels in the uterine wall. Alterations in respiratory exchange in the maternal–fetal interface at the level of the placenta will result in differing responses of the fetus to interruption of maternal blood flow secondary to uterine contractions. If such contractions result in episodic fetal hypoxia, this will be demonstrated by the appearance of late decelerations of the fetal heart rate.

The CST is performed over a period of 30–40 minutes with the patient in the lateral recumbent position while both the fetal heart rate and uterine contractions are simultaneously recorded utilizing an external fetal monitor. A frequency of at least three 40 second or longer contractions in a 10-minute period of monitoring is required and these contractions can be either spontaneous or induced with nipple stimulation or resulting from the intravenous infusion of oxytocin.

The results of the CST are negative (no late or significant variable decelerations), positive (late decelerations following 50% or more of contractions), equivocal (intermittent late or significant variable decelerations or late decelerations following prolonged contractions of 90 seconds or more or with a contraction frequency of more than every 2 minutes), or unsatisfactory. A major problem associated with the CST is the relatively high frequency of equivocal test results.

The relative contraindications to the CST are those conditions associated with a significant increased risk of preterm labor, preterm rupture of membranes, placenta previa with bleeding or history of classical cesarean delivery or extensive uterine surgery.

The CST has a remarkably low false-negative rate of 0.04% (antepartum stillbirth within 1 week of a negative test) but up to 30% of positive tests when followed by induction of labor do not require intrapartum interventions for continued abnormalities of the fetal heart rate or adverse neonatal outcome. Because of the fact that the CST is more labor intensive, takes more time and has a high rate of equivocal test results, this test has generally been abandoned as the primary means of antepartum fetal surveillance. In some centers, the CST remains the primary test for women with type I diabetes. However, the CST remains a very reliable means of either primary or backup fetal surveillance for any number of high-risk pregnancy conditions.

Indications for antepartum fetal surveillance

The American College of Obstetricians and Gynecologists recommends testing in the following situations:

- Women with high-risk factors for fetal asphyxia and stillbirth should undergo antepartum fetal surveillance.
- Maternal conditions: antiphospholipid syndrome, hyperthyroidism, hemoglobinopathies, cyanotic heart disease, systemic lupus erythematosus, chronic renal disease, type I diabetes mellitus and hypertensive disorders.
- Pregnancy-related conditions: pre-eclampsia, gestational hypertension, chronic hypertension, decreased fetal movements, oligohydramnios, poly-hydramnios, intrauterine growth restriction, post-term pregnancy, isoimmunization, previous fetal demise, multiple gestation (with significant growth discrepancy), preterm premature rupture of membranes and uterine bleeding.
- Testing may be initiated at 32–34 weeks for most patients. However, it may begin as early as 26 weeks of gestation in pregnancies with multiple risk factors, when fetal compromise is suspected. However, the fetal reactivity may be diminished due to early gestational age and not necessarily reflect fetal compromise.
- A reassuring test should be repeated on a weekly or a twice-weekly basis.
- Test should be repeated in the event of significant deterioration in the clinical status regardless of the time elapsed since the last test.

Newer indications for antenatal testing

Clinicians should consider utilizing fetal testing in pregnancies at increased risk of fetal demise. Beyond the traditional indications listed above, several recent publications have correlated an increased risk of stillbirth with various additional and common maternal conditions. These include maternal age greater than 35 years, nulliparity, grand multiparity, obesity, abnormalities of first trimester and second trimester genetic risk assessments, pregnancy following assisted reproductive techniques, multifetal gestations even in the absence of fetal growth concerns and various antenatally identified maternal hereditary and acquired thrombophilias. Utilizing such an expanded list of indications would markedly increase the frequency of fetal testing in any population with its attendant costs and consequences. Further, it has not been demonstrated that the use of any form of antenatal fetal surveillance has been associated with a reduction in the incidence of stillbirth in women with such conditions. Consequently, beyond those indications currently listed by the American College of Obstetricians and Gynecologists, the clinician should determine utilization of some form of antenatal testing for other conditions.

Suggested reading

American College of Obstetricians and Gynecologists. Antepartum fetal surveillance. Practice Bulletin Number 9, October 1999 (replaces Technical Bulletin number 188, January 1994; reaffirmed 2012).

Baschat AA, Gembruch U, Harman CR. The sequence of changes in Doppler and biophysical parameters as severe growth restriction worsens. *Ultrasound Obstet Gynecol* 2001;18:571.

Evertson LR, Gauthier RJ, Schifrin BS, Paul RH. Antepartum fetal heart rate testing. I. Evolution of the nonstress test. *Am J Obstet Gynecol* 1979;133:29.

Freeman RK, Anderson G, Dorchester W. A prospective multi-institutional study of antepartum fetal heart rate monitoring. I. Risk of perinatal mortality and morbidity according to antepartum fetal heart rate test results. *Am J Obstet Gynecol* 1982;143:771.

Manning FA, Platt LW, Sipos L. Antepartum fetal evaluation: development of a biophysical profile. *Am J Obstet Gynecol* 1980;136:787.

Miller DA, Rabello YA, Paul RH. The modified biophysical profile: antepartum testing in the 1990s. *Am J Obstet Gynecol* 1996;174:812.

Nageotte MP, Towers CV, Asrat T, Freeman RK. Perinatal outcomes with the modified biophysical profile. *Am J Obstet Gynecol* 1994;170:1672.

Signore C, Freeman RK, Spong CY. Antenatal testing-a reevaluation. Executive summary of the Eunice Kennedy Shriver National Institute of Child Health and Human Development Workshop. *Obstet Gynecol* 2009;113:687.

PROTOCOL 8

Fetal Blood Sampling and Transfusion

Alessandro Ghidini
Perinatal Diagnostic Center, Inova Alexandra Hospital, Alexandria, VA, USA

Clinical significance

Fetal blood sampling (FBS) refers to three techniques used to gain access to fetal blood: cordocentesis (also known as percutaneous umbilical blood sampling), intrahepatic blood sampling, and cardiocentesis. The last two techniques are considered less preferable options because they carry a higher risk of procedure-related fetal loss; they are thus generally reserved for cases in which cordocentesis fails or cannot be performed due to fetal position.

Pathophysiology

Although fetal blood represents a rich source of cells suitable for a variety of diagnostic tests, new technologies can now provide the same information from chorionic villus sampling or amniocentesis, procedures which can be performed at an earlier gestational age and with lower rates of fetal loss than FBS. The most common indications are outlined below.

Cytogenetic diagnosis

Diagnostic FBS for karyotype analysis is indicated when results are required within a few days, such as when the time limit for legal termination is near or when delivery is imminent. In addition, FBS can be used for confirmation of fetal involvement of a true mosaicism, abnormalities at amniocentesis for trisomy 8, 9, 13, 18, 21, or sex chromosomes. However, the absence

Protocols for High-Risk Pregnancies: An Evidence-Based Approach, Sixth Edition.
Edited by John T. Queenan, Catherine Y. Spong and Charles J. Lockwood.
© 2015 John Wiley & Sons, Ltd. Published 2015 by John Wiley & Sons, Ltd.

of abnormal cells in fetal blood does not exclude the possibility of a mosaic cell line in fetal tissues other than blood.

Congenital infection

FBS has a limited role in the prenatal diagnosis of congenital infections such as toxoplasmosis, rubella, cytomegalovirus, varicella, parvovirus, and syphilis. Amniocentesis is currently the primary tool used to diagnose fetal infection and guide parental counseling, since polymerase chain reaction (PCR) and traditional microbiological techniques allow isolation of the infectious agent in amniotic fluid, ascites and pleural fluid without the need to access fetal blood. FBS may still be useful in the presence of fetal hydrops following parvovirus infection, which is usually due to severe anemia.

Suspected fetal anemia

The diagnosis of fetal anemia is suspected in the presence of specific ultrasound findings (e.g., hydrops, pericardial effusions, echogenic bowel, or large chorioangiomas) or laboratory findings (e.g., positive indirect Coombs test, recent maternal parvovirus infection, unexplained high maternal serum alpha-fetoprotein, or sinusoidal fetal heart rate pattern). Peak systolic velocity in the middle cerebral artery is commonly used in such cases as an initial screening step, as it has been found to reliably detect fetal anemia in cases of hemolysis (e.g., RBC isoimmunizations), parvovirus infection, homozygous alpha-thalassemia, and feto-maternal hemorrhage. Moderate/severe anemia is diagnosed in the presence of a decrease in Hb of more than 5 SD below the mean or a decrease in Hb to less than 0.65 MoM, and it is usually an indication for delivery or fetal transfusion.

Coagulopathies

The majority of inherited hematological disorders can be diagnosed by molecular genetic testing on amniocytes or chorionic villi. FBS has a role in the prenatal diagnosis of some congenital hemostatic disorders with a risk of intrauterine or early postnatal hemorrhage, such as severe von Willebrand disease (homozygous cases) and the rare hemophilia cases in which genetic testing is not possible (i.e., those in which the involved mutations are not identified and the family is not informative for linkage). Fresh frozen plasma should be available for fetal transfusion at the time of FBS since excessive bleeding has been reported after sampling in fetuses with coagulopathies.

Platelet disorders

Whereas FBS has been largely supplanted by DNA markers on amniocytes or chorionic cells for the diagnosis of genetic alterations in platelet count or function, FBS can still play a role in the prenatal diagnosis and management of immunological thrombocytopenias. Because exsanguination after cordocentesis has been reported in fetuses affected with alloimmune thrombocytopenia (ATP) and Glanzmann thrombasthenia, it is important to have concentrated platelets available for transfusion prior to needle withdrawal. The most common immune-mediated thrombocytopenias of importance to the obstetrician are idiopathic thrombocytopenic purpura (ITP) and ATP. The risk of neonatal intracranial hemorrhage is 1% for infants of mothers with ITP. No association between the incidence of intracranial hemorrhage and mode of delivery has been reported. Nonetheless, some physicians recommend FBS and that a fetal platelet transfusion or atraumatic cesarean delivery be performed to reduce the risk of neonatal intracranial bleeding if the fetal platelet count is less than $50 \times 10^9/L$. Neonatal ATP is a diagnosis considered after the birth of an affected infant to an immunized mother. The most serious consequence of ATP is intracranial hemorrhage in the baby, which occurs in 10–30% of cases (with 25–50% of these occurring in utero). In families with an affected fetus/infant, the rate of recurrence is in excess of 75–90% and the thrombocytopenia in the second affected child is always as or more severe than in the previous infant. In such cases, paternal platelet-specific antigens should be typed. Fathers homozygous for the specific platelet antigen involved in the ATP will necessarily have affected offspring. In cases of paternal heterozygosity, fetal platelet typing can be performed by PCR on amniotic fluid. Only fetuses incompatible for the relevant platelet antigen are at risk for severe thrombocytopenia from alloimmunization.

Fetal growth restriction

FBS was traditionally used in such cases to identify possible causes of early-onset severe growth restriction, such as karyotype anomalies or fetal infection. The risk of aneuploidy is higher with more severe growth disorders, earlier gestational age at diagnosis, and when growth restriction is associated with polyhydramnios, structural anomalies, or both. Availability of new diagnostic techniques on amniotic fluid (e.g., FISH analysis), which provide results for the most common aneuploidies within few days has obviated much of the need for FBS. Blood gas analysis may show hypoxemia and acidemia; although it has been proposed to assist in the identification of the optimal timing for delivery, FBS carries a 9% to 14% risk of procedure-related loss among growth-restricted fetuses, thus its value for longitudinal assessment of fetal well-being is unproven. Moreover, it is unknown what level of acidemia can be tolerated by the fetus with little or no neurological sequelae, and the effect of gestational age on this level. Therefore, interruption of pregnancy based upon blood gas analysis appears to have a limited role below 32 weeks of gestation since the risks of preterm birth are well known, while those of acidemia are poorly understood.

Suspected fetal thyroid dysfunction

Fetal hyperthyroidism can be diagnosed by FBS in women with a history of Graves disease, high levels of thyroid-stimulating antibodies, and sonographic signs of fetal hyperthyroidism, such as tachycardia, fetal growth restriction, goiter or craniosynostosis. Serial FBS after initiation of maternal administration of PTU is needed to titrate the dose of maternal therapy. Fetal hypothyroidism can be diagnosed by FBS in the presence of fetal goiter usually with polyhydramnios. Serial FBS after initiation of fetal therapy with weekly intra-amniotic injections of levothyroxine are needed to document fetal response and titrate the dose of fetal therapy.

Technique

After ascertaining viability, FBS should be performed near an operating room since an emergency cesarean delivery may be required. Typical steps include:
- Obtain a sample of maternal blood before the procedure for quality control of the fetal samples obtained.
- Intravenous access is optional, but useful to permit administration of analgesics (e.g., Dilaudid® 0.5 mg IV, fentanyl 50–100 μg, midazolam 1–2 mg, or Phenergan 12.5 mg) and antibiotics. Broad-spectrum antibiotic prophylaxis is often administered 30 to 60 minutes prior to the procedure because up to 40% of procedure-related fetal losses are associated with intrauterine infection. Antenatal corticosteroids may be given at least 24 hours prior to the procedure to enhance fetal lung maturity in fetuses at less than 34 weeks of gestation.
- Perform an ultrasound examination to identify either a fixed segment of the cord or the insertion site of the umbilical cord in the placenta (preferable), as these sites will be the target of most procedures.
- Clean the maternal abdomen with an antiseptic solution and drape it.
- Local anesthesia (e.g., 1% lidocaine) to needle insertion site is optional for diagnostic procedures, while it is useful for therapeutic procedures (e.g., transfusions).

- Either a "free-hand technique" or a needle-guiding device attached to the transducer can be employed. A 20–22-gauge spinal needle is generally used. The length of the needle should take into account the thickness of the maternal panniculus, location of the target segment of cord, and the possibility that intervening events, such as uterine contractions, may increase the distance between the skin and target. The standard length of a spinal needle is 8.9 cm, but longer needles (15 cm) are available.
- Amniocentesis, if indicated, should be performed prior to cordocentesis to avoid blood contamination of the fluid specimen.
- The needle is imaged continuously from skin insertion to approach to the target. It is easier and safer to sample the umbilical vein than an artery (puncture of the artery has been associated with a greater incidence of bradycardia and longer post-procedural bleeding).
- Upon entering the umbilical vessel, the stylet is removed and backflow of blood is usually observed. Fetal blood is withdrawn into a syringe attached to the hub of the needle. If free blood is not obtained, the needle can be rotated by a few degrees or gently withdrawn in small increments. Proper positioning of the needle can be confirmed by injection of saline solution into the cord and observation of turbulent flow along the vessel. An initial sample should be submitted to distinguish fetal from maternal cells. Contamination with maternal blood or amniotic fluid can alter the diagnostic value of the specimen. The purity of the fetal blood sample is commonly assessed using the mean corpuscular volume of red blood cells (RBC) since fetal RBCs are larger than maternal RBCs. Dilution with amniotic fluid can be inferred by a similarly proportional decrease in the number of RBCs, white blood cells and platelets in the specimen; diluted samples are still valuable for genetic testing. Blood samples are placed into tubes containing EDTA or heparin and mixed well to prevent clotting. The maximal amount of blood removed should not exceed 6–7% of the fetoplacental blood volume for the gestational age, which can be calculated as 100 mL/kg of estimated fetal weight.
- After the sample, the needle is withdrawn and the puncture site monitored for bleeding.

Transfusion

If an intrauterine transfusion of packed red blood cells (PRBC) is performed after sampling, typical steps include:
- Fetal paralytic agents are rarely used (e.g., pancuronium bromide 0.1–0.3 mg/kg of estimated fetal weight IV), generally if the segment of cord sampled is prone to fetal movements and a transfusion is planned.

- Transfuse warmed, group O negative, CMV-negative, irradiated, PRBCs at a rate below 10 mL/kg/min. The total volume of blood transfused (mL) can be calculated using published tables or the formula:

$$\frac{\text{Estimated fetal blood volume (mL)} \times [\text{desired Hct} - \text{initial fetal Hct}]}{\text{Hct of PRBC to be transfused (usually 80\%--90\%)}}$$

Estimated fetal blood volume is 125 mL/kg of estimated fetal weight at 18–24 weeks, 100 mL/kg at 25–30 weeks, and 90 mL/kg at greater than 30 weeks.
- If an intravascular fetal transfusion fails or is not possible, intraperitoneal transfusion can be performed by injecting PRBC into the peritoneal cavity (any ascitic fluid is aspirated before transfusion): PRBC (mL) = (weeks gestation – 20) × 10 mL.

  If a transfusion of platelets is performed, the platelets are usually obtained from maternal thrombocytopheresis to minimize the risks of transfusion-related infections with pooled donor platelets. A transfusion of 15–20 mL of platelet concentrate increases the fetal platelet count by $70 \times 10^9/L$ to $90 \times 10^9/L$, which is adequate to prevent cord bleeding. It is prudent to slowly transfuse the platelets while awaiting the fetal platelet count, as dislodgement of the needle before transfusion can have fatal consequences for the fetus.
- The fetal heart rate should be monitored intermittently by interrogating an umbilical artery near the sampling area using pulse Doppler. The fetal heart rate of a viable fetus should be monitored for 1–2 hours after the FBS.

Complications

Fetal complications related to FBS include:
- Bleeding from the puncture site is the most common complication of cordocentesis, occurring in up to 50% of cases.
- Cord hematoma is less common and generally asymptomatic, but can be associated with a sudden fetal bradycardia. Expectant management is recommended in the presence of reassuring fetal monitoring and a nonexpanding hematoma.
- Bradycardia is usually transient, but more commonly noted among growth-restricted fetuses.
- Fetal losses – an excess of 1% rate of losses before 28 weeks has been reported after FBS. The most important risk factors for procedure-related loss include operator experience, indication for the procedure (the risk of fetal loss is substantially higher in the presence of fetal growth restriction or nonimmune hydrops) and presence of twins.

Suggested reading

Agrawal P, Ogilvy-Stuart A, Lees C. Intrauterine diagnosis and management of congenital goitrous hypothyroidism. *Ultrasound Obstet Gynecol* 2002;19:501.

Boulot P, Deschamps F, Lefort G, *et al.* Pure fetal blood samples obtained by cordocentesis: Technical aspects of 322 cases. *Prenat Diagn* 1990;10:93.

Daffos F, Forestier F, Kaplan C, Cox W. Prenatal diagnosis and management of bleeding disorders with fetal blood sampling. *Am J Obstet Gynecol* 1988;158:939.

Ghidini A, Sepulveda W, Lockwood CJ, Romero R. Complications of fetal blood sampling. *Am J Obstet Gynecol* 1993;168:1339.

Hogge WA, Thiagarajah S, Brenbridge AN, Harbert GM. Fetal evaluation by percutaneous blood sampling. *Am J Obstet Gynecol* 1988;158:132.

Ludomirsky A, Weiner S, Ashmead GG, *et al.* Percutaneous fetal umbilical blood sampling: procedure safety and normal fetal hematologic indices. *Am J Perinatol* 1988;5:264.

Maxwell DJ, Johnson P, Hurley P, *et al.* Fetal blood sampling and pregnancy loss in relation to indication. *Br J Obstet Gynaecol* 1991;98:892.

Miyata I, Abe-Gotyo N, Tajima A, *et al.* Successful intrauterine therapy for fetal goitrous hypothyroidism during late gestation. *Endocr J* 2007;54:813.

Nicolaides KH, Clewell WH, Rodeck CH. Measurement of human fetoplacental blood volume in erythroblastosis fetalis. *Am J Obstet Gynecol* 1987;157:50.

Paidas MJ, Berkowitz RL, Lynch L, Lockwood CJ, *et al.* Alloimmune thrombocytopenia: fetal and neonatal losses related to cordocentesis. *Am J Obstet Gynecol* 1995;172:475.

Tongsong T, Wanapirak C, Kunavikatikul C, *et al.* Fetal loss rate associated with cordocentesis at midgestation. *Am J Obstet Gynecol* 2001;184:719.

Volumenie JL, Polak M, Guibourdenche J, *et al.* Management of fetal thyroid goitres: a report of 11 cases in a single perinatal unit. *Prenat Diagn* 2000;20:799.

Weiner CP. Cordocentesis for diagnostic indications: two years' experience. *Obstet Gynecol* 1987;70:664.

PART III
Maternal Disease

PROTOCOL 9

Maternal Anemia

Alessandro Ghidini

Perinatal Diagnostic Center, Inova Alexandria Hospital, Alexandria, VA, USA

A comprehensive review of all causes of anemia is often intimidating for the general obstetrician. Moreover, most commonly available algorithms are not targeted to the conditions most prevalent in the obstetric population, which consists mainly of healthy young women. The current protocol aims at suggesting an initial evaluation for anemias, which will allow identification and appropriate therapy of the most common anemias encountered in a pregnant population. The few cases that defy the algorithms outlined in this protocol are best managed in consultation with a hematologist.

Definition

The fall in hemoglobin (Hb) levels seen in normal pregnancies (also known as physiological or dilutional anemia of pregnancy) is caused by a relatively greater expansion of plasma volume (50%) compared with the increase in red cell volume (25%). The fall in hematocrit reaches a nadir during the late second to early third trimester (Table 9.1). The Centers for Disease Control and Prevention (CDC) defined anemia as a Hb or hematocrit (Hct) level below the fifth centile for a healthy, iron-supplemented population, i.e., Hb less than 11 g/dL or Hct less than 33% in the first trimester, and Hb less than 10.5 or Hct less than 32% afterwards. Severe anemia is usually defined as Hb level less than 8.5 mg/dL. The two most common causes of anemia during pregnancy and the puerperium are iron deficiency and acute blood loss.

Consequences

In developed countries, anemia has been associated with increased risk of preterm birth, premature rupture of membranes, infections and fetal

Table 9.1   Changes in laboratory values in pregnancy

	Nonpregnant women	Pregnant women
Hemoglobin (g/dL)	12–16	11–14
Hematocrit	36–46%	33–44%
RBC count ($\times 10^6$/mL)	4.8	4.0
MCV (fL)	80–100	=
MCHC	31–36%	=
Reticulocytes ($\times 10^9$/L)	50–150	=
Ferritin (ng/mL)	>25	>20
RDW (red cell distribution width)	11–15%	=

=, unchanged

Source: Adapted from ACOG Practice Bulletin No. 107, 2009. Reproduced with permission of Lippincott Williams & Wilkins

growth restriction. The symptoms of mild anemia are often indistinguishable from those related to pregnancy, and include fatigue, breathlessness, palpitations, difficulty in concentration, and low intellectual and productive capacity.

Diagnostic workup and treatment

Traditionally, evaluation of anemia starts with the mean corpuscular volume (MCV), based on which anemias are defined as microcytic (less than 80 fL), normocytic (80–100 fL) or macrocytic (greater than 100 fL). However, mixed nutritional deficiencies (folate and iron) often lead to normocytic anemia, and most anemias initially present as normocytic. The red cell distribution width (RDW), a marker of increased variability in red cell size or anisocytosis, is a useful indicator of anemias due to nutritional deficiencies (i.e., it increases above 15% in the presence of iron, folate or vitamin B_{12} deficiencies).

Macrocytic anemia

Figure 9.1 shows the appropriate workup for the search of causes in the presence of macrocytic anemia. *Vitamin B_{12} deficiency* is rare, as most healthy individuals have 2–3 years' storage available in the liver. However, vitamin B_{12} deficiency can be encountered in individuals who have undergone bariatric surgery with partial gastric resection and are not compliant with the recommended vitamin B_{12} supplementation (350 micrograms/day

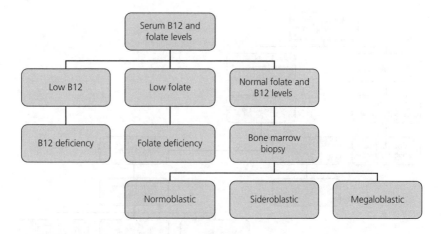

Figure 9.1 Algorithm for evaluation of macrocytic anemia.

sublingually plus 1000 micrograms IM every 3 months if needed), in individuals with pernicious anemia (an extremely uncommon autoimmune disease in women of reproductive age which is diagnosed by the presence of serum intrinsic factor antibodies), and in those with malabsorption (e.g., Crohn's disease or ileal resection). *Folate deficiency* is less common today given the supplementation of foods with folate. In addition to macrocytic anemia, folate deficiency often also causes thrombocytopenia. Recommended folate requirements are 400 micrograms/day during the pregnant state. However, higher dosages are recommended in the presence of multiple gestations, hemolytic disorders such as sickle cell anemia or thalassemia, and in patients taking antiepileptic therapies or sulfa drugs (e.g., sulfasalazine). If a diagnosis of folate deficiency is made or the woman previously had infants with neural tube defects, the recommended dose of folic acid is 4 mg/day. By 4 to 7 days after beginning treatment, the reticulocyte count is increased. In the case of macrocytic anemia with normal folate and vitamin B_{12} levels, a consultation with a hematologist is indicated for bone marrow biopsy.

Normocytic anemia

Figure 9.2 displays the pertinent laboratory workup for normocytic anemia; a low reticulocyte count enables the distinguishing of cases of recent blood loss due to hemolysis (e.g., drug-induced, or immune-based, as witnessed by a positive direct Coombs test) or hemorrhage from the early stage of iron deficiency (see below). Low reticulocyte count with normal or high serum ferritin levels can be seen in the presence of hypothyroidism or chronic disorders, such as inflammatory bowel disease,

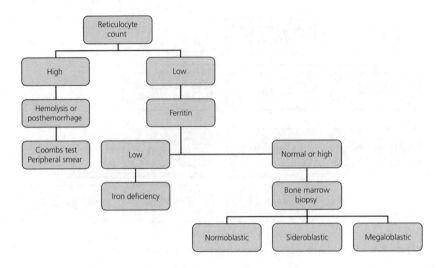

Figure 9.2   Algorithm for evaluation of normocytic anemia.

systemic lupus erythematosus, granulomatous infections, malignant neoplasms and rheumatoid arthritis. Hematology consultation for further assessment is indicated in these circumstances.

Microcytic anemia

Figure 9.3 shows the recommended flow of diagnostic workup for microcytic anemia. Because most cases of microcytic anemia in pregnancy are due to iron deficiency and because serum ferritin is an excellent indicator

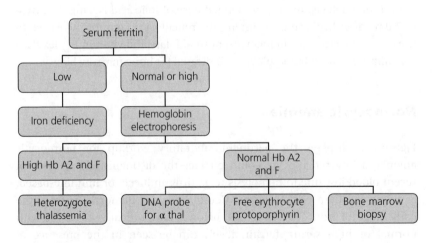

Figure 9.3   Algorithm for evaluation of microcytic anemia.

of body iron stores, the initial step should be assessment of serum ferritin levels. Serum ferritin is the most sensitive screening test for iron deficiency, with a level less than 16 ng/mL indicating depleted iron stores.

Prophylaxis of iron deficiency

In a typical singleton gestation, maternal iron requirements (related to the expansion of the maternal RBC mass, fetal and placental requirements) average 1 gram over the course of pregnancy. In a landmark study of healthy, nonanemic, menstruating young women who agreed to bone marrow biopsy, 66% had inadequate iron stores (Scott and Pritchard). For the above reasons, and because gastrointestinal side effects of oral iron supplementation (constipation, nausea, and diarrhea) are negligible with doses less than 45–60 mg, in the United States, supplementation with elemental iron (30 mg/day) is recommended for all pregnant nonanemic women. The prophylaxis should be continued until 3 months postpartum in areas with high prevalence of anemia. Despite such recommendations, a large study has shown that 50% of women have serum ferritin levels below 16 ng/mL by 26 weeks of pregnancy (Goldenberg et al). A review of randomized clinical trials (most performed in Western countries) shows that routine supplementation in nonanemic women results in higher maternal Hb levels at term and 1 month postpartum, higher serum ferritin levels, lower rates of anemia at term (RR = 0.26) and of iron deficiency anemia in particular (RR = 0.33), and higher serum ferritin levels in the infants (Pena-Rosas and Viteri). However no differences are noted in most clinical outcomes, such as preterm delivery, preeclampsia, or need for transfusion, birth weight, small for gestational age, perinatal mortality or need for NICU admissions.

Treatment of iron deficiency anemia

Higher doses of iron are required for therapy of anemia than for prophylaxis (up to 120–150 mg/day). Table 9.2 lists the most commonly available formulations of *oral iron*. Enteric-coated forms should be avoided because they are poorly absorbed; absorption is increased by intake of iron on an empty stomach and with vitamin C or orange juice. Although several trials have been conducted to compare the types of iron, it is not possible to assess the efficacy of the treatments due to the use of different drugs, doses and routes (Reveiz *et al.*). Gut absorption of iron decreases with increasing doses of iron, therefore it is best to divide the total daily dose into 2–3 doses. A relationship is present between dose of oral iron and gastrointestinal

Table 9.2 Oral preparations for therapy of iron deficiency anemia

Type of iron	Elemental iron (mg)	Brand
Ferrous fumarate	64–200	Femiron, Feostat, Ferrets, Fumasorb, Hemocyte, Ircon, Nephro-Fer, Vitron-C
Ferrous sulfate	40–65	Chem-Sol, Fe50, Feosol, Fergensol, Ferinsol, Ferogradumet, Ferosul, Ferratab, FerraTD, Ferrobob, Ferrospace, Ferrotime, Moliron, Slowfe, Yieronia
Ferrous gluconate	38	Fergon, Ferralet, Simron
Ferrous fumarate and ferrous asparto-glycinate	81	Replica 21/7
Ferric	50–150	Ferrimin, Fe-Tinic, Hytinic, Niferex, Nu-iron

Source: Adapted from ACOG Practice Bulletin No. 107, 2009. Reproduced with permission of Lippincott Williams & Wilkins

side effects. Occurrence of such side effects leads to discontinuation of the therapy in 50% of women. To ensure patients' compliance it is thus important to minimize the side effects: (1) use iron sulfate elixir which allows titration of dosage to the side effects (e.g., 10 mL contain 88 mg of elemental iron, can be taken mixed with orange juice 30 minutes before a meal or 4 hours after a meal); (2) increase the doses of iron gradually; and (3) instruct the patient to take the large doses at bedtime. Stool softeners may be needed to prevent constipation. Serum reticulocyte count can be checked after 7–10 days of therapy to document appropriate response. The rate of increase of Hct is typically slow, and it increases about 1% per week. To replenish iron stores, oral therapy should be continued for 3 months after the anemia has been corrected.

Intravenous (IV) iron is more effective than oral therapy at improving hematological indices, with higher maternal Hb levels at 4 weeks of therapy and lower rates of gastrointestinal side effects. However, randomized trials have not shown significant differences in need for maternal blood transfusion, neonatal birth weight, or neonatal anemia. Therefore, IV therapy is indicated only in patients with severe anemia with intolerance to oral therapy or malabsorption. Different formulations of IV iron are available: those tested in pregnancy or puerperium are shown in Table 9.3. For low-molecular-weight iron dextran, an initial test dose of 25 mL should be given slowly over 5 minutes, observing for possible allergic reactions. For other preparations, test doses are not needed unless allergy to iron dextran is documented or the patient has multiple drug allergies.

Erythropoietin is not indicated in the treatment of iron deficiency anemia unless the anemia is caused by chronic renal failure or other chronic conditions, such as those outlined above among causes of normocytic

Table 9.3 Intravenous preparations for therapy of iron deficiency anemia

Type of intravenous iron	Commercial names	Dose
Iron dextran LMW	INFeD, Cosmofer	1000 mg/60 min (diluted in 250–1000 mL of normal saline)
Ferric gluconate	Ferlecit	125 mg/30 min (diluted in 100 mL of normal saline)
Iron sucrose	Venofer	200 mg/60 min
Ferric carboxymaltose	Ferinject	1000 mg/15 min

Source: Adapted from ACOG Practice Bulletin No. 107, 2009. Reproduced with permission of Lippincott Williams & Wilkins

anemias with low reticulocyte count and normal or high serum ferritin levels. Erythropoietin is an expensive medication with risk of side effects, ranging from flu-like illness to pure red cell aplasia.

Blood transfusion is indicated only for anemia associated with hypovolemia from blood loss or in preparation for a cesarean delivery in the presence of severe anemia.

Suggested reading

Anemia in Pregnancy. ACOG Practice Bulletin No. 95. American College of Obstetricians and Gynecologists. *Obstet Gynecol* 2008;112:201–207.

Centers for Disease Control and Prevention. CDC criteria for anemia in children and childbearing-aged women. *MMWR* 1989;38:400.

Goldenberg RL, Tamura T, DuBard M, *et al.* Plasma ferritin and pregnancy outcome. *Am J Obstet Gynecol* 1996;175:1356.

Kadyrov M, Kosanke G, Kingdom J, *et al.* Increased fetoplacental angiogenesis during first trimester in anaemic women. *Lancet* 1998;352:1747.

Klebanoff MA, Shiono PH, Selby JV, *et al.* Anemia and spontaneous preterm birth. *Am J Obstet Gynecol* 1991;164:59.

Lieberman E, Ryan KJ, Monson RR, *et al.* Risk factors accounting for racial differences in the rate of premature birth. *N Engl J Med* 1987;317:743.

Neural tube defects. ACOG Practice Bulletin No. 44. American College of Obstetricians and Gynecologists. *Obstet Gynecol* 2003;102:203–213.

Pena-Rosas JP, Viteri FE. Effects of routine oral iron supplementation with or without folic acid for women during pregnancy. Cochrane Pregnancy and Childbirth Group. *Cochrane Database Syst Rev* 2009;3.

Reveiz L, Gyte GML, Cuervo LG. Treatments for iron-deficiency anaemia in pregnancy. Cochrane Pregnancy and Childbirth Group. *Cochrane Database Syst Rev* 2011;(10) CD003094.

Scanlon KS, Yip R, Schieve LA, *et al.* High and low hemoglobin levels during pregnancy: differential risk for preterm birth and small for gestational age. *Obstet Gynecol* 2000;96:741.

Scott DE, Pritchard JA. Iron deficiency in healthy young college women. *JAMA* 1967; 199:147.

PROTOCOL 10

Sickle Cell Disease

Marc R. Parrish[1] & John Morrison[2]
[1]Department of Obstetrics and Gynecology, University of Kansas Medical Center, Kansas City, KS, USA
[2]Department of Obstetrics and Gynecology, University of Mississippi Medical Center, Jackson, MS, USA

Clinical significance

Sickle cell anemia is most common in people whose families originate from Africa, South or Central America, the Caribbean Islands, Mediterranean countries (such as Turkey, Greece, and Italy), India, and Saudi Arabia. In the United States, sickle cell anemia affects about 70,000-100,000 people. It mainly affects African Americans but has also been observed in Hispanic Americans. It is a common genetic disease and frequently complicates pregnancy management. Patients with hemoglobin S-S (Hgb S-S), as well as with other genotypic variants, such as hemoglobin S-C (Hgb S-C) and hemoglobin S-β thalassemia (Hgb S-β Thal), are said to have sickle cell disease which is often responsible for adverse effects on the mother, fetus, and newborn. Sickle cell disease has a significant prevalence in the African-American population, with 1 in 12 possessing the sickle cell trait. Among this same population, the frequency of sickle cell anemia (Hgb S-S) is 1 in 500, while Hgb-SC occurs at a rate of 1 in 852. Hemoglobin S-β Thal is somewhat less frequent, with a known prevalence of 1 in 1672.

Approximately 2 million Americans are carriers of the sickle cell trait (Hgb A-S), which has been considered to be an essentially benign condition during pregnancy, with few exceptions. However, its identification is important in offering complete genetic counseling to patients. In addition, it has been associated with twice the rate of urinary tract infections during pregnancy when compared with matched controls. Some investigators have suggested that women with Hgb A-S have an increased risk for placental abnormalities resulting in stillbirth and growth restriction.

Anemia and vaso-occlusive episodes are characteristic of sickle cell diseases. Hemoglobin S-β Thal usually results in only a mild anemia,

Protocols for High-Risk Pregnancies: An Evidence-Based Approach, Sixth Edition.
Edited by John T. Queenan, Catherine Y. Spong and Charles J. Lockwood.
© 2015 John Wiley & Sons, Ltd. Published 2015 by John Wiley & Sons, Ltd.

although its manifestations are variable based on the percentage of Hgb S present. Hemoglobin S-S has been associated with increased complications such as preeclampsia, preterm labor, preterm rupture of membranes, intrauterine growth restriction, antepartum admission, spontaneous abortion and stillbirth. Hemoglobin S-C disease has similarly been linked to intrauterine growth restriction and antepartum admission.

There is significant variability in the course of sickle cell disease, with some experiencing frequent crises, debilitating complications and even death, while others are relatively asymptomatic. The variable clinical symptoms with which these patients present are not fully explained. There is evidence to suggest that this variability may be related to the presence of linked and unlinked genes, which modify the disease expression. Another theory has been that of incomplete penetrance. The life expectancies for sickle cell anemia has also increased, approaching 42 for males and 48 for females, while those with Hgb S-C are significantly higher at 60 and 68 years, respectively. These life expectancies are derived from older data obtained prior to the use of hydroxurea and therefore may have improved compared to the pre-hydroxyurea era.

Pathophysiology

Hemoglobin S-S is characterized by autosomal recessive defects, while Hgb S-β Thal and Hgb S-C are characterized by compound heterozygous defects in the structure and function of the hemoglobin molecule. Sickle hemoglobin results from a gene mutation that substitutes a valine for glutamic acid at the sixth position in the hemoglobin beta-subunit. A missense mutation leading to the substitution of lysine in the sixth position results in hemoglobin C disease. These structurally abnormal molecules function normally in the presence of adequate oxygenation. However, in the presence of relative hypoxia, the substituted amino acid forms a hydrophobic bond with adjacent chains that ultimately yield a dysmorphic and less pliable cellular wall. This structural change is responsible for the characteristic sickle shape of the red blood cell. This structural change is often initiated by states of hypoxia that are associated with infection, extreme temperature changes, acidosis and dehydration. These malformed red blood cells may precipitate microvascular occlusion, resulting in further hypoxia, and ultimately tissue infarction. The hyperviscosity of pregnancy can also exacerbate the process, with consequential maternal–fetal morbidity. The life of the deformed red blood cell is only 12 days, significantly shorter than a normal circulating red cell (120 days). This results in a state of chronic anemia and increased clearance of the cells by the reticuloendothelial system.

Diagnosis

While universal screening of pregnant patients for hemoglobinopathies is not recommended, certain ethnic groups are known to carry a higher risk for these hemoglobinopathies and will benefit from testing. Individuals of African, Southeast Asian and Mediterranean descent should be offered carrier screening. In addition, any patient with a family history of a hemoglobinopathy should be evaluated. Cultural groups considered to be at low risk for hemoglobinopathies include those patients of Japanese, Korean, Native American and northern European descent.

Solubility tests (Sickledex) alone are inadequate for the diagnosis of sickle cell disorders because they cannot distinguish between the heterozygous AS and homozygous SS genotypes. In addition, they fail to detect other pathologic genotypes such as Hgb C trait, thalassemia trait, Hgb E trait, Hgb B trait and Hgb D trait. Those patients who are considered high risk for being carriers of a hemoglobinopathy should undergo a hemoglobin electrophoresis initially. Patients with anemia and a below normal mean corpuscular volume (MCV) should also be evaluated with a hemoglobin electrophoresis if serum iron studies are observed to be normal. If a hemoglobinopathy is identified, the partner should be appropriately tested and counseling by an obstetrician or a genetic counselor should occur. If the partner is found to be either heterozygous or homozygous for a hemoglobinopathy, then antenatal diagnosis may be offered in the form of DNA-based testing utilizing amniocentesis, chorionic villus sampling, or cordocentesis. However, many women turn down the test primarily because of their desire to have a baby in addition to their fear that the fetus will be harmed. Others choose to delay seeking this information until after the delivery, as they would not consider pregnancy interruption based on this diagnosis. With advancing technologies in regard to noninvasive prenatal testing, the commercial availability of an accurate test for fetal sickle cell status is likely on the horizon but currently unavailable. If antenatal diagnosis is not obtained then newborn screening programs in all 50 states ensure that infants with sickle cell disease or sickle cell trait are identified shortly after birth.

Transfusions

Controversy exists concerning the role of prophylactic transfusion in patients with sickle cell disease during pregnancy. While its benefit may be questionable in those sickle cell patients with an uncomplicated pregnancy, transfusions have been shown to lower the incidence of painful crises in pregnancies affected by vaso-occlusive episodes. Simple prophylactic transfusions may be beneficial in women with recurrent pregnancy loss, and those with multiple gestations in order to maintain a hemoglobin level above 9 g/dL. Transfusion should also occur for those patients with severe anemia defined as hemoglobin values 6 g/dL or lower; this threshold has been associated with abnormal fetal oxygenation and fetal death in non-sickle cell populations. In anemic women scheduled to undergo a cesarean delivery, a presurgical transfusion should be considered in order to prepare for blood loss in addition to the benefits achieved in the postsurgical recovery phase. Other indications for simple or exchange transfusions during pregnancy include: acute stroke, acute chest syndrome, acute multi-organ failure, acute symptomatic anemia (e.g., onset of heart failure, dyspnea, hypotension, marked fatigue), reticulocytopenia (most commonly associated with Parvovirus B19 infection, but can occur with any infection), or following hepatic or splenic sequestration. Additionally, women demonstrating continued evidence of preeclampsia despite delivery might also benefit from a blood transfusion.

In the majority of cases, a simple transfusion is appropriate with exchange transfusions typically being reserved for women meeting criteria for transfusion who have higher hemoglobin concentrations and/or those women with a pain crisis who are unresponsive to conservative therapy. If a blood transfusion is warranted we advise the use of cytomegalovirus negative, leukocyte-depleted red blood cells that are phenotypically matched for the C, D, E, and Kell blood groups. Generally, a target hemoglobin concentration of 9–12 g/dL is recommended and if exchange transfusion is being utilized then we recommend the provider set an additional goal of achieving a HgbS concentration of less than 40%. Careful cross matching to minimize minor blood incompatibilities and alloimmunization is critical in avoiding problems later including post-transfusion hemolytic crises.

Complications

The frequency of preconceptual acute vaso-occlusive painful events is usually predictive of the pregnancy course, although some patients may experience an increased incidence of these episodes. Infection must be excluded when a patient presents with pain, and obstetric complications including preterm labor, preeclampsia, abruption, or pyelonephritis must be considered during the evaluation process. Management is similar to nonpregnant patients, including hydration, oxygen therapy and appropriate analgesia. Should infection be suspected, sources should be actively sought and empiric antibiotics used until the etiology of the infection is identified.

Episodic pain associated with sickle cell disease in the pregnant patient is typically attributed to bouts of occlusion in the microcirculation. Many providers caring for pregnant women with sickle cell disease are not familiar with the severe, chronic pain that is associated with longstanding disease. Permanent damage to the microcirculation secondary to years of recurrent sickle injury is the likely etiology for this affliction. Fibrosis and scarring of cartilage and bone can lead to permanent damage and, in some situations, avascular necrosis. Other tissues, by inference, suffer similar insults. In addition to analgesic medications, cognitive/behavioral therapy should be considered in order to enhance coping strategies. Caregivers must also realize that the use of opioids for acute pain relief is not addiction, regardless of the dose or duration of time that opioids are taken. An overrepresentation of a small number of patients in the healthcare system leads many providers to conclude that drug-seeking behavior is a problem for most patients with sickle cell disease. The denial of opioids to patients with sickle cell disease due to fear of addiction is unwarranted and can lead to inadequate treatment. However, the provider must remain cognizant of the potential transient, adverse affects of both a sickle cell crisis (pain or hemolytic) and opioids on the fetus, which can result in abnormal nonstress tests and biophysical profiles. Antenatal assessments usually normalize as the crisis diminishes and as the medication effects subside.

Preterm delivery and intrauterine growth restriction are more common in patients with sickle cell disease. Stillbirths are also more common in this subgroup of patients. However, this devastating complication is much less likely to occur with the utilization of serial maternal-fetal assessments and appropriate interventions.

Many other maternal organ systems can be adversely affected by sickle cell disease, leading to other significant morbidities. These ramifications include cholestasis, cholelithiasis, cholecystitis, osteomyelitis, high-output cardiac failure, cardiomegaly, left ventricular hypertrophy and pulmonary hypertension. A low threshold for consultation with appropriate specialists to assist in the management of these patients throughout their pregnancies is warranted.

The sickle cell status of the fetus does not appear to adversely affect birth outcomes. This is because sickling events do not occur until the production of fetal hemoglobin is replaced by the production of hemoglobin S, which usually begins shortly after 3 months of age.

Follow up

Following delivery, continued surveillance for crises, thrombotic events and infection (i.e., urinary tract infections and endometritis) is imperative. The use of contraceptives should be encouraged in those women who are not planning on conceiving. A 2012 systematic review including eight studies found no evidence that hormonal contraception use in women with sickle cell disease increased their risk of clinical complications. Additionally, the Centers for Disease Control modified the World Health Organization recommendations for medical eligibility criteria for contraceptive use. This modification promotes the use of contraceptive options such as progestin only pills, combined oral, transdermal or vaginal ring hormonal contraception, depot medroxyprogesterone acetate, and levonorgestrel releasing implants or nonhormonal intrauterine devices in sickle cell patients.

Future directions

Research goals include improvement of diagnostic and treatment capabilities and a continued search for a safe and efficient cure. Pre-implantation genetic diagnosis has been successful in diagnosing affected embryos, allowing affected parents with the trait or disease the option to forego embryo implantation. During the antepartum period, free fetal DNA found in the maternal circulation is being investigated as a source for fetal genetic testing for hemoglobinopathies that would replace invasive procedures such as chorionic villus sampling, amniocentesis or cordocentesis. Unfortunately, the commercial availability of an accurate test for fetal sickle cell status is currently unavailable.

Gene therapy is a continual source of investigation, attempting to introduce genes into the hematopoietic system capable of producing HgbA molecules. Currently bone marrow transplants are the only cure and are mostly performed on patients younger than 16 years of age; though the complications are significant and matched donors rare. Improvements in the process of bone marrow donation and transplantation continue. This includes the collection of sibling donor cord blood for stem cell transplantation, allowing marrow transplants without undergoing painful marrow harvesting. Therefore, the option of cord blood banking for subsequent allogeneic hematopoietic cell transplantation is encouraged and should be discussed early in pregnancy.

Families should be advised that cord blood banking is available at no cost, even with private cord blood banks, if a family history of a transplant treatable disease (e.g., sickle cell disease) is present.

Management protocol for pregnancies complicated by sickle cell disease (applies to all sickle cell disease genotypes)

Antepartum (outpatient)
1 Confirm the diagnosis and recommend testing for the partner.
2 Genetic counseling should be offered and the patient should be apprised of the expected course of pregnancy.

3 Consultation with Maternal-Fetal Medicine, Hematology and other specialists as warranted.

4 Discontinue hydroxyurea ideally prior to conception. While known to be teratogenic in animals, little data exist regarding its use during human pregnancy.

5 Obtain a CBC every 4 weeks. Perform iron studies to determine if iron deficiency is a contributing factor to the anemia. Exogenous iron should be given only if indicated by iron studies. The patient should take supplemental folic acid (4 mg/day) due to high red blood cell turnover.

6 Perform a urinalysis with culture and sensitivity in each trimester and in the presence of clinical symptomatology. If the patient has at least one positive culture, then repeat cultures should be obtained monthly.

7 Ensure patient has received a pneumococcal and meningococcal vaccination in the past 5 years and a Haemophilus influenzae type b conjugate vaccine if she did not undergo the vaccination series in childhood. These vaccinations are ideally recommended prior to conception although they are safe to administer in pregnancy. Influenza and hepatitis vaccinations should be documented and updated if needed per standard protocol.

8 Obtain an early ultrasound at 11–13 weeks to establish dating and perform aneuploidy screening followed by a detailed ultrasound at 18–20 weeks. Repeat growth ultrasound at 28 weeks, then every 3–4 weeks until delivery.

9 Initiate weekly fetal surveillance in the form of NST, or biophysical profile at 32 weeks.

10 Consider exchange transfusion in the presence of increasing severity or frequency of pain crises and in those symptomatic patients who are unresponsive to conservative management.

11 Office visits should be scheduled every 1–2 weeks with attention placed on evaluation for infection and the onset of a pain crisis. During the latter half of the pregnancy, additional monitoring is warranted for signs of preterm labor and preeclampsia.

12 Cord blood banking should be discussed early in the pregnancy.

Antepartum (inpatient)

1 Management of pain crises consists of prompt evaluation for precipitating factors (i.e., dehydration or hypoxia) and potential causes such as infection. Initiate oral or intravenous fluid resuscitation (if not contraindicated administer 1 L lactated ringers over 2 hours then maintain at 125 mL/hr), supplemental oxygen titrated to keep saturation at 95% or higher and aggressive pain control using opioids and other adjunct analgesics.

2 If infection is suspected then initiate empiric antibiotic therapy with ceftriaxone due to patient's susceptibility to encapsulated organisms. For

those patients with penicillin/cephalosporin allergies, clindamycin is recommended. If meningitis is suspected, vancomycin is preferred.

3 If there is evidence of impaired pulmonary, hepatic, renal, or CNS function then consultation with a critical care specialist should be obtained
immediately as these are signs of an impending life-threatening event.

4 Medical thromboprophylaxis with Lovenox 40 mg, daily, or heparin
5000–10,000 units subcutaneously, twice daily, in hospitalized patients
who are not actively bleeding. Mechanical prophylaxis (e.g., sequential
compression devices) in those hospitalized patients who are actively
bleeding.

Intrapartum

1 Expect routine term delivery with spontaneous onset of labor. Inductions and cesarean deliveries should be reserved for the usual obstetric
indications.

2 Laboring women should be kept well hydrated, warm and well oxygenated with supplemental oxygen administered to keep their oxygen
saturation levels at 95% or higher.

3 Epidural anesthesia is encouraged during labor to decrease cardiac
demands and oxygen consumption. The use of prostaglandins or oxytocin is not contraindicated based on the presence of sickle cell disease
alone.

4 Obtain cord blood to establish if the newborn has evidence of a
hemoglobinopathy and consider collection for cord blood banking if the
parents have been counseled appropriately and wish to proceed with
the banking process.

Postpartum

1 Continued vigilance to avoid hypovolemia, severe anemia (i.e., Hgb less
than 6 g/dL) hypoxia, infection (increased rates of urinary tract infections and endometritis) and venous thrombotic events.

2 Women undergoing a cesarean delivery should receive prophylactic anticoagulation for 6 weeks after the delivery.

3 Postpartum contraceptive counseling is recommended. All methods of
commercially available contraceptives are considered safe in women
with sickle cell disease.

4 Hydroxyurea can be resumed in the postpartum period only if the
mother does not plan on breastfeeding.

Sickle cell trait

In women with the sickle cell trait there is no evidence to suggest a
significant increase in associated pregnancy risks. Assessment of the
partner's hemoglobin genotype and subsequent genetic counseling is

strongly encouraged. Monthly urinalyses are warranted in this group of patients due to an increased risk for infectious uropathy.

Suggested reading

Bates SM, Greer IA, Middeldorp S, *et al.* VTE, thrombophilia, antithrombotic therapy, and pregnancy: Antithrombotic therapy and prevention of thrombosis, 9th ed: American College of Chest Physicians Evidence-Based Clinical Practice Guidelines. *Chest* 2012; 141:e691S.

Benjamin LJ, Dampier CD, Jacox AK, *et al.* Guideline for the Management of Acute and Chronic Pain in Sickle-Cell Disease. Acute Pain Society Clinical Practice Guidelines Series, No. 1. Glenview, IL, 1999.

Haddad LB, Curtis KM, Legardy-Williams JK, *et al.* Contraception for individuals with sickle cell disease: a systematic review of the literature. *Contraception* 2012;85:527.

Hassell K. Pregnancy and sickle cell disease. *Hematol Oncol Clin N Am* 2005;19:903–916.

Hemoglobinopathies in pregnancy. ACOG Practice Bulletin No. 78. American College of Obstetricians and Gynecologists. *Obstet Gynecol* 2007;109:229–237. (Reaffirmed 2013).

Howard RJ, Tuck SM, Pearson TC. Pregnancy in sickle cell disease in the UK: results of a multicentre survey of the effect of prophylactic blood transfusion on maternal and fetal outcome. *Br J Obstet Gynaecol* 1995;102:947.

Kahn SR, Lim W, Dunn AS, Cushman M, Dentali F, Akl EA, Cook DJ, Balekian AA, Klein RC, Le H, Schulman S, Murad MH. Prevention of VTE in nonsurgical patients: Antithrombotic Therapy and Prevention of Thrombosis, 9th ed: American College of Chest Physicians Evidence-Based Clinical Practice Guidelines. *American College of Chest Physicians: Chest* 2012;141(2 Suppl):e195S.

Koshy M, Burd L, Wallace D, *et al.* Prophylactic red-cell transfusions in pregnant patients with sickle cell disease. *A randomized cooperative study. N Engl J Med* 1988;319:1447.

Okusanya BO, Oladapo OT. Prophylactic versus selective blood transfusion for sickle cell disease in pregnancy. *Cochrane database syst rev* 2013;12:CD010378.

Rees DC, Olunjohungbe AD, Parker NE, Stephens AD, Telfer P, Wright J. Guidelines for the management of the acute painful crisis in sickle cell disease. British Committee for Standards in Haematology. General haematology task force by the sickle cell working party. *Br J Haematol* 2003;120:744–752.

Solomon LR. Treatment and prevention of pain due to vaso-occlusive crises in adults with sickle cell disease: an educational void. *Blood* 2008;111:997.

The management of sickle cell disease. National Institutes of Health; National Heart, Lung, and Blood Institute, Division of Blood Diseases and Resources. NIH publication 04-2117, revised 2004. www.nhlbi.nih.gov/health/prof/blood/sickle/ (Accessed on April 21, 2014).

Umbilical Cord Blood Banking. ACOG Committee Opinion No. 399. American College of Obstetricians and Gynecologists. *Obstet Gynecol* 2008;111:475–457.

U.S. Medical Eligibility Criteria for Contraceptive Use, 2010. Adapted from the World Health Organization Medical Eligibility Criteria for Contraceptive Use, 4th edition MMWR 2010; 59. Available at www.cdc.gov/mmwr/preview/mmwrhtml /rr59e0528a1.htm. (Accessed April, 2014).

Villers MS, Jamison MG, De Castro LM, James AH. Morbidity associated with sickle cell disease in pregnancy. *Am J Obstet Gynecol* 2008;199:125.e1–125.5.

Zempsky WT. Treatment of sickle cell pain: fostering trust and justice. *JAMA* 2009; 302:2479.

PROTOCOL 11

Isoimmune Thrombocytopenia

*Richard L. Berkowitz & Sreedhar Ghaddipati**
Department of Obstetrics and Gynecology, Division of Maternal Fetal Medicine,
Columbia University Medical Center, New York, NY, USA

Overview

Isoimmune or idiopathic thrombocytopenic purpura (ITP) is an autoimmune disorder characterized by antibody-mediated destruction of platelets by the reticuloendothelial system (RES). Acute ITP is usually self-limited and occurs predominantly in children, most often following a viral illness. The chronic form is more common in women than men and the peak incidence occurs in the third decade of life. It is estimated that ITP complicates 1–2 of every 1000 pregnancies.

Pathophysiology

Relevant autoantibodies are usually immunoglobulin G (IgG) and are directed against platelet-specific membrane glycoproteins. Antigen–antibody complexes are removed from the circulation by the RES, primarily the spleen, resulting in decreased circulating platelets. Inhibition of megakaryocyte platelet production is also a component of the disease. When the rate of platelet destruction exceeds the rate of platelet production, thrombocytopenia results.

Since platelet counts have been included in automated complete blood count (CBC) reports that are routine in pregnancy, and perhaps because of the physiological increase in platelet turnover during pregnancy, an increased incidence of thrombocytopenia has been noted in pregnant patients. Many women with mild thrombocytopenia noted late in gestation are misdiagnosed as having ITP when they actually have gestational thrombocytopenia. In this mild disorder, C3 (activated complement) rather than IgG binds to platelets. Platelet counts usually

* Dr. Sreedhar Ghaddipati has regrettably passed away prior to the publication of this protocol.

Protocols for High-Risk Pregnancies: An Evidence-Based Approach, Sixth Edition.
Edited by John T. Queenan, Catherine Y. Spong and Charles J. Lockwood.
© 2015 John Wiley & Sons, Ltd. Published 2015 by John Wiley & Sons, Ltd.

remain above 70,000/microliter and normalize within 2–12 weeks post-partum. These patients are generally asymptomatic without a previous history of decreased platelet counts except perhaps in previous pregnancies. The recurrence risk of gestational thrombocytopenia is unknown and risk for neonatal thrombocytopenia negligible.

While the majority of women with ITP will have a history of easy bruising, petechiae, epistaxis, and gingival bleeding, some are asymptomatic. Maternal hemorrhage rarely occurs unless the platelet count is less than 20,000/microliter. Pregnancy is not thought to increase the incidence of, or to worsen, ITP. However, ITP may have a profound impact on pregnancy as severe thrombocytopenia places the mother at risk for hemorrhage in both the antepartum and postpartum periods. ITP may also affect the fetus, as there is a small risk that it may be associated with neonatal thrombocytopenia, which places the neonate at risk for poor outcomes such as intracranial hemorrhage and subsequent long-term adverse neurological outcomes.

Maternal antiplatelet IgG antibodies can cross the placenta, bind to fetal platelets, and enhance the destruction of fetal platelets resulting in transient neonatal thrombocytopenia. There is an approximately 10% risk that the neonate will have a platelet count less than 50,000/microliter and a less than 5% risk that the neonate will have a platelet count of less than 20,000/microliter. Neonatal platelet counts of less than 50,000/microliter can result in minor bleeding such as purpura, ecchymoses, and melena. Rarely, fetal thrombocytopenia associated with ITP can lead to intracranial hemorrhage irrespective of mode of delivery. Serious bleeding complications are thought to be less than 3%, and the rate of intracranial hemorrhage is thought to be less than 1%, which is greater than the risk among neonates born to women without ITP. The actual incidence of neonatal thrombocytopenia and associated hemorrhage is uncertain as no large-scale studies exist. The correlation between maternal and fetal platelet count is poor, and no noninvasive method is currently available to detect neonates at risk. It is thought that women with a history of splenectomy, a platelet count of less than 50,000/microliter at some time during the pregnancy, and a previous child with neonatal thrombocytopenia are at increased risk for fetal/neonatal thrombocytopenia. Circulating antibodies also may be associated with increased fetal risk. Maternal administration of steroids and or intravenous gamma globulin has no demonstrable therapeutic effect on the fetal platelet count.

Diagnosis

ITP is a diagnosis of exclusion as there are no specific diagnostic tests or pathognomic signs or symptoms for the disorder. Work-up requires

exclusion of other causes of decreased platelet counts in pregnancy such as:
- HELLP
- Drug reaction
- Lab error
- Systemic lupus erythematosus
- Antiphospholipid antibody
- Lymphoproliferative disorder
- Human immunodeficiency virus infection
- Hypersplenism
- Disseminated intravascular coagulation
- Thrombotic thrombocytopenic purpura
- Hemolytic uremic syndrome
- Congenital thrombocytopenia
- Gestational thrombocytopenia

Diagnostic criteria include:
- Normal CBC with the exception of persistent thrombocytopenia (platelet count less than 100,000/microliter)
- Peripheral smear may show decreased number of platelets, with presence of large platelets
- Normal coagulation studies
- Absence of splenomegaly
- No other causes of thrombocytopenia
- Antiplatelet antibodies may or may not be detectable
- Bone marrow aspirate (not essential for diagnosis) shows normal or increased number of megakaryocytes.

Antepartum management

Pregnant women with a history of ITP require serial assessment of their platelet counts as these counts many fluctuate during pregnancy. Monthly testing is suggested for the first two trimesters. In the third trimester, patients should be tested every other week and then weekly as they approach term. Consultation with a physician who is experienced with ITP is suggested. Pregnant women with ITP and thrombocytopenia should be encouraged to restrict their activity and to avoid trauma, alcohol, aspirin, and all platelet inhibitor medications. They should also avoid intramuscular injections, and treat fevers with acetaminophen.

The goal of therapy in pregnant patients with ITP is to decrease the risk of bleeding complications associated with severe thrombocytopenia. Platelet function is usually normal despite decreased numbers of platelets. Thus, maintaining a normal platelet count in these patients is not necessary.

The general consensus is that treatment is not required unless the platelet count is significantly less than 50,000/microliter, or if the patient is symptomatic. However, counts greater than 50,000/microliter may be desired at the time of delivery and for regional anesthesia. It is important to note that treatment is indicated for the maternal status and not for fetal indications, as these therapies have not been proven to decrease the risks of neonatal thrombocytopenia and subsequent hemorrhage. The initial treatment for ITP is prednisone 1 mg/kg orally once per day. Improvement in platelet count is usually noted within 3–7 days. The maximal response is usually noted within 2–3 weeks. The dose can be increased as necessary. Once the platelet count has increased to an acceptable level, the dosage can be tapered by 10–20% until the lowest dose required to maintain the platelet count at an acceptable level is determined.

Intravenous immune globulin (IVIG) may be warranted if the patient remains refractory to oral steroids, the platelet count is less than 10,000/microliter, or if the platelet count is less than 30,000/microliter and the patient is symptomatic or delivery is likely within a week. A response may be noted anywhere from 6 to 72 hours following administration of IVIG. If IVIG is being considered, consultation with a physician familiar with this treatment is recommended. In cases of continued resistance, high-dose IV steroids (methyl-prednisolone) in conjunction with IVIG or azothioprine may be considered. In nonpregnant adults additional treatment modalities for steroid-resistant patients include anti-Rh immunoglobulin in Rh-positive patients and the anti-CD20 antibody, rituximab. However, the former therapy could induce hemolysis in Rh-positive fetuses and there is limited experience with rituximab in pregnancy, although the agent has been associated with B-cell lymphocytopenia persisting beyond 6 months in some exposed infants. Rituximab is classified as a class C drug in pregnancy by the US Food and Drug Administration.

If there is no response to IVIG, splenectomy should be considered. Removal of the spleen removes the primary site of platelet destruction and antibody production. Splenectomy has been associated with complete remission of ITP in some patients, but has not consistently been found to be beneficial in those patients who fail IVIG therapy. While splenectomy can be performed safely in pregnancy, the procedure should be avoided if possible as it is technically difficult and may trigger preterm delivery. The procedure may be warranted in pregnancy if platelet counts are less than 10,000/microliter and the patient has failed both prednisone and IVIG therapy. The optimal timing for splenectomy is the second trimester. If deemed necessary in the third trimester, cesarean delivery followed by the splenectomy should be considered. In addition to the flu vaccine, pregnant women with a history of splenectomy should be vaccinated against pneumococcus, menigococcus, and Haemophilis influenzae.

Platelet transfusion should only be utilized as a temporizing measure for severe hemorrhage or to help prepare a patient for surgery. Donor platelets do not survive for long periods of time in women with ITP. The medications commonly used to treat ITP in nonobstetric patients such as colchicines, vinca alkaloids, cyclophosphamide, danazol and other potentially terato- genic agents are avoided in pregnancy as they are thought to have adverse effects on the fetus.

Intrapartum management

The most significant clinical dilemma relating to ITP is the fact that the fetus may be at risk for developing fetal/neonatal thrombocytopenia and severe bleeding complications. The risk is small, and unfortunately, there is no test that can accurately discern if a fetus is at risk for severe thrombocytopenia. At the present time, obtaining a fetal platelet count prior to delivery is not thought to be necessary. Scalp sampling during labor is often inaccurate and technically challenging. Cordocentesis prior to labor involves a 1–2% risk of emergent cesarean delivery secondary to complications of that proce- dure. Vaginal delivery is not contraindicated in these women and cesarean delivery is not thought to protect these patients from fetal bleeding com- plications. Thus, routine obstetric management is appropriate for pregnant women with ITP. However, fetal scalp electrodes and delivery by vacuum should be avoided. Antiplatelet medications such as nonsteroidal inflam- matory drugs (NSAIDs) should not be prescribed to these patients during the postpartum period. Breast-feeding is safe for women with a history of ITP.

Consultation with an anesthesiologist is recommended for patients with ITP. Neuraxial anesthesia (spinal or epidural) is generally safe in women with platelet counts more than 80,000/microliter provided that coagula- tion studies are normal. The risk of epidural hematoma with neuraxial anesthesia is exceedingly low in patients with functional platelets and platelet counts more than 100,000/microliter. The risk does not increase significantly until the platelet count falls below 50,000–75,000/microliter. A summary of observational studies has not revealed an increase in the risk of hemorrhagic complications following accruing neuraxial anesthesia with platelet counts between 50,000 and 100,000/microliter. Generally, this form of anesthesia should be avoided in patients with platelet counts less than 50,000/microliter as the risk of hematoma is believed to be greater than acceptable. Consistency of the platelet count weighs significantly in the decision to proceed with neuraxial anesthesia. Thromboelastogram testing is not routinely available and thus has a limited role in assessing adequate clot formation. In patients with platelet counts between 50,000 and 100,000/microliter, there should be consultation between the obstetrician and anesthesiologist and a unified risk/benefit analysis should be presented to the patient.

It is recommended that these women deliver in a hospital where all physicians caring for the patient including the obstetrician, anesthesiologist, and pediatrician are familiar with ITP, and where potential maternal and neonatal complications can be adequately handled. The infant's platelet count should be monitored through the first few days of life as thrombocytopenia may develop in the postpartum period. Head ultrasound should be performed if the neonate was born with, or develops, thrombocytopenia.

Conclusion

In summary, ITP is a relatively rare disease in pregnancy and is often a diagnosis of exclusion. For the most part, maternal and fetal outcomes are favorable. Serial platelet counts are suggested. Consultation with a physician familiar with the care of these patients is often warranted. Platelet counts significantly less than 50,000/microliter should be considered for treatment, especially in preparation for intrapartum management. Likewise, symptomatic patients require treatment. Prednisone is the first-line therapy. IVIG may be necessary for refractory cases. Splenectomy is reserved for severe cases refractory to other treatments. While up to 10% of neonates may be diagnosed with neonatal thrombocytopenia, the risk for neonatal intracranial hemorrhage is thought to be less than 1%. Delivery at a center familiar with this disorder and the potential maternal and neonatal complications is advised. Vaginal delivery is not thought to place these patients at increased risk for fetal intracranial hemorrhage and elective cesarean delivery has not been proven to be protective. As a result, routine obstetric management is appropriate for the majority of these patients. However, fetal scalp electrodes and delivery by vacuum should be avoided. The use of medications affecting platelet function such as NSAIDs is not recommended.

Suggested reading

American College of Obstetricians and Gynecologists. Practice Bulletin. *Thrombocytopenia in Pregnancy.* Practice Bulletin #6, September 1999. Reaffirmed in 2009.

Burrows R, Kelton J. Low fetal risks in pregnancies associated with idiopathic thrombocytopenic purpura. *Am J Obstet Gynecol* 1990;163:1147–1150.

Burrows R, Kelton J. Fetal thrombocytopenia and its relation to maternal thrombocytopenia. *N Engl J Med* 1993;329:1463–1467.

Cines DB, McMillan R. Management of adult idiopathic thrombocytopenic purpura. *Annu Rev Med* 2005;56:425–442.

Choi S, Brull, R. Neuraxial techniques in obstetric and non-obstetric patients with common bleeding diatheses. *Anesth Analgesia* 2009;109:648–660.

Clark AL, Gall SA. Clinical uses of intravenous immunoglobulin in pregnancy. *Am J Obstet Gynecol* 1997;176:241–253.

Payne SD, Resnik R, Moore TR, Hedriana HL, Kelly TF. Maternal characteristics and risk of severe neonatal thrombocytopenia and intracranial hemorrhage in pregnancies complicated by autoimmune thrombocytopenia. *Am J Obstet Gynecol* 1997;177:149–155.

Samuels P, Bussel J, Baitman L, *et al.* Estimation of the risk of thrombocytopenia in the offspring of pregnant women with presumed immune thrombocytopenic purpura. *N Engl J Med* 1990;323:229–235.

Valet AS, Caulier MT, Devos P, *et al.* Relationships between severe neonatal thrombocytopenia and maternal characteristics in pregnancies associated with autoimmune thrombocytopenia. *Br J Haematol* 1998;103:397–401.

Webert KE, Mittal R, Sigouin C, *et al.* A retrospective 11-year analysis of obstetric patients with idiopathic thrombocytopenic purpura. *Blood* 2003;102:4306–4311.

PROTOCOL 12

Autoimmune Disease

Charles J. Lockwood
Department of Obstetrics and Gynecology, University of South Florida, Morsani College of Medicine, Tampa, FL, USA

Systemic lupus erythematosus

Overview

Systemic lupus erythematosus (SLE) complicates 1 in 2000 to 1 in 5000 pregnancies, with a fivefold increase in prevalence among African American women. It is associated with multiple pregnancy complications, including spontaneous abortion, fetal loss, intrauterine growth restriction, fetal distress, preeclampsia and both spontaneous or indicated preterm birth.

Pathophysiology

The disease is triggered by an abnormal humoral antibody response that causes the production of antibodies that cross-react with a variety of tissues in genetically susceptible individuals. These antibodies cause damage by: (1) forming nonspecific antibody–antigen complexes, whose resultant inflammation causes glomerulonephritides, arthritis, dermatitis, central nervous system (CNS) involvement, pericarditis, pneumonitis and hepatitis; or (2) antibodies directed against cell-specific antigens that cause isolated cell or tissue damage (e.g., autoimmune thrombocytopenia, hemolytic anemia, antiphospholipid antibody (APA) syndrome, leukopenia, vasculitis and/or neonatal congenital heart block (CHB). The risk of developing a specific manifestation is linked to a patient's HLA-DR and HLA-DQ histocompatability loci.

Diagnosis

Patients generally present with intermittent, unexplained fevers, malaise, arthralgias, myositis, serositis, thrombocytopenia, nephritis, and/or CNS abnormalities. A positive antinuclear antibody (ANA) is found in 98% of patients (and 10–20% of uncomplicated pregnant patients). The diagnosis

Protocols for High-Risk Pregnancies: An Evidence-Based Approach, Sixth Edition.
Edited by John T. Queenan, Catherine Y. Spong and Charles J. Lockwood.
© 2015 John Wiley & Sons, Ltd. Published 2015 by John Wiley & Sons, Ltd.

is established when *four or more* of the following American College of Rheumatology criteria are present:

1 Malar rash.
2 Discoid rash.
3 Photosensitivity.
4 Oral ulcers.
5 Nonerosive arthritis.
6 Serositis (Pleuritis or pericarditis).
7 Renal disease manifested by proteinuria greater than 500 mg/day, 3+ urine protein, and/or cellular casts on urinalysis.
8 Neurological abnormalities including seizures or psychosis.
9 Hematological abnormalities including hemolytic anemia with reticulocytosis, immune thrombocytopenia with platelet counts less than $100,000/mm^3$ in the absence of offending drugs, or two or more occurrences of leukopenia less than 4000 cells/mm^3 or lymphopenia less than 1500/mm^3.
10 Laboratory findings including anti-dsDNA, anti-Sm, or antiphospholipid antibodies (APA) (Table 12.1).
11 Positive ANA in the absence of drug therapy.

Effect of SLE on pregnancy

The prognosis for a live birth depends on four factors: the activity of the disease at conception and the occurrence of subsequent flares during pregnancy, the coexistence of lupus nephritis, development of APA, and the presence of anti-SSA (Ro) antibodies. Overall, SLE is associated with higher rates of various adverse outcomes. Wallenius *et al.* analyzed data from a Norwegian national registry covering pregnancies between 1998 and 2009 to identify outcomes among SLE patients having 95 first and

Table 12.1 SLE-associated laboratory findings

Antibody	HLA	Clinical feature
Anti-ds DNA	DR2	Nephritis
	DQB1	Vasculitis
Anti-SM	DR2	Nephritis
	DQw6	CNS disease
Anti-RNP	DR4	Arthritis
	DQw8	Myositis and Raynaud's
Anti-SSA (Ro)	DR3	CHB
	DQw2.1	Sjögren syndrome
Anti-SSB (La)		Negatively associated with renal disease in SSA(1) patients
Anti-centromere		CREST syndrome
Anti-U1-RNP		Mixed connective tissue disease
LAC and ACA		APAS

145 subsequent births. Compared with control patients, affected patients had a twofold higher cesarean delivery rate in both first and subsequent births. Affected patients had higher rates of low birth weight infants in their first (adjusted odds ratio of 5.00; 95% CI: 3.02–8.27) and subsequent (aOR 4.33; 95% CI: 2.64–7.10) births; and higher preterm birth rates in their first (aOR 4.04; 95% CI: 2.45–6.56) and subsequent (aOR 3.13; 95% CI: 1.97–4.98) births. Congenital anomalies were around threefold more common in first and subsequent pregnancies, but stillbirth rates were increased only in first pregnancies (aOR 7.34; 95% CI: 2.69–20.03).

A meta-analysis by Smyth *et al.* of 37 studies conducted between 1980 and 2009 involving 1,842 SLE patients having 2,751 pregnancies reported rates of lupus flare of 25.6%, hypertension (16.3%), nephritis (16.1%), preeclampsia (7.6%), and eclampsia (0.8%). The rate of spontaneous abortion was 16.0%, stillbirth (3.6%), neonatal deaths (2.5%), and intrauterine growth restriction (12.7%). The preterm birth rate was 39.4%. Meta-regression analysis displayed positive associations between preterm birth and active nephritis as well as an increased incidence of hypertension and preeclampsia in patients with active or a history of lupus nephritis. Antiphospholipid antibodies were also associated with hypertension, preterm birth, and an increased rate of induced abortion. While it remains uncertain as to whether flares are more common in pregnancy, patients with a history of lupus flare in the prior 6 months have an increased risk of adverse outcome and recurrent flare, and contraception should be employed. Other risk factors for perinatal and maternal morbidity and mortality include pulmonary hypertension, chronic active renal disease with creatinine levels greater than 2.8 mg/dl, history of cerebrovascular accident and cardiomyopathy.

Evaluation

Many patients with underlying renal disease may be on an angiotensin-converting enzyme (ACE) inhibitor to control hypertension and slow the progress of renal disease. These and related agents should be stopped prior to or immediately after conception as they are teratogenic. The following laboratory studies should be obtained at the first visit and in each trimester:

1 APA screen with lupus anticoagulant (LAC) and anticardiolipin antibody (ACA) assays – patients with SLE and APA appear to be at a twofold to threefold higher risk of fetal death after 9 weeks of gestation compared with SLE patients without such antibodies.

2 24-hour urine collection for creatinine clearance and total protein, and urinalysis – as noted lupus nephritis and renal failure are poor prognostic indices.

3 Complete blood count – useful to rule-out autoimmune hemolysis and thrombocytopenia and as an aid in the detection of subsequent diagnoses of flares and superimposed preeclampsia and HELLP syndrome.
4 Anti-Ro/SSA and anti-La/SSB antibodies – 2% of patients with such antibodies are at risk for neonatal lupus and congenital heart block (CHB). Their presence also suggests the child has a 2% risk of ultimately developing SLE as an adult. Recurrence risk for CHB is 15%.
5 Anti-double-stranded DNA antibodies, complement (CH50, or C3 and C4) levels – these are relatively sensitive markers of a flare. Liver function tests may also be helpful in differentiating flares from superimposed preeclampsia (see Table 12.2).

Fetal surveillance should include:
1 Baseline dating scan.
2 Anatomy scan at 20 weeks.
3 Serial fetal echocardiograms and weekly assessment of heart rate if SSA or SSB antibodies are detected or if there is a history of a prior infant with CHB. These patients should be managed with a pediatric cardiologist or maternal–fetal medicine specialist with expertise in this area.
4 Monthly growth scans and assessment of amniotic fluid volume.
5 Nonstress tests and/or biophysical profiles, weekly beginning at 36 weeks in uncomplicated cases or at 28 weeks and beyond given the presence of fetal growth restriction, APA, lupus flare, worsening renal function, or hypertension.

Treatment

1 Predinisone remains the mainstay of therapy for active disease in pregnancy. If patients are refractory to glucocorticoid therapy add azathioprine.
2 Hydroxychloroquine appears safe in pregnancy and may be associated with reduced rates of CHB.
3 Low-molecular-weight heparin and low-dose aspirin should be used in SLE patients with APA. If there is no history of thrombosis or other major thrombotic risk factors, use prophylactic doses (e.g., enoxaparin 40 mg, subcutaneously, every 12 hours, adjusted to maintain antifactor Xa levels at 0.1–0.2 units/mL, 4 hours after an injection). If there is a history of maternal thrombosis, or a prior fetal loss on prophylactic low-molecular-weight heparin, use therapeutic does (e.g., enoxaparin 1 mg/kg, subcutaneously, every 12 hours to maintain antifactor Xa levels of 0.6–1 units/mL, 4–6 hours after injection). Anticoagulant therapy should be continued for 6 weeks postpartum (patients with recurrent thrombosis generally receive long-term, oral, anticoagulant therapy when not pregnant).

Table 12.2 Differentiating a lupus flare from preeclampsia

Lupus flare	Superimposed PIH
Any gestational age	Third trimester
Diffuse SLE symptoms	Preeclampsia symptoms (headache, etc.)
Increased anti-DNA titer	Stable anti-DNA titer
Stable platelets (if no immune thrombocytopenia or APA)	Thrombocytopenia
Normal AST, ALT	Elevations in AST, ALT
Normal plasma fibronectin	Increased plasma fibronectin
Exacerbation postpartum	Resolution postpartum

Antepartum SLE flare

The occurrence of a lupus flare should be treated with prednisone, 60 mg/day orally for 3 weeks, with gradual tapering of the dose to 10 mg/day. Alternatively, intravenous methylprednisolone, 1000 mg given over 90 minutes once a day for 3 days may permit rapid control of a flare. Patients with evidence of membranous or diffuse glomerulonephritis should be treated with even higher doses of prednisone up to 200 mg/day and/or plasmapheresis (with intravenous immunoglobulin or fresh frozen plasma) or azathioprine. Given the osteopenic effects of glucocorticoids, patients treated with prednisone should receive calcium supplementation. In addition, they should undergo repeated glucose screens. Stress dose steroids must be given at delivery in all SLE patients treated with more than 20 mg/day of prednisone or its equivalent for more than 3 weeks during the pregnancy or for more than 1 month in the past year. Hydroxychloroquine may also be employed. Rituximab crosses the placenta and can induce B-cell lymphocytopenia lasting up to 6 months in exposed infants. Its use should be limited to maternal life-threatening conditions refractory to other therapies.

Timing of delivery

Uncomplicated SLE

In patients with SLE in the absence of SSB/SSA antibodies, APA, worsening nephritis or hypertension, fetal growth restriction, oligohydraminos, or superimposed preeclampsia, delivery can be delayed until 40 weeks provided that the twice-weekly fetal testing initiated at 36 weeks is reassuring.

In the presence of deteriorating maternal or fetal health:

Beyond 34 weeks of gestation

Patients beyond 34 weeks with worsening renal, liver, or CNS function; hypertension; fetal growth restriction with oligohydraminos, absent or reversal of diastolic Doppler flow, cessation of fetal growth, or nonreassuring fetal testing should be promptly delivered. Cesarean delivery is reserved for usual obstetric indications. Intravenous magnesium sulfate prophylaxis should be used in the presence of superimposed preeclampsia.

At 28–34 weeks of gestation

Patients between 28 and 34 weeks with worsening renal or liver function, development of or exacerbation of hypertension, CNS symptoms, or uteroplacental vascular compromise should be immediately hospitalized and given appropriate medical therapy (e.g., prednisone, antihypertensives) as well as a course of betamethasone to enhance fetal lung maturity, and daily fetal heart rate testing or biophysical profiles. Delivery is indicated for uncontrolled maternal hypertension, the development of severe preeclampsia, or fetal distress. The cessation of fetal growth (evaluated every 2 weeks) may be an indication for delivery after 28 weeks in the presence of severe oligohydraminos, persistent reverse diastolic Doppler flow, or both. Cesarean delivery is reserved for usual obstetric indications. Intravenous magnesium sulfate prophylaxis should be used as indicated in the presence of suspected preeclampsia or for neonatal neuroprotection.

At 24–28 weeks of gestation

Patients between 24 and 28 weeks with deteriorating maternal or fetal health should be immediately hospitalized with daily fetal testing using nonstress testing or biophysical profile, treated with prednisone and antihypertensives if indicated, and given antenatal steroids to enhance fetal lung maturity. Delivery is indicated for deteriorating maternal renal, cardiac, liver, or CNS function unresponsive to therapy, the development of severe preeclampsia, or for fetal distress. Again, attempts at a vaginal delivery are indicated in the absence of acute fetal distress. Intravenous magnesium sulfate prophylaxis can be used as needed.

At less than 24 weeks of gestation

Patients at less than 24 weeks with a rapidly deteriorating maternal or fetal condition that is refractory to medical therapy and bed rest should be given

the option of pregnancy termination since the prognosis is poor in this setting. Patients should be cautioned, however, that the maternal condition
may not improve after pregnancy termination.

Postpartum care
Because some experts believe a lupus flare after delivery may be more
likely, patients require careful monitoring during the puerperium. Patients
should be counseled to promptly report any concerning symptoms. Estrogen containing contraceptives should be avoided in the presence of APA
as they may contribute to the risk of thrombosis; long-term progestin-only
contraceptives are excellent alternatives.

Rheumatoid arthritis

Overview
Rheumatoid arthritis (RA) is the most common autoimmune disease in
women of childbearing age, with a prevalence of 1 in 2,000 pregnancies.
Its peak incidence is at 35–40 years of age.

Pathophysiology
Rheumatoid arthritis is associated with a HLA-D4 haplotype. It is marked
by specific induction of an immune response by CD4+ T cells, with
subsequent release of cytokines and recruitment of lymphocytes and
monocytes into the synovia of small joints (e.g., wrist and hand) and
within other tissues. An anti-IgM or IgG rheumatoid factor (RF) complex
deposition is also noted in 90% of patients. The resultant joint pain
and effusions are mediated by local prostaglandin generation, and result
in proteolytic degradation of the cartilage via neutrophil and synovial
collagenases.

Diagnosis
The diagnosis of RA requires the following clinical features to be present:
1 Inflammatory arthritis involving three or more joints.
2 Duration of symptoms is more than 6 weeks.
3 Positive rheumatoid factor (RF) and/or antibodies citrullinated protein
   antibody (e.g., anti-cyclic citrullinated peptide).
4 Elevated C-reactive protein levels or an elevated erythrocyte sedimenta-
   tion rate.
5 Exclusion of other diseases involving joints (e.g., SLE, gout).

Additional features may include:

1 Rheumatoid nodules: 1–4 cm subcutaneous lumps over the elbows, various pressure points, lungs, and heart valves.
2 Symmetric involvement that occurs simultaneously in similar joint areas on both sides of the body.
3 Radiographic findings: characteristic changes seen on posteroanterior hand and wrist radiographs.
4 Felty's syndrome (a rare complication seen in long-standing RA and is associated with splenomegaly and granulocytopenia), rheumatoid vasculitis, pleuritis, pericarditis and anemia.

Effect of pregnancy on rheumatoid arthritis

In affected patients 40–80% improve in pregnancy, while 90% experience postpartum exacerbations. There is conflicting evidence whether breast-feeding is associated with flares; conversely breastfeeding may lower the risk of developing RA. There appears to be no increased rate of spontaneous abortion, perinatal mortality, or fetal growth restriction in the presence of RA uncomplicated by APA or anti-SSA/SSB antibodies.

Management

Initial treatment in pregnancy should include local steroid injections into affected joints. If the response to local measures proves inadequate, begin prednisone 5 mg every morning and 2.5 mg every evening. The utility and/or safety of other drugs are listed below:

1 Acetominophen is the analgesic of choice.
2 Nonsteroidal anti-inflammatory agents (NSAIDs) should be avoided after 20 weeks.
3 Hydroxychloroquine may be effective and appears safe.
4 Azathioprine can be used if the patient is refractory to steroids.
5 Tumor necrosis factor-alpha (TNF) inhibitor therapy appears to be an acceptable approach to refractory cases in pregnancy and the periconceptional period. While initial reports suggested a higher risk of VACTERL-associated birth defects, this link has not been formally or consistently established. Cush and colleagues noted that among 454 RA patients who conceived on such treatment, there were 378 normal deliveries, 9 premature babies, 5 therapeutic abortions, and 25 miscarriages.
6 Intramuscular gold salts may cross the placenta creating a theoretical risk but may be useful in postpartum period to reduce exacerbations.
7 Methotrexate, d-Penicillamine and cyclophosphamide are all contraindicated in pregnancy.

Scleroderma

Overview

Scleroderma is a rare autoimmune disease associated with progressive fibrosis and vasculitides that primarily affects the skin and can be further classified into diffuse cutaneous and limited cutaneous forms. When there are systemic manifestations, it is called systemic sclerosis. The course of scleroderma is unaffected by pregnancy. It does not appear to cause a higher incidence of spontaneous abortion, but is associated with a modestly higher risk of stillbirth and preterm delivery, particularly in the setting of renal disease and hypertension.

Pathophysiology

Scleroderma is characterized by an autoimmune reaction causing fibroblast stimulation that coordinates the overproduction, deposition and remodeling of collagen and other extracellular matrix proteins. This excess collagen causes thickening and hardening of the skin and other organs. Important features of the tissue lesions include early microvascular damage, mononuclear cell infiltrates into the perivascular space, and slowly developing fibrosis. Later stages of scleroderma include densely packed collagen in the dermis, loss of cells and atrophy. Clinical manifestations include:

1 Raynaud's phenomenon
2 sclerodactyly
3 telangiectasia
4 cardiomyopathy, myocardial infarctions, and cardiac conduction abnormalities
5 calcinosis
6 dysphagia and gastrointestinal motility disorders
7 renal failure

Effect of pregnancy on scleroderma

There does not appear to be a clear effect from pregnancy on disease activity with the majority of patients having no change in symptoms. Conversely, prospective studies suggest most pregnancies have a favorable outcome unless progressive disease is present. The most serious complication is renal crisis, which generally occurs with early diffuse disease. However, retrospective and prospective studies by Steen found this condition occurred in only 2–11% of pregnancies. While there were early reports of maternal mortality associated with such crises, use of aggressive antihypertensive therapy or dialysis, or both, renders such untoward outcomes rare. Maternal prognosis is, however, greatly worsened by the presence of pulmonary and malignant systemic hypertension. Use of ACE inhibitors, a cornerstone of therapy in the setting of renal disease, is contraindicated in pregnancy. Likewise, targeted treatments for other stigmata of the disease are also contraindicated in pregnancy including prostaglandin analogues for Raynaud's, and the endothelin receptor antagonist, bosentan, for pulmonary hypertension and digital ulcers. Thus, affected patients with pulmonary hypertension, severe restrictive lung disease, or severe gastrointestinal involvement should avoid pregnancy. Autologous hematopoietic stem cell transplantation (HSCT) has shown promise as a new treatment for severe disease. Most subsequent pregnancies in women so treated for other conditions result in live births, though the likelihood of reduced longevity in women with such severe disease should be considered when counseling them prior to conception.

Effect of scleroderma on pregnancy

Earlier reports suggested that scleroderma was associated with high rates of perinatal mortality due to preeclampsia (35%), preterm deliveries (30%), and stillbirths (30%). However, ascertainment bias may have inflated these rates and perinatal mortality appears to have lessened with the advent of improved fetal surveillance and neonatal intensive care.

Management

The progress of mothers should be followed for evidence of deteriorating renal function and worsening hypertension. The presence of coexisting APA and anti-SSA antibodies should be assessed and, if detected, managed as described for SLE patients. Fetal surveillance should follow the paradigm outlined for SLE above. The hallmarks of scleroderma management in pregnancy include:

1 Serial assessment of 24-hour urine collection for creatinine clearance and total protein.
2 Physiotherapy for hand contractures.
3 Antihypertensive therapy (calcium channel blockers) – avoid ACE inhibitors.
4 Prednisone for concomitant myositis.
5 Antacids and metoclopramide to prevent severe reflux esophagitis.
6 Dialysis in the setting of renal failure.
7 Institution of fetal surveillance as is described for patients with SLE, including early dating ultrasonography, serial scans for growth, and non-stress tests and/or biophysical profiles weekly beginning at 36 weeks in uncomplicated cases or 28 weeks and beyond given the presence of IUGR, worsening renal function, or hypertension.

Suggested reading

SLE:

Petri M. The Hopkins Lupus Pregnancy Center: ten key issues in management. *Rheum Dis Clin North Am.* 2007;33(2):227–235.

Smyth A, Oliveira GH, Lahr BD, Bailey KR, Norby SM, Garovic VD. A systematic review and meta-analysis of pregnancy outcomes in patients with systemic lupus erythematosus and lupus nephritis. *Clin J Am Soc Nephrol.* 2010;5(11):2060–2068.

Wallenius M, Salvesen KA, Daltveit AK, Skomsvoll JF. SLE and outcomes in first and subsequent births based on data from a national birth registry. *Arthritis Care Res (Hoboken).* 2014;16. doi: 10.1002/acr.22373. [Epub ahead of print]

Rheumatoid arthritis

Cush JJ. Biological drug use: US perspectives on indications and monitoring. *Ann Rheum Dis* 2005;64 Suppl 4:iv18–iv23.

Makol A, Wright K, Amin S. Rheumatoid arthritis and pregnancy: safety considerations in pharmacological management. *Drugs* 2011;71(15):1973–1987.

Scleroderma

Steen VD. Pregnancy in scleroderma. *Rheum Dis Clin North Am* 2007;33(2):345–358.

Steen VD, Conte C, Day N, Ramsey-Goldman R, Medsger TA Jr., Pregnancy in women with systemic sclerosis. *Arthritis Rheum* 1989;32(2):151–157.

PROTOCOL 13

Antiphospholipid Antibody Syndrome

Charles J. Lockwood

Department of Obstetrics and Gynecology, University of South Florida, Morsani College of Medicine, Tampa, FL, USA

Overview

Pregnancy is a hypercoaguable state by virtue of hormone-induced increases in vitamin K-dependent clotting factors, reduced anticoagulant free protein S levels and decreased fibrinolysis, coupled with venous stasis of the lower extremities and vascular injury due to placentation. Thus, the risk of venous thromboembolism (VTE) increases at least fivefold in pregnancy compared to age-matched nonpregnant women. In the United States, VTE complicates about 1 per 1,600 pregnancies, roughly divided between deep venous thrombosis (75%) and acute pulmonary embolism (25%); the latter accounts for about 10% of maternal deaths.

The major acquired thrombophilia is antiphospholipid antibody (APA) syndrome. These are antibodies directed against proteins bound to negatively charged phospholipids. They are present in up to 20% of individuals with VTE, and affected patients have a 5% risk of VTE during pregnancy and the puerperium despite treatment. However, APA-related thrombosis can occur in any tissue or organ and can be either venous or arterial. In addition, APA syndrome is linked to higher rates of preeclampsia, abruption, fetal growth restriction, and fetal loss.

Pathophysiology

There are several pathological mechanisms by which APAs induce VTE and adverse pregnancy outcomes. These include antibody-mediated impairment of endothelial annexin V, thrombomodulin and activated protein C-mediated anticoagulation; induction of endothelial tissue factor expression; impairment of fibrinolysis; and increased platelet activation.

Protocols for High-Risk Pregnancies: An Evidence-Based Approach, Sixth Edition.
Edited by John T. Queenan, Catherine Y. Spong and Charles J. Lockwood.
© 2015 John Wiley & Sons, Ltd. Published 2015 by John Wiley & Sons, Ltd.

In addition, APA appears to induce complement-mediated inflammation of the decidua and placenta.

Diagnosis

The diagnosis of APA syndrome requires one of the following clinical and laboratory criterion:

1 Thrombosis diagnosed by diagnostic imaging or histology involving one or more venous, arterial, or small vessels but not including superficial venous thrombosis; <u>or</u>
2 Adverse pregnancy outcome including unexplained fetal death at 10 weeks of gestation or more of a morphologically normal fetus, *or* 1 or more preterm birth(s) prior to 34 weeks due to preeclampsia or placental insufficiency, or 3 or more unexplained embryonic losses; and
3 At least one of the following laboratory criteria on two or more occasions at least 12 weeks apart and no more than 5 years prior to clinical manifestations:
   A. IgG and/or IgM anticardiolipin antibodies (ACA) (greater than 40 GPL or MPL units or more than 99th percentile for the testing laboratory); <u>or</u>
   B. Antibodies to β2-glycoprotein-1 of IgG or IgM more than 99th percentile for the testing laboratory; <u>or</u>
   C. Lupus anticoagulant activity detected according to published guidelines.

Effect on pregnancy

The presence of a lupus anticoagulant and high ACA IgG levels present the highest risk of adverse pregnancy outcomes. Moreover, APA are present in about 20% of women with recurrent pregnancy loss. Most losses occur after fetal cardiac activity is noted. That these antibodies do not appear to be associated with very early pregnancy loss is suggested by a meta-analysis of seven studies by Hornstein *et al.*, reporting a lack of effect from APA on in vitro fertilization (IVF) outcomes. Moreover, APA can be found in approximately 2% of the general obstetric population.

Antepartum management

Baseline information
1 24-hour urine collection for creatinine clearance and total protein to establish a baseline for the early detection of preeclampsia and since APA has been linked to glomerulonephritis.

2 Maternal echocardiogram to rule out Libman-Sachs endocarditis.
3 Liver function tests since APA have been linked to primary biliary cirrhosis and Budd-Chiari syndrome prior to pregnancy and HELLP syndrome before 20 weeks of gestation.

Anticoagulation therapy

Low-dose aspirin plus:
1 (if prior VTE) therapeutic doses of unfractionated or low-molecular-weight heparin (e.g., enoxaparin 1 mg/kg subcutaneously every 12 hours, adjusted to achieve anti-factor Xa level at 0.6–1 U/mL 4 hours after an injection).
2 (if no prior VTE) prophylactic doses of unfractionated or low-molecular-weight heparin (e.g., enoxaparin 30–40 mg subcutaneously every 12 hours).
3 If low-molecular-weight heparin is used in the antepartum period, I recommend switching to unfractionated heparin (10,000 units subcutaneously every 12 hours for prophylaxis) at 36 weeks or earlier if preterm delivery is expected since it has a shorter half-life than low-molecular-weight heparin. If the aPTT for patients on unfractionated heparin is normal or vaginal or cesarean delivery occurs more than 12 hours after the last dose of unfractionated LMWH, patients should not experience anticoagulation-related problems with delivery. Protamine may fully reverse the anticoagulant effects of unfractionated heparin.

Pregnancy monitoring
1 Level II ultrasonography at 18 weeks.
2 Fetal growth should be monitored every 4–6 weeks beginning at 20 weeks for any patient on anticoagulation; ultrasonographic assessment should be more frequent if fetal growth restriction is suspected or documented; in such a case, Doppler flow studies may be useful in determining the optimal timing of delivery.
3 Office visits as often as every 2 weeks beginning at 20 weeks to screen for preeclampsia.
4 Nonstress tests (NST) and/or biophysical profiles (BPP) weekly beginning at 36 weeks in uncomplicated cases or earlier as clinically indicated.

Timing of delivery
If the pregnancy is complicated by fetal growth restriction or preeclampsia, antenatal testing and maternal status will guide the timing of delivery. If the pregnancy is uncomplicated, delivery can be delayed until 39 completed weeks provided that antenatal surveillance (NST/BPP) is reassuring.

Postpartum

Pneumatic compression boots should be used during labor and delivery or at cesarean delivery. Either unfractionated heparin or low-molecular-weight heparin can be restarted 6 hours after vaginal delivery or 12 hours after cesarean delivery. This should be continued until at least 6 weeks postpartum. If the patient has a history of VTE, long-term prophylaxis is required as there is as high as a 30% recurrence risk for VTE in an APA-positive patient with a prior VTE. In this case, warfarin is to be started on day 2, and both heparin and warfarin are to be continued for 5 days <u>and</u> until the INR is therapeutic (2–3) for 2 consecutive days.

Summary

The combination of VTE, obstetric complications, and APA defines the antiphospholipid syndrome. The three APA classes most commonly associated with clinical problems are lupus anticoagulant, IgG anticardiolipin antibodies, and IgG anti-β-2-glycoprotein-I antibodies. These antibodies are associated with an elevated risk of thromboembolism (venous and arterial) and obstetric complications including fetal loss, abruption, severe preeclampsia, and fetal growth restriction. Treatment includes low-dose aspirin and heparin.

Suggested reading

Galli M, Luciani D, Bertolini G, Barbui T. Anti-beta 2-glycoprotein I, antiprothrombin antibodies, and the risk of thrombosis in the antiphospholipid syndrome. *Blood* 2003;102:2717–2723.

Hornstein M, Davis OK, Massey JB, Paulson RJ, Collins JA. Antiphospholipid antibodies and in vitro fertilization success: a meta-analysis. *Fertil Steril* 2000;73:330–333.

Miyakis S, Lockshin MD, Atsumi T, Branch DW, Brey RL, Cervera R, Derksen RH, De Groot PG, Koike T, Meroni PL, Reber G, Shoenfeld Y, Tincani A, Vlachoyiannopoulos PG, Krilis SA. International consensus statement on an update of the classification criteria for definite antiphospholipid syndrome (APS). *J Thromb Haemost* 2006;4(2): 295–306.

Rand JH, Wu XX, Andree HA, Lockwood CJ, Guller S, Scher J, Harpel PC. Pregnancy loss in the antiphospholipid-antibody syndrome – a possible thrombogenic mechanism. *N Engl J Med* 1997;337:154–160.

PROTOCOL 14

Inherited Thrombophilias

Andra H. James
Division of Maternal-Fetal Medicine, Department of Obstetrics & Gynecology, Duke University,
Durham, NC, USA

Overview

Thrombophilia is a term that can refer to almost any risk factor (such as the postoperative state), which could predispose to thrombosis. More specifically, the term has been used to describe hemostatic factors that predispose to thrombosis. Pregnancy already increases the risk of thrombosis four-fold to fivefold. Thrombophilia, when superimposed on pregnancy, has implications for both mother and fetus. Thrombophilia can be inherited or acquired. The most significant acquired thrombophilia impacting pregnancy is the antiphospholipid syndrome (Protocol 14). The purpose of this protocol is to review the inherited thrombophilias, their association with thrombosis, their association with adverse pregnancy outcomes, and the evaluation and treatment of inherited thrombophilias in pregnancy.

Hemostasis

The normal response to blood vessel injury is formation of a clot. Platelets adhere to damaged endothelium at the site of injury via von Willebrand factor, are activated, aggregate and form an initial platelet plug. The aggregated platelets are enmeshed by fibrin, which has been converted from soluble fibrinogen by the enzyme thrombin, to form a more stable clot. Factor XIII, also activated by thrombin, cross-links the fibrin monomers, further stabilizing the evolving clot. Thrombin is converted from its precursor, prothrombin, in the presence of activated factor X (FXa) and its cofactor, activated factor V (FVa). Both factor X and factor IX are activated by factor VII, which has been activated by tissue factor exposed at the time of blood vessel injury. Factor X can also be activated by activated factor IX

Protocols for High-Risk Pregnancies: An Evidence-Based Approach, Sixth Edition.
Edited by John T. Queenan, Catherine Y. Spong and Charles J. Lockwood.
© 2015 John Wiley & Sons, Ltd. Published 2015 by John Wiley & Sons, Ltd.

and its cofactor, activated factor VIII (FVIIIa), which is also activated by thrombin.

The natural anticoagulants, protein C, protein S, antithrombin, and tissue factor pathway inhibitor regulate clot formation and localize the clot to the site of injury. During hemostasis, excess thrombin binds to thrombomodulin and the thrombin–thrombomodulin complex activates protein C. Activated protein C and its cofactor, protein S, inactivate FVIIIa and FVa. (Heparin complexes with antithrombin to inactivate thrombin and FXa.)

In normal hemostasis, a clot is temporary and undergoes fibrinolysis or degradation rather than propagation. Plasmin, which is converted from plasminogen in the presence of fibrin, is responsible for fibrin degradation. The process is up-regulated by tissue plasminogen activator and down-regulated by thrombin-activatable fibrinolysis pathway inhibitor (TAFI) and plasminogen activator inhibitor type-1 (PAI-1).

Mechanisms of thrombosis

Thrombosis can occur in the arterial or venous circulation, but the mechanisms and major risks factors, while overlapping, are different. The major risk factor for arterial thromboembolism (e.g., myocardial infarction and stroke) is endothelial damage most commonly due to atherosclerosis. Endothelial damage causes turbulence, altered blood flow, and platelet activation. In contrast, the primary mechanism in venous thromboembolism (VTE), which accounts for 80% of the thromboembolic events in pregnant women, is activation of coagulation factors.

Genetic risk factors for thrombosis

Increased levels of coagulation factors, decreased levels of the natural anticoagulants, decreased levels of fibrinolytic factors, or increased levels of fibrinolytic inhibitors can each increase the risk of thrombosis and such changes can be inherited. There are many different genetic mutations responsible for the deficiencies of antithrombin, protein C or protein S, whereas most cases of resistance to activated protein C result from a single nucleotide polymorphism (SNP) in the factor V gene (1691A). The consequence of this SNP is a single amino acid difference that eliminates one of the cleavage sites of FVa. Absence of this cleavage site confers the altered protein, known as factor V Leiden (FVL), with resistance to activated protein C and with prolonged activity compared to that of normal FVa. The factor V 1691A mutation has been found to be present in 25% of patients with VTE. In 1996, another SNP was discovered in the untranslated portion of the prothrombin (FII) gene (20210A) that was also associated with an increased risk of thrombosis. This prothrombin (FII) 20210A mutation has been found to be present in 6% of patients with VTE.

VTE is a multifactorial condition potentially involving multiple environmental and genetic factors. Whether VTE occurs is contingent upon an individual's combined risk factors at the time, but some genetic risk factors confer a higher risk than others (Table 14.1). Deficiencies of the natural anticoagulants (antithrombin, protein C, and protein S) are relatively rare, high-risk thrombophilias (relative risk for heterozygotes about 10). As there is no one mutation for these conditions, deficiencies of the natural anticoagulants are diagnosed by a low level of the clotting proteins. There is a cut-off below which the condition is thought to be present, but there is a spectrum in the degree of deficiency. A recent study has documented that even mild deficiencies of antithrombin confer an increased risk of VTE (threefold to fourfold for levels less than 70% of normal and twofold to threefold for levels between 70% and 80% of normal). FVL and FII 20210A are more common and confer a moderate risk (fivefold for FVL and twofold to threefold for FII 20210A). Homozygosity for the fibrinogen gamma (FGG) 10034T gene confers a twofold increased risk. Multiple

Table 14.1 Inherited thrombophilia and the risk of venous thromboembolism

Thrombophilia	Increased risk of VTE	Prevalence	Approximate prevalence among VTE patients
Antithrombin	Approximate 10-fold	0.02%	1–4%*
Protein C	Approximate 10-fold	<1%	3–5%*
Protein S	Approximate 10-fold	<1%	1%
Factor V Leiden (FVL)	Fivefold (50-fold in homozygotes)	5% of Caucasians	25%
Prothrombin gene (20210) mutation	Twofold to threefold (20-fold in compound FVL heterozygotes)	1% of Caucasians	6%
Fibrinogen gamma (FGG) 10034T variant	Twofold (in homozygotes)	6%	12%
Non-O blood group	Twofold	>50%	70%
Sickle cell trait	Twofold	3% among African Americans	7% of African American VTE patients
Sickle cell disease	3.5- to 100-fold	0.2% of African Americans	

VTE, venous thromboembolism.
*Different prevalences depending on criteria used for diagnosis.

other SNPs have been discovered in genes for coagulation factors, the natural anticoagulants, the fibrinolytic factors and the fibrinolytic inhibitors that are associated with an increased risk of VTE, but all would be considered weak risk factors. The methylenetetrahydrofolate reductase SNPs C677T and A1298C, previously thought to be associated with an increased risk for thrombosis, are not.

There are other genetic risk factors for thrombosis that are not usually regarded as inherited thrombophilias, which do meet the definition. The most common genetic risk factor for VTE is non-O blood group. Non-O blood group is associated with higher levels of von Willebrand disease, is present in more than 50% of individuals, and confers a twofold risk of VTE. Sickle cell trait, which is present in 3% of African Americans, also confers a twofold risk. Sickle cell disease, which affects 0.2% of African Americans, confers a high risk of VTE. While sickle cell disease is not usually regarded as a thrombophilia, 25% of adult patients with sickle cell disease have experienced VTE by a median age of 30 years, which is comparable to the proportion of adult patients with high-risk thrombophilias who have experienced VTE by young adulthood. Multiple mechanisms, including activation of coagulation factors, have been postulated. Family history of VTE alone confers a twofold increased risk and the risk is independent of other risk factors.

Adverse pregnancy outcome

Early and retrospective studies found associations between thrombophilia and adverse pregnancy outcome – recurrent miscarriage and placental-mediated adverse pregnancy outcomes such as fetal growth restriction, placental abruption, stillbirth and preeclampsia. Prospective studies have found no associations between thrombophilia and adverse pregnancy outcome or only weak ones.

The use of anticoagulation to mediate against adverse pregnancy outcome based on the presence of thrombophilia alone no longer appears justified. Anticoagulation with heparins may reduce the risk of placental-mediated adverse pregnancy outcome, however, not because they are anticoagulants, but because they are anti-inflammatory and anti-complement agents. Small, nonrandomized studies of women with a history of adverse pregnancy outcome and thrombophilia have found improved outcomes in subsequent pregnancies with anticoagulation using heparins. Elegant research using an antiphospholipid mouse model demonstrated that fondaparinux, an anticoagulant which contains the pentasaccharide sequence responsible for the anti-factor Xa, antithrombotic property of heparins, did not rescue fetal mice from loss, but heparins, which have anti-inflammatory and anti-complement properties, did rescue fetal mice from loss. A very recent randomized controlled trial of dalteparin in women with thrombophilia who had a history of adverse pregnancy outcome or a history of thrombosis found no improvement in pregnancy outcomes with treatment; nor have randomized controlled trials of anti-coagulation using low-molecular-weight heparin in women with a history of recurrent miscarriage, independent of inherited thrombophilia status, found improvement in pregnancy outcomes with treatment. However, randomized controlled trials of anticoagulation in women with a history of severe placental-mediated adverse pregnancy outcome, independent of their inherited thrombophilia status, have found improvement in pregnancy outcomes with treatment.

Evaluation and treatment

Every woman who is pregnant or planning pregnancy should be asked about a personal or family history of thrombosis and about the details of previous pregnancies. Her risk factors for thrombosis, inherited and otherwise should be identified, as should her risk factors for adverse pregnancy outcome. Women of African, Southeast Asian, and Mediterranean ancestry should be offered screening for hemoglobinopathies. Testing for other inherited thrombophilias should be performed only if the results would alter management of a pregnancy. The American College of Obstetricians and Gynecologists' Practice Bulletin 138, Inherited Thrombophilias in Pregnancy, suggests consideration of testing only in women with a history of unprovoked thrombosis, or a family history of high-risk thrombophilia. There is general consensus that testing, when performed, should be limited to the high-risk and moderate-risk thrombophilias as outlined in Table 14.2.

The tests that measure protein levels (antithrombin, protein C, and protein S) can be influenced by pre-analytic variables such as time to processing of the specimen which can lead to protein degradation and artificially reduced levels. These tests should be processed within 4 hours of collection. Protein S levels are reduced in pregnancy due to binding by C4b-binding protein. A functional level below 35% would be two standard deviations or more below normal for pregnancy and suspicious for a true protein S deficiency. Many laboratories reflexively perform testing for free protein S when the functional level is below the laboratory normal. A free protein S level of less than 30% in the second trimester and less than 24% in the third trimester would be considered abnormal.

Treatment for thrombophilia, in most cases should be based on the clinical phenotype. There are no large randomized trials to guide treatment and

Table 14.2 Testing for inherited thrombophilia

Inherited thrombophilia	Abnormal test	Comments
Antithrombin deficiency	Antithrombin activity <60%	
Protein C deficiency	Protein C activity <60%	
Protein S deficiency	Protein S activity of <35% is below 2 standard deviations in pregnancy	Reflex testing with a free protein S level of less than 30% in the second trimester or less than 24% in the third trimester would be considered to be abnormal
Factor V Leiden mutation	Presence of the mutation: One copy = heterozygote Two copies = homozygote	Screening may be performed by testing for activated protein C resistance, and then performing the definitive DNA test reflexively. In many laboratories, the cost of DNA testing is comparable and DNA testing is performed as the only test
Prothrombin (FII) gene (20210A) mutation	Presence of the mutation	

recommendations for anticoagulation are based on the opinion of experts. In general, if a woman does not have a high-risk thrombophilia, has no history of thrombosis or has no history of adverse pregnancy outcome, she likely needs no anticoagulation treatment. The exception is after delivery (vaginal or cesarean) when the risk of thrombosis increases from the fourfold to fivefold increased risk above background during pregnancy to 20-fold to 80-fold above background. Since half of postpartum thrombosis occurs within the first 3 weeks postpartum, pneumatic compression devices during labor or at the time of cesarean delivery and a minimum of 3 weeks of prophylactic or low-dose anticoagulation may be sufficient. The other exception is the woman with a very high-risk thrombophilia (homozygosity for FVL; homozygosity for the FII 20210A mutation; or compound heterogyzosity for FVL and the FII 20210A mutation) who should receive at least prophylactic or low-dose anticoagulation during pregnancy and for at least 6 weeks postpartum. If a woman has a history of a single unprovoked thrombosis, and is not currently on anticoagulation, she will likely need prophylactic or low-dose anticoagulation during pregnancy. If a woman is already on anticoagulation or has a history of recurrent thrombosis, she will likely need full-dose anticoagulation during pregnancy with full-dose anticoagulation continued indefinitely after delivery (Table 14.3). For detailed recommendations about the management of thromboembolism during pregnancy see Protocol 18. Women with antithrombin deficiency who are receiving anticoagulation during

Table 14.3 Protocols for anticoagulation

Intensity	Regimen
Prophylactic LMWH*	Enoxaparin, 40 mg SC once daily
	Dalteparin, 5,000 units SC once daily
Therapeutic LMWH[†]	Enoxaparin, 1 mg/kg every 12 hours
	Dalteparin, 200 units/kg once daily
	Dalteparin, 100 units/kg every 12 hours
	May target an anti-Xa level in the therapeutic range of 0.6–1.0 units/mL for twice daily regimen
Minidose prophylactic UFH*	UFH, 5,000 units SC every 12 hours
Prophylactic UFH*	UFH, 5,000–10,000 units SC every 12 hours
	UFH, 5,000–7,500 units SC every 12 hours in first trimester
	UFH, 7,500–10,000 units SC every 12 hours in second trimester
	UFH, 10,000 units SC every 12 hours in third trimester, unless the aPTT is elevated
SC therapeutic UFH[†]	UFH, 144 units/kg SC every 8 hours or 216 units/kg SC every 12 hours in doses adjusted to target aPTT in the low end of the therapeutic range mid-interval
Postpartum anticoagulation	Prophylactic LMWH/UFH* for 4–6 weeks or vitamin K antagonists for 4–6 weeks with a target INR of 2.0–3.0, with initial UFH or LMWH therapy overlap until the INR is 2.0 or more for 2 days
	There is no published postpartum experience with the new oral anticoagulants and unlike warfarin, they have not yet been shown to be safe in breastfeeding

aPTT, activated partial thromboplastin time; INR, international normalized ratio;
LMWH, low-molecular-weight heparin; SC, subcutaneously; UFH, unfractionated heparin.
*Also referred to as low-dose anticoagulation. Modification of dose may be required at extremes of body weight.
[†]Also referred to as weight-adjusted, full treatment dose.
Source: Adapted from Practice Bulletin No. 138, 2013. Reproduced with permission of Lippincott Williams & Wilkins.

pregnancy may benefit from replacement with antithrombin concentrate when anticoagulation is held intrapartum.

A meta-analysis of recent randomized controlled trials suggested that women with a history of severe placenta-mediated adverse pregnancy outcome (severe or early preeclampsia, small for gestational age, placental abruption or stillbirth) have improved pregnancy outcomes with a single daily prophylactic dose of subcutaneous low-molecular-weight heparin. The relative risk was 0.5 for any preeclampsia and small for gestational age less than the 5th percentile; 0.4 for abruption, stillbirth and small for gestational age less than the 10th percentile; and 0.2 for severe or early preeclampsia less than 34 weeks of gestation. Although 25% of the women enrolled in the randomized controlled trials had thrombophilia, the benefits of low-molecular-weight heparin did not appear to be limited to women with thrombophilia. While possibly modified by thrombophilia, the benefits appeared to be independent of thrombophilia. While many women have been tested for thrombophilia because of a history of adverse pregnancy outcome and have been prescribed anticoagulation based on expectations of improved pregnancy outcomes, it appears that any improvement may have been due to the anti-inflammatory and anti-complement properties of heparins, and not their anticoagulant properties. Low-molecular-weight heparin appears to be a promising therapy to prevent recurrent severe placenta-mediated adverse pregnancy outcome, but further research is required.

Recommendations for fetal surveillance and timing of delivery in most cases of thrombophilia should be based on the pregnancy history and other pertinent clinical history.

Low-dose aspirin is sometimes prescribed to women with inherited thrombophilia in an attempt to reduce their risk of pregnancy-related thrombosis or to reduce their risk of adverse pregnancy outcome. When started after 12 weeks of gestation, doses of 50–150 mg per day have been shown to be safe and reduce the risk of adverse pregnancy outcome, specifically preeclampsia, by approximately 15%, independent of the presence of inherited thrombophilia. After initial treatment for thrombosis, low-dose aspirin has been shown to reduce the risk of recurrence by one-third, but there are no specific data in pregnant women. Low-dose aspirin, in combination with heparin, has been shown to reduce the risk of adverse pregnancy outcome in women with the antiphospholipid syndrome, but the same benefit has not been demonstrated specifically in women with inherited thrombophilia. Therefore, low-dose aspirin may reduce the risk of pregnancy-related thrombosis and adverse pregnancy outcome in women with inherited thrombophilia, but there are insufficient data.

Suggested reading

Austin H, Key NS, Benson JM, Lally C, Dowling NF, Whitsett C, Hooper WC. Sickle cell trait and the risk of venous thromboembolism among blacks. *Blood* 2007;110: 908–912.

Bates SM, Greer IA, Middeldorp S, Veenstra DL, Prabulos AM, Vandvik PO. VTE, thrombophilia, antithrombotic therapy, and pregnancy: Antithrombotic Therapy and Prevention of Thrombosis, 9th ed: American College of Chest Physicians Evidence-Based Clinical Practice Guidelines. *Chest* 2012;141:e691S–736S.

Bezemer ID, van der Meer FJ, Eikenboom JC, Rosendaal FR, Doggen CJ. The value of family history as a risk indicator for venous thrombosis. *Arch inter med* 2009;169: 610–615.

Di Minno MN, Dentali F, Lupoli R, Ageno W. Mild antithrombin deficiency and the risk of recurrent venous thromboembolism: a prospective cohort study. *Circulation* 2013.

Esmon C. Regulatory mechanisms in hemostasis. In: Hoffman R, Benz EJ, Silberstein LE, Heslop HE, Weitz JI, Anastasi J, eds. *Hematology: Basic Principles and Practice*, 6th edn. 3rd ed. Philadelphia, PA: Elsevier Saunders, 2013:1842–1846. e1843.

Inherited thrombophilias in pregnancy. Practice Bulletin No. 138 American College of Obstetricians and Gynecologists. *Obstet Gynecol* 2013;122:706–717.

Jackson E, Curtis KM, Gaffield ME. Risk of venous thromboembolism during the postpartum period: a systematic review. *Obstet Gynecol* 2011;117:691–703.

Larsen TB, Johnsen SP, Gislum M, Moller CA, Larsen H, Sorensen HT. ABO blood groups and risk of venous thromboembolism during pregnancy and the puerperium. A population-based, nested case-control study. *Journal of thrombosis and haemostasis: JTH* 2005;3:300–304.

Mann KG. Thrombin formation. *Chest* 2003;124:4S–10S.

Naik RP, Streiff MB, Haywood C, Jr., Nelson JA, Lanzkron S. Venous thromboembolism in adults with sickle cell disease: a serious and under-recognized complication. *Am J Med* 2013;126:443–449.

Rodger MA, Betancourt MT, Clark P, Lindqvist PG, Dizon-Townson D, Said J, Seligsohn U, Carrier M, Salomon O, Greer IA. The association of factor V Leiden and prothrombin gene mutation and placenta-mediated pregnancy complications: a systematic review and meta-analysis of prospective cohort studies. *PLoS med* 2010;7:e1000292.

Rodger MA, Carrier M, Le Gal G, Martinelli I, Perna A, Rey E, de Vries JI, Gris JC. Meta-analysis of low-molecular-weight heparin to prevent recurrent placenta-mediated pregnancy complications. *Blood* 2014;123:822–828.

Rodger MA, Hague WM, Kingdom J, Kahn SR, Karovitch A, Sermer M, Clement AM, Coat S, Chan WS, Said J, Rey E, Robinson S, Khurana R, Demers C, Kovacs MJ, Solymoss S, Hinshaw K, Dwyer J, Smith G, McDonald S, Newstead-Angel J, McLeod A, Khandelwal M, Silver RM, Le Gal G, Greer IA, Keely E, Rosene-Montella K, Walker M, Wells PS. Antepartum dalteparin versus no antepartum dalteparin for the prevention of pregnancy complications in pregnant women with thrombophilia (TIPPS): a multinational open-label randomised trial. *Lancet* 2014.

Rosendaal FR, Reitsma PH. Genetics of venous thrombosis. *Journal of thrombosis and haemostasis: JTH* 2009;7 Suppl 1:301–304.

Thromboembolism in pregnancy. Practice Bulletin No. 123. American College of Obstetricians and Gynecologists. *Obstet Gynecol* 2011;118:718–729. (Reaffirmed 2014).

PROTOCOL 15

Cardiac Disease

Katharine D. Wenstrom
Division of Maternal-Fetal Medicine, Women & Infants' Hospital of Rhode Island and Brown Alpert
Medical School, Providence, RI, USA

Overview

Cardiac disease is among the leading causes of maternal mortality during pregnancy and the relative proportion of maternal deaths attributable to cardiac disease has been increasing. A thorough evaluation of the woman with preexisting heart disease is ideally initiated before pregnancy, so that she can be counseled regarding the risks and advisability of pregnancy based on her specific cardiac lesion. Counseling should include a discussion of her cardiac anomaly and baseline functional status, the possibility of optimizing her cardiac status by medical or surgical means, any additional risk factors, and, if the mother has a congenital heart defect, her risk of having a child with the same or different cardiac lesion. Perhaps the most difficult counseling issue is the woman's physical ability to care for a child and her life expectancy, which must be addressed. During pregnancy, consultation with appropriate subspecialists as part of a team approach to antepartum and postpartum care is likely to improve both maternal and fetal outcome. Table 15.1 categorizes the risk of maternal death associated with the most common cardiac lesions. Pregnancy is not recommended for women with severe pulmonary arterial hypertension (PAH; pulmonary pressure more than 70% of systemic pressure) and those with significant left to right shunts; such women should consider sterilization or long-term progestin-only contraception.

Pathophysiology

In a normal pregnancy, the cardiovascular system undergoes significant physiological changes that may not be tolerated by the pregnant woman with heart disease. Increases in plasma volume, oxygen demand, and

Table 15.1 Pregnancy-associated maternal mortality in cardiac disease

Mortality 25–50%
Significant left heart obstruction*
Marfan syndrome (with aortic root dilation greater than 4 cm)
Pulmonary hypertension
Severe ventricular dysfunction (ejection fraction less than 40%)

Mortality 5–15%
Aortic stenosis
Mitral stenosis, New York Heart Association (NYHA) classes III and IV
Mitral stenosis with atrial fibrillation
Coarctation of aorta (without valvular involvement)
Uncorrected tetralogy of Fallot
Marfan syndrome with normal aorta
Artificial valve (mechanical)
Previous myocardial infarction

Mortality less than 1%
Atrial septal defect
Ventricular septal defect
Pulmonic or tricuspid disease
Patent ductus arteriosus
Artificial valve (bioprosthetic)
Mitral stenosis, NYHA classes I and II
Corrected tetralogy of Fallot

*Mitral valve area less than 2 cm^2; aortic valve area less than 1.5 cm^2; or peak left ventricular outflow gradient less than 30 mmHg

cardiac output may stress an already compromised cardiovascular system. As summarized in Fig. 15.1, by mid-gestation there is a 50% increase in both blood volume and cardiac output and a 20% decrease in systemic vascular resistance. By the end of the second trimester, the heart rate has increased by 20% and blood pressure has reached its nadir. Maternal position further affects these parameters (Fig. 15.2); cardiac output decreases by 20% when the woman is supine and by 16% when in dorsal lithotomy position. Cardiac output increases by another 30% during labor, and further increases occur during contractions, Valsalva maneuver, and with pain. At delivery, central blood volume may drop as the result of blood loss. Immediately afterward, however, sustained uterine contraction results in an acute 500 ml autotransfusion from the uterine to the systemic circulation, and increased venous return due to relief of vena caval compression. With loss of the placental circulation and hormones, peripheral resistance increases, and at the same time extravascular fluid is mobilized. All these peripartum changes lead to a high output state that may persist for up to 4 weeks. The hemodynamic

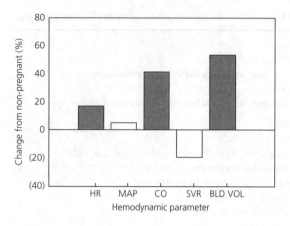

Figure 15.1 Cardiovascular adaptation to pregnancy. HR, heart rate; MAP, mean arterial pressure; CO, cardiac output; SVR, systemic vascular resistance; BLD VOL, blood volume.

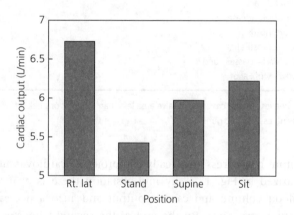

Figure 15.2 Cardiac output changes with maternal position.

effects of these pregnancy-induced changes on specific cardiac lesions, along with recommendations for management, are shown in Table 15.2.

Diagnosis and Workup

After excluding an acute pulmonary embolus, cardiac disease should be suspected in any pregnant woman who develops dyspnea, chest pain, palpitations, arrhythmias, or cyanosis, or who experiences a sudden limitation of activity. Particular attention should be given to the woman who has a history of exercise intolerance, a heart murmur predating pregnancy, or a

Table 15.2 Management of specific cardiac lesions in pregnancy

Cardiac lesion	Hemodynamic defect	Effect on pregnancy	Management
Mitral/aortic stenosis	↓ LV filling ↑ PVR; eventual pulmonary HTN	Fixed CO; tachy- or bradycardia will ↓ LV filling and ↓ CO Left atrial dilation leading to pulmonary congestion Arrhythmias Thrombus formation	Maintain preload, but avoid ↑ central blood volume Avoid ↓ SVR Avoid tachycardia and bradycardia Beta-blocker for persistent HR >90–100 beats/min
Mitral valve insufficiency	Component of regurgitation LV hypertrophy Eventual LV failure Eventual pulmonary HTN	Complications occur late in life; generally asymptomatic during pregnancy The ↓ SVR of pregnancy improves forward flow ↑ SVR during labor increases regurgitation	Treat symptomatic prolapse with beta-blocker Avoid ↑SVR Avoid myocardial depressants Treat arrhythmias
Aortic insufficiency	LV volume overload, left heart failure, pulmonary congestion	The ↓ SVR and ↑ HR of pregnancy reduce regurgitant flow During labor, ↑ intravascular volume, ↑ SVR, and stress of labor can lead to LV dysfunction	Avoid ↑ SVR Avoid bradycardia Avoid myocardial depressants
Marfan syndrome (aortic root <4 cm*)	Aortic regurgitation, LV dilation, LV failure, pulmonary congestion Spontaneous aortic dissection or rupture	The ↓ SVR and ↑ HR of pregnancy reduce regurgitant flow During labor, ↑ intravascular volume, ↑ SVR, and stress of labor can lead to LV dysfunction or aortic dissection	Prophylactic beta blockade throughout pregnancy recommended Adequate analgesia during labor; avoid wide surges in blood pressure and heart rate Shorten second stage
Prosthetic valve	Component of regurgitation	Risk of embolization Valvular dysfunction Endocarditis	Full-dose anticoagulation for mechanical valve
Left-to-right shunt (septal defects)	↑ Pulmonary flow, eventual pulmonary HTN and LV failure	Small lesions: asymptomatic Large VSD associated with aortic insufficiency CHF Arrhythmia Pulmonary HTN	Avoid ↑ SVR Avoid ↑ HR If pulmonary HTN, treat as right-to-left shunt; avoid ↓ SVR

(continued overleaf)

Table 15.2 *(continued)*

Cardiac lesion	Hemodynamic defect	Effect on pregnancy	Management
Right-to-left shunt (tetralogy of Fallot, Eisenmenger syndrome)	Blood shunted away from lungs, cyanosis	↓ SVR worsens shunt ↑ PVR during labor worsens shunt Increased hypoxia, cyanosis	Avoid hypotension Maintain preload; avoid ↓ SVR Avoid decreases in blood volume Avoid myocardial depressants Give oxygen Air filters on IV lines
Cardiomyopathy	LV dysfunction Global chamber dilation	Increased cardiac demand may lead to decompensation	↓ Afterload Careful volume administration and diuresis Inotropic support to maximize cardiac output

SVR, systemic vascular resistance; PVR, pulmonary vascular resistance; LV, left ventricle; RV, right ventricle; CO, cardiac output; HR, heart rate; VSD, ventricular septal defect; CHF, congestive heart failure; HTN, hypertension; ↓, decrease; ↑, increase.
*Women with Marfan syndrome with aortic root >4 cm should be advised against pregnancy

history of rheumatic fever. Cardiac disease should preferably be diagnosed and/or fully characterized before pregnancy, or as early in the pregnancy as possible, so that the level of maternal and fetal risk can be determined and a therapeutic plan developed. The evaluation should begin with a thorough history and physical examination, which allow classification of the woman's disease on a functional basis (Table 15.3). A 12-lead EKG and a transthoracic echocardiogram should be performed, and women with cyanosis should undergo percutaneous oximetry and/or arterial blood gas analysis. Stress testing, magnetic resonance imaging, or cardiac catheterization may be indicated in some patients. Any associated factors that could increase risk, such as a history of heart failure, a prosthetic valve, or a

Table 15.3 Functional status in cardiac disease (New York Heart Association classification

Class I	Asymptomatic with greater than normal activity
Class II	Symptomatic* with greater than normal activity (stair climbing, etc.)
Class III	Symptomatic with normal activity (walking, etc.)
Class IV	Symptomatic at rest

*Dyspnea, chest pain, orthopnea.

history of thromboembolism should be noted. While women determined to have functional New York Heart Association Class I or II heart disease generally tolerate pregnancy well, those with Class III or IV disease are at increased risk of adverse maternal and fetal outcomes; these women should reconsider pregnancy. Women determined to be candidates for pregnancy but who are at increased risk should be managed by a team that includes a maternal–fetal medicine specialist, a cardiologist, an anesthesiologist, and a pediatrician.

Management

General principles

Key principles in the antepartum management of heart disease focus on minimizing cardiac work while optimizing perfusion of the tissues including the uteroplacental bed. Any factors that could increase cardiac work, such as anxiety, anemia, infection, arrhythmia, or nonphysiological edema should be identified and eliminated or minimized as soon as possible. Any pregnancy-induced, exacerbated or associated complication such as hypertension, infection, anemia or thromboembolism should be treated promptly. Women with cardiac disease should avoid strenuous activity during pregnancy; those choosing to continue a pregnancy whose underlying cardiac lesion involves ventricular dysfunction, who are cyanotic, or who are functional class III or IV will need to significantly limit their physical activity and have specified daily rest periods. The woman's functional status should be closely monitored as pregnancy progresses. Any diminution in cardiac function or worsening of maternal functional class should prompt consideration of hospitalization. Oxygen, diuretics, and inotropes such as digitalis can be used as necessary to optimize cardiac function. Fetal growth should be monitored closely and a fetal echocardiogram performed between 18 and 22 weeks of gestation if the mother has a congenital heart lesion. Depending on the maternal functional class and fetal status, weekly or biweekly evaluation of fetal well-being should be considered, beginning in the third trimester.

Anticoagulation

Pregnancy is a hypercoagulable state, and pregnant women with mechanical heart valves or cardiac failure are at especially high risk of thromboembolism. Unfortunately, there are little data regarding the efficacy of and best protocol for anticoagulation of such patients during pregnancy. The most effective anticoagulant, warfarin, readily crosses the placenta and has adverse fetal effects throughout pregnancy. If used in the first trimester, it increases the risk of early pregnancy loss or may result in a specific embryopathy including abnormal cartilage and hypoplastic midface; if used in the second or third trimesters, it increases the risk of pregnancy loss, growth restriction, and abnormalities caused by vascular disruption such as cerebral bleeding or limb reduction defects. There are some data suggesting that these complications are less likely if the daily dose is 5 mg or less per day. The various forms of heparin do not cross the placenta, and are thus safe for the fetus, but are not completely effective in preventing thrombosis; several reports indicate a 12–30% incidence of thromboembolic complications and a 4–15% incidence of mortality for pregnant women with mechanical valves taking heparin. Antiplatelet drugs are not recommended unless the patient also has significant coronary artery disease.

The American College of Cardiology and American Heart Association recommend that all women with mechanical heart valves undergo therapeutic anticoagulation during pregnancy. Women with mechanical heart valves should be counseled about management options and should participate in creating a therapeutic plan that, ideally, achieves a balance between risks and benefits for both mother and fetus.

Managing anticoagulation during pregnancy and delivery

1 Many women will elect to discontinue warfarin immediately after conception and receive heparin or low-molecular-weight heparin until 12 weeks of gestation.

2 From 12 to 36 weeks, the patient must choose either warfarin or heparin. The risks of warfarin may be acceptable if the patient requires 5 mg or less per day. If the patient chooses unfractionated heparin, it should be given twice daily at a dose that keeps the aPTT at twice the normal control value when tested 6 hours after administration; if the patient chooses low-molecular-weight heparin, it should be given twice daily at a dose that keeps the anti-Xa level between 1.0 and 1.2 U/mL, 4 to 6 hours after administration. Some advocate maintaining a therapeutic anticoagulant level until just prior to the next injection of low-molecular-weight heparin (i.e., at 12 hours). The patient may also take low-dose aspirin in the second and third trimesters as further prophylaxis against valvular thrombosis.

3 Management is easiest if the patient is switched to therapeutic unfractionated heparin at 35–36 weeks; unfractionated heparin has a short half-life (1.5 hours), its effects can be rapidly reversed with protamine sulfate, and an aPTT can rapidly confirm that its effects have resolved.

4 Patients on unfractionated heparin should be instructed to withhold their injections at the onset of labor or 8–12 hours prior to a planned induction of labor or cesarean, primarily so they can receive neuraxial anesthesia (see points).

5 Therapeutic heparin (either unfractionated or low-molecular-weight) and warfarin should be restarted 4–6 hours after vaginal delivery or 6–12 hours after cesarean delivery, as long as the patient has no significant bleeding. It is crucial to maintain therapeutic doses of unfractionated heparin or low-molecular-weight heparin until the INR is in the therapeutic range (2–3), for 2 successive days, which is usually at least 5 days.

Prophylactic antibiotics

Women with a history of acute rheumatic fever and endocarditis who are taking penicillin prophylaxis should continue it throughout pregnancy. Whether women with other kinds of heart disease should receive antibiotic prophylaxis during pregnancy is controversial. The American College of Cardiology and the American Heart Association Task Force on Practice Guidelines have stated that, in general, intrapartum antibiotics are not necessary for women undergoing vaginal or cesarean delivery unless infection is suspected. However, prophylactic antibiotics should be considered at the time of membrane rupture or prior to delivery for certain high-risk patients (Table 15.4). These include: women with prosthetic heart valves or prosthetic material used for valve repair; heart defects repaired with prosthetic material (within 6 months of the procedure); heart defects repaired with prosthetic material with residual defects adjacent to the prosthetic material (any time); a previous history of endocarditis; or an unrepaired or palliated cyanotic heart defect, including those with a surgically constructed shunt or conduit. Therapeutic antibiotics should be given when bacteremia is suspected or there is an active infection.

Anesthesia

Conduction anesthesia is the preferred method of providing intrapartum pain control for the woman with cardiac disease. However, it is important to avoid hypotension when establishing regional anesthesia. Careful administration of intravenous crystalloid before placement of the catheter, close monitoring of fluid status, and slow administration of the anesthetic agent help to prevent this complication. Ephedrine is usually the agent

Table 15.4 Prophylactic antibiotic regimens in pregnancy

Standard regimen	Ampicillin 2 g IV* or Cefazolin or ceftriaxone 1 g IV*
Allergic to penicillin/ampicillin	Cefazolin or ceftriaxone 1 g IV* or Clindamycin 600 mg IV* †
Oral	Amoxicillin 2 g PO*

*Given 30–60 minutes before delivery
†Use vancomycin if enterococcus is a concern

of choice for the treatment of hypotension associated with regional anesthesia, because it does not constrict the placental vessels. However, because ephedrine increases the maternal heart rate, phenylephrine may be more appropriate for patients in whom tachycardia and increased myocardial work must be avoided (e.g., those with mitral and aortic stenosis, left to right shunt, etc.). A single-dose spinal technique is relatively contraindicated in patients with significant cardiac disease because hypotension frequently occurs during establishment of the spinal block. A narcotic epidural is an excellent alternative method and may be particularly effective for patients in whom systemic hypotension must be avoided (e.g., those with pulmonary hypertension, etc.).

Because the US Food and Drug Administration has reported cases in which nonpregnant patients on low-molecular-weight heparin had spinal or epidural anesthesia and suffered spinal or epidural hematomas, some of which caused neurological injury, the most prudent strategy is to switch patients to unfractionated heparin several weeks before anticipated delivery, as outlined above. For patients with a normal aPTT and platelet count, epidural anesthesia is generally considered safe.

Route of delivery

Vaginal delivery is preferred for the patient with cardiac disease. Cesarean delivery results in blood loss that is at least twice that associated with vaginal delivery, hemodynamic fluctuations that are significantly greater, and an increased risk of infection, thromboembolism and other postoperative complications, all of which could compromise care of the gravida with cardiac disease. However, women with certain severe cardiac conditions may benefit from elective cesarean delivery. These include women with severe congestive heart failure or recent myocardial infarction, severe aortic stenosis, dilated aortic root (greater than 4 cm), warfarin use within 2 weeks of delivery, and those who require valve replacement immediately after delivery.

Heart rate, stroke volume, cardiac output, and mean arterial pressure increase further during labor and in the immediate postpartum period, and should be monitored closely. Fluid intake and output and pulse oximetry readings should also be carefully reviewed. Lateral positioning and adequate pain control can reduce maternal tachycardia and increase cardiac output (Fig. 15.2). There is no consensus on intrapartum invasive hemodynamic monitoring, but women with New York Heart Association class III or IV disease may be candidates. Operative assistance with the second stage of labor is recommended to decrease maternal cardiac work. The immediate postpartum period is especially critical for the patient with cardiovascular disease. Blood loss must be minimized and blood pressure maintained, but congestive failure from fluid overload must also be avoided.

Follow up

Approximately 4–6 weeks after delivery, most of the cardiovascular changes of pregnancy will have resolved and the patient should be re-evaluated by a cardiologist. The infant's pediatrician can decide whether or not to perform a cardiac evaluation of the neonate, depending on the results of the targeted fetal ultrasonographic examination or echocardiogram and the newborn examination. Based on the outcome of the pregnancy and the results of the cardiac re-evaluation, the patient can be counseled regarding the risks of subsequent pregnancy, and appropriate contraception provided if indicated.

Suggested reading

ACA/AHA Guidelines for the management of adults with congenital heart disease: Executive summary: A report of the American College of Cardiology/American heart Association Task Force on Practice Guidelines (writing committee to develop guidelines for the management of adults with congenital heart disease) *Circulation* 2008;118(23):2395–2451.

Bates SM, Greer IA, Hirsh J, Ginsburg JS. Use of antithrombolic agents during pregnancy: the seventh ACCP conference on antithrombotic and thrombolytic therapy. *Chest* 2004;126:627S–644S.

D'Alton MD, Diller G-P. Pulmonary hypertension in adults with congenital heart disease and Eisenmenger syndrome: current advanced management strategies. *Heart* 2014, doi:10.1136/heartjnl-2014-305574.

Drenthen W, Boersma E, Balci A, Moons P, Roos-Hesselink JW, Mulder BJM, *et al.* Predictors of pregnancy complications in women with congenital heart disease. *European Heart J* 2010;31:2124–2132.

Ruys TPE, Roos-Hesselink JW, Hall R, Subirana-Domenech MT, Grando-Ting J, Estensen M *et al.* heart failure in pregnant women with cardiac disease: data from the ROPAC. *Heart* 2014;100:231–238.

Simpson LL. Maternal Cardiac Disease: Update for the clinician. Clinical expert series. *Obstet Gynecol* 2012;119:345–359.

Siu SC, Colman JM. Heart disease and pregnancy. *Heart* 2001;85:710–715.

Regitz-Zagrosek V, Bloomstrom Lundqvist C, Borghi C, *et al.* Guidelines on the managements of cardiovascular diseases during pregnancy: the Task Force on Management of Cardiovascular Diseases during pregnancy of the European Society of Cardiology (ESC). *Europ Heart J* 2011;32(24):3147–3197.

Roos-Hesselink JW, Ruys PTE, Johnson MR. Pregnancy in Adult congenital heart disease. *Curr Cardiol Rep* 2013;15:410.

Ruys TPE, Cornette J, Roos-Hesselink JW. Pregnancy and delivery in cardiac disease. *J Cardiology* 2013;61:107–112.

Thorne SA. Pregnancy in heart disease. *Heart* 2004;90:450–456.

Thromboembolism in pregnancy. Practice Bulletin No. 123. American College of Obstetricians and Gynecologists. *Obstet Gynecol* 2011;118:718–729.

Tsiaras S, Poppas A. Cardiac disease in pregnancy: value of echocardiography. *Curr Cardiol Rep* 2010;12:250–256.

Use of prophylactic antibiotics in labor and delivery. Practice Bulletin No. 120. American College of Obstetricians and Gynecologists. *Obstet Gynecol* 2011;117:1472–1483.

Vitale N, de Feo M, De Snato LS, Pollice A, Tedesco N, Cotrufo M. Dose-dependent fetal complications of warfarin in pregnant women with mechanical heart valves. *J Amer Coll Cardiol* 1999;33:1637–1641.

PROTOCOL 16

Peripartum Cardiomyopathy

F. Garry Cunningham

Department of Obstetrics and Gynecology, University of Texas Southwestern Medical Center, Dallas, TX, USA

Clinical significance

Peripartum cardiomyopathy refers to otherwise unexplained heart failure during late pregnancy after an evaluation that excludes known causes of cardiomyopathy that commonly include hypertension, thyrotoxicosis, or valvular heart disease. It is likely this disorder does not differ from idiopathic cardiomyopathy that is encountered in any previously healthy nonpregnant young adult, and thus it is not unique to pregnancy. Its incidence during pregnancy is inversely proportional to the diligence used to exclude known causes of heart failure and in the United States averages about 1 in 4000 births. Its importance is underscored by its contribution to maternal mortality; it is estimated to cause 10% of maternal-related deaths by the Centers for Disease Control and Prevention. Moreover, some form of cardiomyopathy accounts for 1–2 hospitalizations per 1,000 pregnancies, and about a third of these are for peripartum cardiomyopathy.

Etiopathogenesis

While the cause of peripartum cardiomyopathy remains unknown, there are a number of risk factors that include gestational hypertension (especially preeclampsia), high parity, and multifetal pregnancy, and there is a predilection for obese black women. A number of etiological mechanisms have been proposed, however, none has been proven. In up to half of women in whom endomyocardial biopsy is done, there is evidence for myocarditis associated with identification of viral genomic material to include parvovirus B19, Epstein–Barr virus, herpesvirus 6, and cytomegalovirus. Another hypothesis is activation of autoantibodies to cause immune destruction of myocardial tissue targeted in response to fetal antigenic material. In some women, oxidative stress, as in preeclampsia, is posited to activate cardiac cathepsin D, which cleaves prolactin into antiangiogenic subfragments that impair cardiomyocyte function. Importantly, it may be that these causes are multifactorial and there may be different forms of the disease.

Diagnosis

Because peripartum cardiomyopathy is idiopathic, it is a diagnosis of exclusion. The National Heart, Lung, and Blood Institute established the following diagnostic criteria:

1 Development of heart failure in the last month of pregnancy, or within 5 months of delivery;
2 Absence of an identifiable cause for the heart failure;
3 Absence of recognizable heart disease prior to the last months of pregnancy; and
4 Left ventricular systolic dysfunction with an ejection fraction less than 45% or fractional shortening less than 30%, or both.

Typical chest X-ray findings include impressive cardiomegaly with pulmonary edema, and there is single- to four-chamber dilatation with ventricular dysfunction evident on echocardiography.

Management

Treatment of heart failure is the cornerstone of management and vigorous diuresis with furosemide is begun promptly. Afterload reduction is accomplished with hydralazine prior to delivery and an angiotensin-converting-enzyme inhibitor is given postpartum. Digoxin can be given for its inotrophic properties and treatment of dangerous arrhythmias that cause rate-related dysfunction. Because left ventricular dysfunction has a high concurrence with pulmonary embolism, anticoagulation is usually warranted. In a small proportion of women, implantable cardiac devices are required to maintain an ejection fraction to sustain the circulation. Cardiac transplantation is rarely required.

Complications

Spontaneous labor commonly follows pulmonary edema and hypoxemia caused by heart failure. If hypoxemia is severe or prolonged, fetal death may ensue. There is no evidence that delivery improves the prognosis, but it may help manage heart failure. Immediate maternal mortality has been reported as high as 5–10% with deaths caused by intractable heart failure, malignant arrhythmias, and pulmonary embolism. Complications of delivery, especially cesarean delivery, contribute to mortality because they may add the burden of sepsis syndrome, hemorrhage and anemia, and anesthesia.

Follow up

The long-term prognosis following peripartum cardiomyopathy depends on the extent of residual heart muscle damage. In general, those women who regain normal ventricular function within 6 months have a good prognosis. This includes perhaps half of affected women. In the other half with ventricular dysfunction that persists there is a high incidence of chronic heart failure, including end-stage disease requiring cardiac transplantation. It follows that subsequent pregnancy outcomes also depend on residual cardiac function. Half of women with persistent ventricular dysfunction develop congestive heart failure during a subsequent pregnancy. And although women with apparent resolution of cardiomyopathy have a 20% incidence of heart failure with a subsequent pregnancy, it is usually less severe.

Prevention

There currently are no known preventive measures for peripartum cardiomyopathy. Efforts are concentrated on determining the prognosis if the woman desires a subsequent pregnancy. If there is evidence of substantively persistent ventricular dysfunction as measured by a diminished ejection fraction, or by exercise or drug-induced ventricular dysfunction, then pregnancy likely should not be undertaken. For women who choose to have a subsequent pregnancy, close follow-up with frequent assessment of cardiac function is imperative. For these women, management is the same as for heart failure of any cause.

Conclusions

In its purest form, peripartum cardiomyopathy likely represents idiopathic cardiomyopathy of young adults with at least half of cases caused by inflammatory myocarditis usually from viral infections. It is a diagnosis of exclusion. Standard treatment is given for heart failure and close observation for its complications. Evaluation is continued after delivery and persistence of ventricular dysfunction at 6 months carries a poor long-term prognosis for recovery.

Suggested reading

Cunningham FG. Peripartum cardiomyopathy: we've come a long way .... but. *Obstet Gynecol* 2012;120:992–994.

Berg CJ, Callaghan WM, Syverson C, *et al.* Pregnancy-related mortality in the United States:1980-2007. *Obstet Gynecol* 2010;116:1302–1309.

Elkayam U. Clinical characteristics of peripartum cardiomyopathy in the United States. *J Am Coll Cardiol* 2011;58:659–670.

Harper MA, Meyer RE, Berg CJ. *Obstet Gynecol* 2012;120:1013–1019.

Hilfiker-Kleiner D, Kaminski K, Podewski E, *et al.* A cathepsin D-cleaved 16 kDa form of prolactin mediates postpartum cardiomyopathy. *Cell* 2007;128:589–600.

Kuklina EV, Callaghan WM. Cardiomyopathy and other myocardial disorders among hospitalizations for pregnancy in the United States: 2004–2006. *Obstet Gynecol* 2010; 115:93–100.

PROTOCOL 17

Thromboembolism

Alan Peaceman
Division of Maternal-Fetal Medicine, Northwestern University Feinberg School of Medicine, Chicago, IL, USA

Thromboembolism remains a leading cause of obstetric morbidity and mortality in the United States. It is estimated that the risk of venous thrombosis is approximately five times higher during pregnancy than in the nonpregnant state due to the hypercoagulable nature of pregnancy as well as venous stasis and vascular injury. While previously thought to be more prevalent in the third trimester, it is now recognized to occur at similar frequencies throughout pregnancy. Day for day, it is more common in the postpartum period than during pregnancy. Despite its risk, thromboembolism during pregnancy is a poorly studied area and significant controversy remains over the management of pregnant women at risk for this disorder.

Pathophysiology

Normal pregnancy is associated with an increase in the level or activity of many of the vitamin K-dependent clotting factors, and is accompanied by reduced anticoagulant protein S activity and increases in the anti-fibrinolytic agents, type 1 and 2 plasminogen activator inhibitor (PAI). These changes provide a defense against hemorrhage during placentation and after delivery, but promote clot formation during pregnancy. Under normal circumstances, the increased levels of clotting factors do not result in thrombus formation, but some clinical situations such as trauma or vascular injury and stasis predispose toward lower extremity clotting. Once formed, portions of the thrombus can embolize to the pulmonary vasculature, with resultant symptoms ranging from mild hypoxia to cardiovascular collapse and death. Other risk factors for thrombosis during pregnancy include inactivity, obesity, prior thrombosis, antiphospholipid syndrome, and inherited thrombophilias such as factor V Leiden.

Protocols for High-Risk Pregnancies: An Evidence-Based Approach, Sixth Edition.
Edited by John T. Queenan, Catherine Y. Spong and Charles J. Lockwood.
© 2015 John Wiley & Sons, Ltd. Published 2015 by John Wiley & Sons, Ltd.

Diagnosis

The diagnosis of deep venous thrombosis (DVT) is often difficult to make clinically, especially in pregnancy. Patients presenting with asymmetric lower extremity swelling, associated with pain and erythema should be evaluated. The left leg is far more often affected (17-fold) than the right. Assays for serum D-dimer are useful for detecting thrombosis outside of pregnancy because of its high negative predictive value, but of limited value in pregnancy because most women have increased levels by the second trimester. However, a negative D-dimer test is reassuring. Venography was once the gold standard for making the diagnosis, even in pregnancy, but is rarely performed now because of its invasive nature and its use of radiation. Compression venous ultrasound is now the primary tool for evaluation of clinical symptoms in the lower extremities for pregnant women (Fig 17.1). Magnetic resonance imaging has utility for evaluating possible pelvic vein thrombosis.

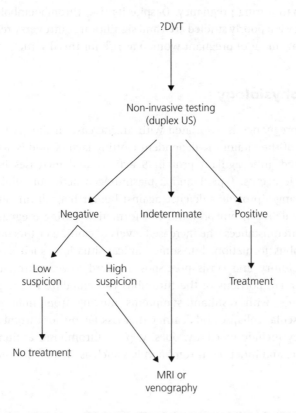

Figure 17.1 Diagnostic protocol for suspected deep venous thrombosis (DVT). US, ultrasound; MRI, magnetic resonance imaging.

The presenting signs and symptoms of pulmonary embolism (PE) include shortness of breath, chest pain, tachypnea, tachycardia, and decreased oxygen saturation by pulse oxymeter. Initial evaluation traditionally included an arterial blood gas to determine the presence of hypoxia and increased A-a gradient, both suggestive of an embolic event. However, this test is now recognized as having limited value in that many pregnant patients with PE are without such an abnormality. Two tests are used to diagnose acute PE in pregnancy: ventilation/perfusion (V/Q) scanning and computerized tomographic pulmonary angiograms (CTPA). The increased cardiac output and plasma volume accompanying pregnancy dilute the contrast medium and result in decreased pulmonary arterial visualization with CTPA leading to higher rates of inadequate studies. In addition, CTPA presents a significantly greater amount radiation burden to the mother's breast than does V/Q scanning. Conversely, young otherwise healthy pregnant women tend not to have other pulmonary pathology enhancing the efficacy of V/Q scanning. In view of these findings the American Thoracic Society recommends the following approach to diagnosing acute PE in pregnancy, which minimizes radiation exposure and maximizes diagnostic efficacy. Patients with left lower extremity symptoms should undergo lower extremity compression ultrasound. Those without such symptoms should undergo chest radiography (CXR). If the CXR is normal, V/Q scanning is performed. If the CXR is abnormal, CTPA is performed. In unstable patient, anticoagulation should be promptly initiated before such studies are commenced. If V/Q scans are not available at a given institution proceed directly to CTPA after compression ultrasound if indicated.

Treatment of acute thromboembolism

Because of the lack of clinical trials, all recommendations regarding treatment for or prevention of thromboembolism during pregnancy are based on expert opinion. Nonetheless, consensus does exist on some of the approaches to treatment. Acute DVT or PE should be treated with full anticoagulation using either intravenous heparin or subcutaneous low-molecular-weight heparin, and it is important to achieve therapeutic doses very early to prevent extension of clot (Table 17.1). The patient is then transitioned to either subcutaneous heparin or enoxaparin (or other forms of low-molecular-weight heparin) injections every 12 hours, which are continued for the remainder of the pregnancy and postpartum period to prevent recurrence. It is thought that the use of heparin injections requires monitoring to maintain the activated partial thromboplastin time (aPTT) at least 1½ times control throughout the dosing interval.

Table 17.1 Management of thromboembolism

Condition	Heparin	Enoxaparin
DVT or PE during current pregnancy	IV heparin (aPTT 2–3 times control) for 5–10 days, followed by q 8–12 h injections to prolong midinterval aPTT 1 ½ times control for remainder of the pregnancy; warfarin can be used postpartum	Enoxaparin 1 mg/kg (up to 100 mg maximum) q 12 h; monitoring of anti-factor Xa levels at 4–6 hours post injection
Patient who requires long-term therapeutic anticoagulation	Heparin q 8–12 h to prolong mid interval aPTT 1 ½ times control	1 mg/kg (up to 100 mg maximum) q 12 h; monitoring of anti-factor Xa levels at 4–6 hours post injection
Previous DVT or PE before current pregnancy (prophylactic treatment)	5000 units q 12 h first trimester 7500 units q 12 h second trimester 10,000 units q 12 h third trimester; monitoring unnecessary	40 mg q 12 h; monitoring unnecessary for patients under 100 kg

DVT, deep vein thrombosis; PE, pulmonary embolism; IV, intravenous; aPTT, activated partial thromboplastin time.

However, with the more rapid metabolism of heparin during pregnancy, it is usually difficult to achieve prolongation of the aPTT throughout the dosing interval without an excessive peak level, even when administered three times a day. Enoxaparin injections are also given twice daily because of the rapid metabolism, and can be started at 1 mg/kg for each injection. Monitoring of enoxaparin when given outside of pregnancy is thought to be unnecessary for most patients, but its pharmacokinetics in pregnancy are incompletely studied. If monitoring is to be performed, anti-factor Xa levels are followed, with the target being 0.6–1.0 IU/mL 4 hours after injection. Both heparin and low-molecular-weight heparins do not cross the placenta, but warfarin does due to its smaller size. Warfarin is contraindicated in pregnancy among patients with venous thromboembolism unrelated to artificial heart valves due to its fetopathic effects in the first trimester (stippled epiphyses and nasal and limb hypoplasia) and the risk of fetal bleeding complications in the second and third trimesters. However, warfarin does not enter breast milk in sufficient quantities to anticoagulate the newborn, and is safe to use in the breastfeeding mother. If used, careful monitoring is necessary during initial warfarin administration since warfarin results in reduced anticoagulant protein C levels prior to reduced levels of vitamin K-dependent clotting factors. Thus, it is important to maintain therapeutic doses of unfractionated heparin or low-molecular-weight heparin for 5 days *and* until the INR reaches the therapeutic range between 2 and 3, for 2 successive days.

Prevention of thromboembolism

The use of anticoagulation to prevent thromboembolism is more controversial. Traditionally, chemoprophylaxis has been recommended to pregnant patients with a history of thrombosis with the idea that pregnancy significantly increases the risk of recurrence. Anticoagulant doses lower than needed to prolong the aPTT have been used (Table 17.1), unless the patient is thought to be of such increased risk that full anticoagulation is necessary. Because it is now recognized that a significant portion of these thrombotic events occur as early as the first trimester, it is prudent to start treatment soon after the pregnancy is recognized and viability confirmed, and continue it until 6 weeks after delivery.

One study suggested that prophylactic anticoagulation may not be necessary in some patients with a history of venous thromboembolism. In this study of women with a single previous episode of thrombosis associated with a temporary risk factor (e.g., oral contraceptives, surgery, trauma), and no recognized thrombophilia, no recurrences were seen without treatment during pregnancy. However, in my opinion the number of patients in this study was relatively small and larger studies are required to support withholding prophylaxis for this type of patient.

Risks to the mother of heparin therapy include a rare thrombocytopenia and the possibility of heparin-induced osteoporosis. These risks are thought to be lower with the use of low-molecular-weight heparin. Heparin-induced thrombocytopenia (HIT) occurs within the first week of treatment, so checking the platelet count 5-10 days after beginning therapy will provide reassurance. Up to one-third of women may demonstrate subclinical bone loss and the reversibility of this process is not assured. Significant maternal hemorrhage is a possibility in patients that are over-anticoagulated.

Special considerations

Patients with artificial heart valves are at a high risk for thromboembolism, stroke, and valve failure and, therefore, must be therapeutically anticoagulated throughout pregnancy. If low-molecular-weight heparin is thought to be insufficient for this purpose for long periods of time, restarting a patient on warfarin after the first trimester may be a consideration. See Protocol 16.

Patients with a history of a documented clot or a first-degree relative with a documented high-risk thrombophilia should be evaluated. Testing includes assessment for antiphospholipid antibodies, as well as factor V Leiden mutation, prothrombin gene mutation G20210A, and deficiencies of protein C, protein S, and antithrombin-III. Factor V Leiden homozygosity, prothrombin gene 20210A mutation homozygosity, compound heterozygosity of these mutations, or the presence of antithrombin-III deficiency are thought to be high-risk thrombophilias. Anticoagulant prophylaxis should be used when high-risk thrombophilias are identified in the absence of prior thrombosis, especially in the postpartum period. I would recommend therapeutic anticoagulation in patients with high-risk thrombophilias having a prior thrombosis. All patients with two or more prior thrombosis and receiving long-term anticoagulation therapy also should receive therapeutic anticoagulation regardless of thrombophilic state. Prophylactic dose anticoagulation should be used when there is a personal history of thrombosis and another (lower risk) thrombophilia is identified. It is more difficult to diagnose protein S deficiency in pregnancy since levels normally decrease beginning in the first trimester; prophylaxis may be appropriate if protein S deficiency is suspected. Patients with a prior thromboembolic event who have been diagnosed with antiphospholipid antibody syndrome should be given low-dose aspirin plus unfractionated or low-molecular-weight heparin prophylaxis at a minimum, with consideration of full anticoagulation for those thought to be at significant risk (e.g., prior thrombosis or pregnancy loss on prophylactic doses of anticoagulants). Screening for factor V Leiden and prothrombin mutation should not be performed in patients without a personal or close family history of prior thrombosis.

There is concern regarding the use of epidural anesthesia during labor and delivery in patients treated with anticoagulants. To reduce the risk of epidural hematoma, regional anesthesia is usually avoided for 12–24 hours from the last injection of low-molecular-weight heparin. Because of its more rapid disappearance, a shorter waiting time is used for patients on unfractionated heparin, and these patients can receive regional anesthesia when laboratory tests confirm a normal aPTT result. For this reason, switching from low-molecular-weight to unfractionated heparin at 36 weeks of gestation may increase the number of patients eligible for regional anesthesia.

Suggested reading

Barbour L, Kick S, Steiner J, *et al.* A prospective study of heparin-induced osteoporosis in pregnancy using bone densitometry. *Am J Obstet Gynecol* 1994;170:862–869.

Bates SM, Greer IA, Pabinger I, Sofaer S, Hirsh J. Venous thromboembolism, thrombophilia, antithrombotic therapy, and pregnancy: American College of Chest Physicians evidence-based clinical practice guidelines (8th Edition). *Chest* 2008;133:844S–886S.

Brill-Edwards P, Ginsberg JS, Gent M, *et al.* Safety of withholding heparin in pregnant women with a history of venous thromboembolism. *N Eng J Med* 2000;343:1439–1444.

Cross JL, Kemp PM, Walsh CG, Flower CDR, Dixon AK. A randomised trial of spiral CT and ventilation perfusion scintography for the diagnosis of pulmonary embolism. *Clin Radiol* 1997;53:177–182.

Dahlman TC. Osteoporotic fractures and the recurrence of thromboembolism during pregnancy and the puerperium in 184 women undergoing thromboprophylaxis with heparin. *Am J Obstet Gynecol* 1993;168:1265–1270.

Dizon-Townson DS, Nelson LM, Jang H, Varner MW, Ward K. The incidence of the factor V Leiden mutation in an obstetric population and its relationship to deep vein thrombosis. *Am J Obstet Gynecol* 1997;176:883–886.

Eldor A. The treatment of thrombosis during pregnancy. *Hematology* 1999;483–490.

Inherited thrombophilias in pregnancy. Practice Bulletin No. 138 American College of Obstetricians and Gynecologists. *Obstet Gynecol* 2013;122:706–717.

Leung AN, Bull TM, Jaeschke R, Lockwood CJ, Boiselle PM, Hurwitz LM, James AH, McCullough LB, Menda Y, Paidas MJ, Royal HD, Tapson VF, Winer-Muram HT, Chervenak FA, Cody DD, McNitt-Gray MF, Stave CD, Tuttle BD; ATS/STR Committee on Pulmonary Embolism in Pregnancy. American Thoracic Society documents: an official American Thoracic Society/Society of Thoracic Radiology Clinical Practice Guideline–evaluation of suspected pulmonary embolism in pregnancy. *Radiology* 2012;262(2):635–646.

Maternal and Neonatal Haemostasis Working Party of the Haemostasis and Thrombosis Task. Guidelines on the presentation, investigation, and management of thrombosis associated with pregnancy. *J Clin Pathol* 1993;46:489–496.

Thromboembolism in pregnancy. Practice Bulletin No. 123. American College of Obstetricians and Gynecologists. *Obstet Gynecol* 2011;118:718–729.

PROTOCOL 18

Renal Disease

Susan Ramin

Department of Obstetrics and Gynecology, Baylor College of Medicine, Texas Children's Hospital
Pavilion For Women, Houston, TX, USA

Overview

Renal disease during pregnancy is relatively uncommon, occurring in approximately 0.03–0.12% of all pregnancies. Obstetricians are more likely to encounter pregnant women with renal disease given improvements in reproductive success in women with underlying renal disease. The management of pregnant women with this complication presents a challenge to obstetricians, maternal–fetal medicine physicians, nephrologists, anesthesiologists and neonatologists. Thus, a multidisciplinary approach should be taken in managing pregnant women with underlying renal disease. As the degree of renal impairment increases, there is a concomitant increase in both maternal and fetal complications. Maternal morbidity includes preeclampsia, eclampsia, worsening renal impairment, chronic hypertension, placental abruption, anemia, and cesarean delivery. The associated fetal complications include preterm birth, low birth weight, and fetal/neonatal death.

Clinicians should have a basic understanding of normal physiology in pregnant women when considering renal disorders in pregnancy. Within the first month of conception, glomerular filtration rate (GFR) is increased by approximately 50% while renal plasma flow (RPF) is increased 50–80%. These physiological changes result in a normal reduction in levels of serum creatinine and urea nitrogen to mean values of 50 micromoles/L (0.6 mg/dL) and 3 mmol/L (9 mg/dL), respectively; thus, serum creatinine values of 80 micromoles/L (0.9 mg/dL) and blood urea nitrogen values of 6 mmol/L (14 mg/dL) may represent underlying renal disease in pregnancy. During the third trimester of pregnancy, the GFR may decrease by 20% with little effect on serum creatinine. Pre-pregnancy levels are achieved within 3 months after delivery.

Protocols for High-Risk Pregnancies: An Evidence-Based Approach, Sixth Edition.
Edited by John T. Queenan, Catherine Y. Spong and Charles J. Lockwood.
© 2015 John Wiley & Sons, Ltd. Published 2015 by John Wiley & Sons, Ltd.

Table 18.1 Severity of renal disease and prospects for pregnancy*

Prospects	Category†		
	Mild (%)	Moderate (%)	Severe (%)
Pregnancy complications	25	47	86
Successful obstetric outcome	96 (85)	90 (59)	25 (71)
Long-term sequelae	<3 (9)	47 (8)	53 (92)

*Estimates are based on 1862 women/2799 pregnancies (1973–1992) and do not include collagen diseases.
†Numbers in parentheses refer to prospects when complication(s) develop before 28 weeks of gestation.

There is a paucity of scientific data regarding the management of pregnant women with chronic renal disease. However, fertility and the ability to sustain an uncomplicated pregnancy generally relate to the degree of functional renal impairment and the presence or absence of hypertension rather than to the nature of the underlying renal disorder (Table 18.1). Pregnant women with underlying renal insufficiency are arbitrarily divided into three categories based on serum creatinine values: those with (1) preserved or only mildly impaired renal function (serum creatinine less than 1.4 mg/dL); (2) moderate renal insufficiency (serum creatinine 1.4 to 2.4–2.8 mg/dL); and (3) severe renal insufficiency (serum creatinine greater than 2.4–2.8 mg/dL).

Women with mild renal dysfunction usually have successful obstetric outcomes and pregnancy does not appear to adversely affect their underlying renal condition. About half of the pregnant women with mild renal impairment experience worsening proteinuria, which can progress to severe range along with nephrotic edema. Perinatal outcome is compromised by the presence of uncontrolled hypertension and nephrotic proteinuria in early pregnancy. Perinatal outcome for women with mild renal disease is minimally affected, and the risk of irreversible renal function loss in the mother is low. This generalization, however, may not hold true for certain kidney diseases (Table 18.2). For instance, pregnant women with severe scleroderma and periarteritis nodosa, disorders often associated with hypertension, often do poorly. Conception in some of these women with severe disease may be contraindicated. Women with lupus nephritis do not do as well as women with primary glomerulopathies, especially if the disease has flared within 6 months of conception. Controversy exists regarding adverse pregnancy effect on the natural history of the disease process that exists with other kidney diseases such as immunoglobulin A (IgA) nephritis, focal glomerular sclerosis, membranoproliferative nephritis, and reflux nephropathy. However, it

Table 18.2 Specific kidney diseases and pregnancy

Renal disease	Effects and outcome
Chronic glomerulonephritis	Usually no adverse effect in the absence of hypertension. One view is that glomerulonephritis is adversely affected by the coagulation changes of pregnancy. Urinary tract infections may occur more frequently
IgA nephropathy	Risks of uncontrolled and/or sudden escalating hypertension and worsening of renal function
Pyelonephritis	Bacteriuria in pregnancy can lead to exacerbation. Multiple organ system derangements may ensue, including adult respiratory distress syndrome
Reflux nephropathy	Risks of sudden escalating hypertension and worsening of renal function
Urolithiasis	Infections can be more frequent, but ureteral dilatation and stasis do not seem to affect natural history. Limited data on lithotripsy thus best avoided
Polycystic disease	Functional impairment and hypertension usually minimal in childbearing years
Diabetic nephropathy	Usually no adverse effect on the renal lesion, but there is increased frequency of infection, edema and/or preeclampsia
Systemic lupus erythematosus (SLE)	Controversial; prognosis most favorable if disease in remission >6 months before conception. Steroid dosage should be increased postpartum
Periarteritis nodosa	Fetal prognosis is dismal and maternal death often occurs
Scleroderma (SS)	If onset during pregnancy, rapid overall deterioration can occur. Reactivation of quiescent scleroderma may occur postpartum
Previous urinary tract surgery	Might be associated with other malformations of the urogenital tract. Urinary tract infection common during pregnancy. Renal function may undergo reversible decrease. No significant obstructive problem but cesarean delivery often needed for abnormal presentation and/or to avoid disruption of the continence mechanism if artificial sphincter present
After nephrectomy, solitary kidney and pelvic kidney	Might be associated with other malformations of urogenital tract. Pregnancy well tolerated. Dystocia rarely occurs with pelvic kidney
Wegener granulomatosis	Limited information. Proteinuria (± hypertension) is common from early in pregnancy. Cytotoxic drugs should be avoided if possible
Renal artery stenosis	May present as chronic hypertension or as recurrent isolated preeclampsia. If diagnosed then transluminal angioplasty can be undertaken in pregnancy if appropriate

is generally agreed that as functional impairment progresses along with hypertension, maternal and fetal risks significantly increase.

There is limited information on women with moderate or severe renal dysfunction who conceive. Fetal outcome is still good in 80–90% of the pregnancies in women with moderate renal dysfunction after exclusion of spontaneous abortions. Women with severe renal insufficiency have a live birth rate of 64%. Progression of maternal renal disease is of greater concern in women with moderate or severe renal dysfunction because approximately 50% of pregnant women with an initial serum creatinine 1.4 mg/dL or greater experienced an increase in serum creatinine during gestation to a mean serum creatinine of 2.5 mg/dL in the third trimester. The greatest risk for accelerated progression to end-stage renal disease is seen in women with a serum creatinine above 2.0 mg/dL (177 micromoles/L) in early pregnancy. Within 6 months postpartum, 23% of these women progress to end-stage renal disease. Maternal problems appear greater with severe renal dysfunction even before dialysis is required. The diagnosis of "superimposed preeclampsia" is often difficult to make because hypertension and proteinuria may be manifestations of the underlying renal disorder; however, superimposed preeclampsia may be diagnosed in up to 80% of cases. Thus, it is primarily the maternal risk in women with moderate renal insufficiency, and the added likelihood of a poor fetal outcome when renal impairment is severe, that leads the clinician to the counseling of women regarding the advisability of pregnancy.

Prepregnancy counseling

Women should be counseled that elevated serum creatinine levels greater than 1.5 mg/dL (132 micromoles/L) and hypertension are important predisposing risk factors for permanent exacerbation of underlying renal disease. Fertility is diminished as renal impairment progresses. Normal pregnancy is unusual when preconception serum creatinine is above 3 mg/dL (265 micromoles/L or GFR less than 25 mL/min). The reported frequency of conception among women requiring dialysis is 0.3–1.5% per year. Fetal demise is markedly increased; however, recent improvements in management of these pregnant women have led to improved live birth rates (approximately 50% of cases). With well-controlled blood pressures and mild renal insufficiency, pregnancy outcome is similar to that of normotensive pregnant women with renal disease. Ideally, diastolic blood pressure before conception should be less than 90 mmHg. Women should be counseled to wait 1 year before attempting pregnancy after a living-related donor transplantation and 2 years after unrelated deceased donor transplantation to avoid problems with immunotherapy and rejection. Pregnancy has little, if any, effect on kidney function in women with renal allograft.

Management

A multidisciplinary approach is best at a tertiary care center under the coordinated care of an obstetrician, maternal–fetal medicine subspecialist and a nephrologist. Renal ultrasonography can be used to evaluate a pregnant woman with renal disease. The initial laboratory tests should include specialized tests, which help in the early detection of renal impairment as well as superimposed preeclampsia. Thus, besides the usual prenatal screening tests, the following baseline parameters should be determined:

1 Serum creatinine, blood urea nitrogen, albumin, and electrolytes.
2 24-hour urine collection for volume, protein, and creatinine clearance. Quantification of urine protein can also be done by a random protein-to-creatinine ratio.
3 Urinalysis and urine culture (to detect and treat asymptomatic bacteriuria).
4 Uric acid level, aspartate and alanine aminotransferases, complete blood count, and platelet count.
5 Lactic dehydrogenase, prothrombin time, and partial thromboplastin time may also be considered in the baseline assessment.

The number and frequency of prenatal visits should be based on the severity of renal disease and the presence of other complications such as hypertension and fetal growth restriction. Generally, women can be followed every 2 weeks until 30 to 32 weeks of gestation and weekly thereafter. Maternal renal parameters should be assessed every 4 weeks throughout pregnancy unless more frequent evaluations become necessary. More frequent screening for asymptomatic bacteriuria should be performed throughout pregnancy.

Fetal surveillance such as biophysical profile testing is best started at approximately 30–32 weeks of gestation, especially in nephrotic patients with hypoalbuminemia. Ultrasonographic examinations for pregnancy dating, fetal anatomy and monitoring fetal growth are also an integral part of surveillance.

In general, diuretics should be avoided. This is especially important in nephrotic gravidas, as these women already have reduced plasma volume and further intravascular volume depletion may impair uteroplacental perfusion. Furthermore, since blood pressure normally declines during pregnancy, saluretic therapy could conceivably precipitate circulatory collapse or thromboembolic episodes. This recommendation, however, is relative, because we have observed occasional patients whose kidneys were retaining salt so avidly that diuretics had to be used, albeit cautiously. This is especially true for women with diabetic nephropathy, in whom excessive salt retention may lead to volume-dependent hypertension during pregnancy. Prophylactic anticoagulation (i.e., mini-heparin) in nephrotic pregnant women has been recommended by some specialists, but there are few, if any, data to prove the efficacy of such treatment.

Dietary consultation is recommended for the pregnant women requiring dialysis or with nephrotic syndrome. Adequate protein and caloric intake should be ensured in these women. The diet should be supplemented with water-soluble vitamins and zinc.

Anemia is a common clinical issue in pregnant women requiring dialysis. Treatment of anemia includes blood transfusions as indicated and administration of erythropoietin to maintain hemoglobin of at least 10 or 11 g/dL. Vitamin supplementation is also part of the dialysis regimen.

Dialysis should be utilized to maintain the blood urea nitrogen less than 50 mg/dL (17 mmol/L) to prevent polyhydramnios and improve fetal outcomes. With peritoneal dialysis during pregnancy, the frequency should be increased and the exchange volumes decreased. The frequency of hemodialysis should be increased to 5 to 7 sessions per week to optimize control of uremia and should consist of slow-rate ultrafiltration, bicarbonate buffer and minimal heparinization to avoid dialysis-induced hypotension and volume contraction.

There are a few indications for renal biopsy during pregnancy and these include those women with rapid unexplained renal function deterioration or profound symptomatic nephrotic syndrome prior to 32 weeks of gestation. In experienced clinicians, a renal biopsy, if indicated, can be safely done in pregnant women with controlled blood pressures and normal coagulation studies.

Pregnant women with preexisting renal disease or essential hypertension are more susceptible than control populations to superimposed preeclampsia, which frequently occurs in midpregnancy or early in the third trimester. Superimposed preeclampsia, however, may be difficult to differentiate from aggravation of the underlying disease, especially in women with glomerular disease who are prone to hypertension and proteinuria. In any event, when these situations occur the patient should be hospitalized and managed as if she has superimposed preeclampsia. While there are debates on whether mild hypertension (90–100 mmHg – diastolic pressure, Korotkoff V) should be treated in pregnant women without underlying renal disorders, treatment is recommended for such levels of blood pressures when renal disease is present. The goal diastolic pressure is 80 mmHg. Detection of fetal growth restriction or fetal compromise, or both, is important and, regardless of maternal well-being, will influence the timing of delivery.

Suggested reading

Cunningham FG, Cox SM, Harstad TW, Mason RA, Pritchard JA. Chronic renal disease and pregnancy outcome. *Am J Obstet Gynecol* 1990;163:453–459.

Davison JM. Pregnancy in renal allograft recipients: problems, prognosis and practicalities. *Clin Obstet Gynaecol* 1994;8:501–525.

Executive summary: hypertension in pregnancy. American College of Obstetricians and Gynecologists. *Obstet Gynecol* 2013;122(5):1122–1131.

Fischer MJ, Lehnerz SD, Hebert JR, Parikh CR. Kidney disease is an independent risk factor for adverse fetal and maternal outcomes in pregnancy. *Am J Kidney Dis* 2004;43(3):415–423.

Hou, S. Pregnancy in chronic renal insufficiency and end-stage renal disease. *Am J Kidney Dis* 1999;33:235–252.

Hou SH. Pregnancy in women on haemodialysis and peritoneal dialysis. *Clin Obstet Gynaecol* 1994;8:481–500.

Jones DC, Hayslett JP. Outcome of pregnancy in women with moderate or severe renal insufficiency [published erratum appears in *N Engl J Med* 1997;336:739]. *N Engl J Med* 1996;335:226–232.

Jungers P, Chauveau G, Choukroun G, *et al.* Pregnancy in women with impaired renal function. *Nephrology* 1997;47:281–288.

Lindheimer MD, Grunfeld JP, Davison JM. Renal disorders. In: Baron WM, Lindheimer MD (eds) *Medical Disorders During Pregnancy*, 3rd edn. St. Louis, MO: Mosby Inc, 2000; pp. 39–70.

Mastrobattista JM, Gomez-Lobo V. The Society for Maternal-Fetal Medicine. Pregnancy after solid organ transplantation. *Obstet Gynecol* 2008;112:919–932.

Pertuiset N, Grunfeld JP. Acute renal failure in pregnancy. *Clin Obstet Gynaecol* 1994;8:333–351.

Piccoli GB, Conijn A, Consiglio V, *et al.* Pregnancy in dialysis patients: is the evidence strong enough to lead us to change our counseling policy? *Clin J Am Soc Nephrol* 2010;5:62–71.

Ramin SM, Vidaeff AC, Yeomans ER, Gilstrap LC III,. Chronic renal disease in pregnancy. *Obstet Gynecol* 2006;108:1531–1539.

Thadhani RI, Maski MR. Renal disorders. In: Creasy RK, Resnik R, Iams JD, Lockwood CJ, Moore TR, Greene M (eds) *Creasy and Resnik's Maternal-Fetal Medicine: Principles and Practice*, 7th edn. Philadelphia: Saunders, 2013; pp. 949–964.

PROTOCOL 19

Obesity

Raul Artal
Department of Obstetrics, Gynecology and Women's Health, Saint Louis University, St. Louis, MO, USA

Clinical significance

Since 1980 the worldwide rate of obesity has doubled; in the United States, more than one in three women are obese, more than half of pregnant women are overweight or obese, and 8% or more (depending on geographical distribution) are extremely obese. Major consequences of this obesity epidemic are increased rates of premature mortality and multiple co-morbidities, with attendant increases in health care cost. Obesity is recognized as a chronic relapsing disease that has genetic, environmental, metabolic, and behavioral components. Sedentary lifestyle, lack of sleep, poor diet, and excess gestational weight gain are major contributors to the obesity epidemic. Excessive gestational weight gain, particularly in overweight or obese pregnant women, amplifies their risk for complications particularly diabetes, hypertension, operative deliveries, sleep apnea, congenital malformations, macrosomia, stillbirths, and neonatal complications.

Pathophysiology

Pregnancy is associated with many physiological and endocrine changes. Under normal circumstances, pregnancy is characterized by progressive insulin resistance. Insulin and insulin-like growth factors are essential for regulation of cell proliferation, tissue development and energy metabolism. In overweight and obese pregnant patients, insulin resistance is further increased, which is deleterious. Excessive gestational weight gain results in even further fat storage and further exacerbates insulin resistance. Increased adiposity also leads to an increase in circulating levels of adiponectin and leptin. Adiponectin regulates insulin sensitivity and

Protocols for High-Risk Pregnancies: An Evidence-Based Approach, Sixth Edition.
Edited by John T. Queenan, Catherine Y. Spong and Charles J. Lockwood.
© 2015 John Wiley & Sons, Ltd. Published 2015 by John Wiley & Sons, Ltd.

glucose homeostasis. Other pregnancy-associated contributors to insulin resistance are placental-derived human placental lactogen, progesterone, estrogen, and cytokines (TNFα). All of these changes predispose pregnant women, particularly overweight or obese women, to gestational diabetes, and diabetes beyond pregnancy. Normalizing weight before pregnancy and exercise before and during pregnancy can reverse these adverse endocrine responses. In contrast, additional gestational weight gain in obese pregnant women is counterproductive and potentially harmful.

Diagnosis

For nonpregnant individuals, obesity is diagnosed and classified based on body mass index (BMI). The categories for adults are as follows: BMI under 18.5, underweight; BMI 18.5–24.9, normal weight; BMI 25.0–29.9, overweight; BMI 30.0 and above, obese. A limitation of BMI is that it does not reflect differences in body composition. Given the normal physiological and anthropometric changes associated with pregnancy, including excess edema, the fetus and amniotic fluid, accurate BMI measurements during pregnancy are not possible. Obesity in pregnancy is being assessed strictly by weight and it has been assumed that additional weight gain reflects excessive fat accumulations. In nonobese pregnant women under normal circumstances, pregnancy results in an additional 5–6% of body fat accumulation. Excess gestational weight gain has been associated with multiple co-morbidities, fetal macrosomia, operative deliveries, and neonatal complications.

The current Institute of Medicine (IOM) guidelines for gestational weight gain (Table 19.1) are based on prepregnancy BMI. The IOM summary

Table 19.1 New recommendations for total and rate of weight gain during pregnancy, by prepregnancy BMI

Prepregnancy BMI	Total weight gain		Rates of weight gain* Second and third trimester	
	Range (kg)	Range (lbs)	Mean (range) (kg/week)	Mean (range) (lbs/week)
Underweight (<18.5 kg/m²)	12.5–18	28–40	0.51 (0.44–0.58)	1 (1–1.3)
Normal weight (18.5–24.9 kg/m²)	11.5–16	25–35	0.42 (0.35–0.50)	1 (0.8–1)
Overweight (25.0–29.9 kg/m²)	7–11.5	15–25	0.28 (0.23–0.33)	0.6 (0.5–0.7)
Obese (≥30.0 kg/m²)	5–9	11–20	0.22 (0.17–0.27)	0.5 (0.4–0.6)

*Calculations assume a 0.5–2 kg (1.1–4.4 lbs) weight gain in the first trimester.
Source: Rasmussen & Yaktine AL, 2009. Reproduced with permission of National Academic Press.

report indicates that "utilizing BMI as an approach reflects the imprecision of the estimates on which the recommendations are based, and that many additional factors need to be considered for the individual woman."

The IOM guidelines were originally aimed at reducing the risk of low fetal birth weight and did not address other co-morbidities associated with obesity. Thus, the IOM gestational weight gain guidelines should be used in concert with good clinical judgment as well as a discussion between the woman and her provider about diet and exercise. Recommendations by ACOG emphasize that "individualized care and clinical judgment are necessary in the management of the overweight or obese woman" ... "for the overweight pregnant woman who is gaining less than the recommended amount but has an appropriately growing fetus, no evidence exists that encouraging increased weight gain to conform with the current IOM guidelines will improve maternal or fetal outcomes" (ACOG Committee Opinion, Number 548).

Treatment

The obesity treatment pyramid for nonpregnant patients includes lifestyle modification (diet and physical activity), pharmacotherapy, and surgery. Currently, the management options in pregnancy are limited to lifestyle modification.

Initial Visit

Ideally, overweight or obese patients should have prepregnancy counseling and lifestyle modifications prescribed at that time. However, pregnancy could be considered an ideal time for behavior modification since women are more inclined to adopt behavior modification regimens. Also they benefit from early and frequent access to medical care. At the first prenatal visit, it is important to establish if the patient's obesity is related to a sedentary lifestyle or to a preexisting medical condition. Thus, at the first visit certain rare genetic and other medical causes for obesity should be ruled out such as Prader-Willi Syndrome, Bardet-Biedl Syndrome, Cushing Syndrome, and hypothyroidism. Fifty percent of women with polycystic ovary syndrome (PCOS) are obese, frequently have irregular menstrual cycles, and insulin resistance, and their pregnancies are also more often complicated by gestational diabetes. To manage insulin resistance, such patients are often prescribed metformin treatment prior to pregnancy. This agent can be continued during pregnancy if needed or switched to glyburide if gestational or type 2 diabetes is diagnosed. Antidepressant drugs, which are frequently prescribed, can cause significant weight gain. Early pregnancy screening for undiagnosed type 2 diabetes is recommended to women with a prepregnancy BMI of 30 or greater.

First trimester pregnancy dating by ultrasound and first trimester screening for aneuploidy is recommended by ACOG (Practice Bulletin No. 101 and Practice Bulletin No.77), and particularly essential in overweight or obese patients. At 18–22 weeks, a second ultrasound is recommended to evaluate fetal structures. Maternal size may preclude sonographic visualization of all the structures, and another follow-up ultrasound 2–4 weeks later may be required.

Practitioners should use nonjudgmental language when counseling overweight or obese patients and approach the condition from a multifactorial perspective considering the genetic, biologic, cultural and environmental factors that contribute to excessive weight; motivational interviewing is the most useful patient–physician communication technique.

At the initial prenatal visit, patients should be counseled regarding the benefits of appropriate weight gain or no weight gain, nutrition and exercise, to achieve best pregnancy outcomes.

A judicious diet, caloric restriction and exercise limit gestational weight gain and reduce the risk for diabetes, preeclampsia, fetal macrosomia, and operative deliveries. Ideally, nutrition counseling should be individualized and provided by a dietician. The medical nutrition therapy should be a eucaloric, consistent carbohydrate meal plan that distributes nutrient dense foods over three meals and three snacks. The daily caloric requirements are 25 kcal/kg (BMI 25–29.9 kgm^2), 20 kcal/kg (BMI 30–39.9 kg/m^2), and 15 kcal/kg (BMI more than 40 kg/m^2).

Women are advised not to skip meals and to choose nutrient dense foods consisting of fruits, vegetables, low fat dairy, lean meats, and whole grains. The diet is of improved nutritional quality while decreasing fat, sugar, and sodium intake. Patients are advised to engage in at least 30 minutes of physical activity each day, and since most of them were previously sedentary should be encouraged to walk at a moderate to brisk pace after each meal if possible for a total of 150 minutes or more per week.

Complications

Maternal obesity is associated with multiple fetal and maternal complications; among those with higher prevalence are miscarriages, antepartum fetal death, fetal growth restriction, macrosomia, and neonatal death. Obesity is also a risk factor for maternal mortality. As noted, among maternal complications, preeclampsia, diabetes and operative deliveries are common. Congenital malformations including cardiac defects (OR 1.2), neural tube defects (OR 1.8), and omphalocele (OR 3.3), are more common among obese pregnant women and could potentially be prevented by optimal glucose control at the time of conception and for the first weeks of pregnancy. Timing for initiating antepartum testing depends on the type and severity of complications affecting the patient. Careful consideration should be given to the interpretation of these tests to avoid iatrogenic prematurity as a result of false-positive testing. For certain complications such as fetal growth restriction, testing may be indicated as early as 26–28 weeks of gestation. The large habitus of these patients may hamper the ability for an adequate fetal assessment and suboptimal visualization is cited as a barrier. Recently, available ultrasound equipment appears to be more effective for monitoring or imaging studies.

For labor and delivery pain control lumbar epidural anesthesia (LEA) is not only desirable but medically indicated as LEA attenuates changes in oxygen consumption and cardiac output, and also lessens the risks associated with the administration of drugs to obese patients.

Obese women are at greater risk for operative and cesarean deliveries. Shortening the time of surgery by utilizing high transverse abdominal incision has resulted in less intraoperative and postoperative complications.

With the rise of the obesity epidemic, many obese women have undergone bariatric surgery. The management of these patients once pregnant often relates more to their type of surgery than complications associated with obesity as treated patients, even if they achieve only modest weight loss following surgery, have reduced complications in pregnancy and better outcomes. Depending on the type of surgery, these patients could experience certain complications in pregnancy for which medical or surgical interventions may be necessary, such as hernia formation resulting in bowel ischemia, band slippage, excess nausea, bowel obstruction, staple line strictures, Vit A, B_{12} and folate deficiency, and chronic diarrhea.

Conclusion

- Obesity affects fertility, pregnancy, and offspring.
- Obesity in pregnancy is associated with pathophysiological changes leading to:
  - Increased pregnancy loss (early and late pregnancy).
  - Increase in congenital malformations.
  - Increase in maternal co-morbidities such as:
    1 Preeclampsia, risk doubles with each $5 \, kg/m^2$ BMI.
    2 Thromboembolism, risk doubles.
    3 Gestational diabetes, rate increases 3–4-fold.
  - Increased cesarean delivery rate by approximately 50%.
  - Increase in risk of maternal death, based on above risk factors.

- Judicious lifestyle modifications in pregnancy improve both maternal and neonatal outcomes in obese patients.
- Interpregnancy weight loss improves future maternal and neonatal outcomes.

Suggested reading

Artal R, Bray GA, Champagne CM. Role of Exercise, Diet and Medical Intervention in Weight Management. Precis, Primary and Preventive Care, pgs 50–59. ACOG Publications, 4th edn 2009.

Artal R, Catanzaro RB, Gavard JA, *et al.* A lifestyle intervention of weight-gain restriction: diet and exercise in obese women with gestational diabetes mellitus. *Appl Physiol Nutr Metab* 2007;32:596–601.

Artal R, Lockwood CJ, Brown HL. Weight Gain recommendations in pregnancy and the obesity epidemic. *Obstet Gynecol* 2012;115:152–155.

The California Pregnancy-Associated Mortality Review. Report from 2002 and 2003 Maternal Death Reviews. Sacramento: California Department of Public Health, Maternal Child and Adolescent Health Division; 2011.

Exercise during pregnancy and the postpartum period. Committee Opinion No. 267. American College of Obstetricians and Gynecologists. *Obstet Gynecol* 2002;99:171–173 (reaffirmed 2009).

Gestational diabetes mellitus. Practice Bulletin No. 137. American College of Obstetricians and Gynecologists. *Obstet Gynecol* 2013;122:406–16.

Jacque-Fortunato SY, Khodiguian N, Artal R and Wiswell RA. Body composition in pregnancy, *Semin in Perin* 1996;20(4):340–342.

Obesity in pregnancy. Committee Opinion No. 549. American College of Obstetricians and Gynecologists. *Obstet Gynecol* 2013;121:213–217.

Rasmussen KM, Yaktine AL (eds). *Weight Gain During Pregnancy: Reexamining the Guidelines.* Institute of Medicine and National Research Council Committee to Reexamine IOM Pregnancy Weight Guidelines. Washington, DC: National Academic Press; 2009.

Reddy UM, Abuhamad AZ, Levine D, *et al.* Fetal Imaging, *Obstet Gynecol* 2014;123: 1070–1082.

Smith De, Lewis CE, Caremy JL, *et al.* Longitudinal changes in adiposity associated with pregnancy. The CARDIA study. Coronary Artery risk development in young adults study. *JAMA* 1994;271:1747–1751.

Weight gain during pregnancy. Committee Opinion No. 548. American College of Obstetricians and Gynecologists. *Obstet Gynecol* 2013;121:210–212.

PROTOCOL 20

Diabetes Mellitus

Mark B. Landon & Steven G. Gabbe
Department of Obstetrics and Gynecology, The Ohio State University College of Medicine, Columbus, OH, USA

Overview

Diabetes mellitus complicates approximately 7% of all pregnancies. Gestational diabetes mellitus (GDM), or carbohydrate intolerance detected for the first time during gestation, represents about 90% of all cases, whereas pregestational diabetes mellitus, which includes both type 1 and type 2 diabetes mellitus, accounts for the remaining 10%. Type 2 diabetes is now the most common form of pregestational diabetes.

Pathophysiology

The increased perinatal morbidity and mortality associated with the pregnancy complicated by diabetes mellitus can be attributed directly to maternal hyperglycemia. Glucose crosses the placenta by facilitated diffusion. Therefore, maternal hyperglycemia can produce fetal hyperglycemia. During the first trimester, maternal hyperglycemia is associated with an increased risk for abnormal fetal organogenesis. Major fetal malformations, now the leading cause of perinatal mortality in pregnancies complicated by type 1 and type 2 diabetes mellitus, occur in 6–10% of pregnancies complicated by pregestational diabetes. Poorly controlled patients can have up to a 25% risk for fetal malformations. Chronic fetal hyperglycemia in later gestation leads to fetal hyperinsulinemia, which is associated with excessive fetal growth, as well as delayed fetal pulmonary maturation. Intrauterine fetal death, which is observed in pregnancies complicated by poorly controlled diabetes mellitus, can also be attributed to fetal hyperinsulinemia that results in hypoxia and lactic acidosis. The likelihood that any of these complications will occur is directly related to maternal glucose control, as reflected by mean glucose levels or concentrations

Protocols for High-Risk Pregnancies: An Evidence-Based Approach, Sixth Edition.
Edited by John T. Queenan, Catherine Y. Spong and Charles J. Lockwood.
© 2015 John Wiley & Sons, Ltd. Published 2015 by John Wiley & Sons, Ltd.

of glycosylated hemoglobin. The presence of diabetic vasculopathy may also affect placental function, thereby increasing the risk for fetal growth restriction, preeclampsia, and preterm delivery.

Pregestational diabetes mellitus

Risk assessment
Maternal and perinatal risks are increased in the presence of:
1 vasculopathy, such as retinopathy, nephropathy, and hypertension;
2 poor glucose control;
3 prognostically bad signs of pregnancy, including ketoacidosis, pyelo-nephritis, pregnancy-induced hypertension, and poor clinic attendance or neglect.

Prepregnancy care
Objectives
1 Assess for maternal vasculopathy by an ophthalmological evaluation, electrocardiogram and 24-hour urine collection for creatinine clearance and protein excretion.
2 Improve maternal glucose control (target glycosylated hemoglobin 7% or lower with normal range 6% or lower) to reduce the risk of fetal malformations and miscarriage; assess for hypoglycemic awareness.
3 Provide contraceptive counseling.
4 Educate the patient and her partner about the management plan for diabetes in pregnancy.
5 Determine rubella immune status and check thyroid function studies.
6 Begin folic acid supplementation to reduce risk of fetal neural tube defects.

Detection and evaluation of malformations
1 Identification of women at greatest risk: maternal glycosylated hemoglobin levels in the first trimester.
2 Noninvasive aneuploidy screening and MSAFP.
3 Ultrasonography at 13–14 weeks to detect anencephaly.
4 Comprehensive ultrasonography at 18–20 weeks with careful study of cardiac structure, including great vessels.

Antepartum care: regulation of maternal glycemia
Target capillary glucose levels in pregnancy are listed below:
- Mean level: 100 mg/dL
- Before breakfast: less than 95 mg/dL
- Before lunch, supper, bedtime snack: less than 100 mg/dL

- 1 hour after meals: less than 140 mg/dL
- 2 hours after meals: less than 120 mg/dL
- 2 a.m. to 6 a.m.: greater than 60 mg/dL

1 Capillary glucose monitoring with fasting, prelunch, predinner and bed-time levels daily, as well as 1- or 2-hour postprandial values; glycosylated hemoglobin levels in each trimester, target 6% or less.

2 Insulin therapy
- Multiple insulin injections: prandial insulin (insulin lispro or insulin aspart) with meals, snacks; basal insulin (neutral protamine Hagedorn (NPH)), before breakfast (two-thirds of total NPH dose) and at bedtime (one-third of total NPH dose). If well controlled on insulin glargine or detemir, may continue these basal insulins.
- Continuous subcutaneous insulin infusion (insulin pump): insulin lispro; continuous basal rate and boluses, in highly compliant patients.

3 Dietary recommendations
- Plan: three meals, three snacks.
- Diet: 30–35 kcal/kg normal body weight, 2000–2400 kcal/day.
- Composition: carbohydrate 40–50% complex, high fiber; protein 20%; fat 30–40% (less than 10% saturated).
- Weight gain: per IOM guidelines.

4 General guidelines for insulin use and carbohydrate intake:
- 1 unit of rapid-acting insulin lowers blood glucose 30 mg/dL.
- 10 g of carbohydrate increases blood glucose 30 mg/dL.
- 1 unit of rapid-acting insulin will cover intake of 10 g of carbohydrate.

Fetal evaluation

Assessment of fetal well-being to prevent intrauterine fetal deaths and guide timing of delivery:

1 Biophysical
- Maternal assessment of fetal activity at 28 weeks.
- Nonstress test (NST), weekly at 28–30 weeks for women with vasculopathy; twice weekly at 32 weeks and beyond in all pregestational diabetes; may alternate with biophysical profile (BPP).
- BPP or contraction stress test if NST nonreactive.

2 Sonographic evaluation of fetal growth during the third trimester.

Delivery

Timing

1 Patients at low risk for fetal death (excellent glucose control, no vasculopathy, normal fetal growth, reassuring antepartum fetal testing, no prior stillbirth): may electively deliver after 39 weeks or allow spontaneous labor up to 40 weeks.

2 Patients at high risk for fetal death (poor control, vasculopathy, macrosomia, hydramnios, prior stillbirth): consider delivery prior to 39 weeks. Amniocentesis may be employed to assess for lung maturity.

Method

To reduce birth trauma, counsel regarding elective cesarean delivery if estimated fetal weight is 4500 g or more. For estimated weight 4000–4500 g, mode of delivery will depend on prior obstetric history, sonographic growth characteristics, pelvic examination and patient preference.

Intrapartum glycemic control

1 Check capillary glucose hourly at the bedside; maintain below 110 mg/dL.
2 Glucose control during labor (first stage) (Table 20.1).

Contraception for the patient with type 1 or type 2 diabetes mellitus

Combination oral contraceptives

1 Low-dose pills appear safe in patients without vasculopathy.
2 Contraindicated in presence of smoking, hypertension.

Progestin-only pills

Acceptable for patients with vasculopathy.

Mechanical or barrier methods

Less effective than oral contraceptives but no effect on glucose control or vasculopathy.

Intrauterine device

Acceptable for multiparous patients.

Sterilization

Consider when family has been completed, especially for patients with significant vasculopathy.

Table 20.1 Glucose control during first stage of labor

	Insulin	Glucose
Latent phase	1 unit/hr	5 g/h
Active phase	None	10 g/h

Gestational diabetes

Definition

Gestational diabetes is defined as carbohydrate intolerance of variable severity with onset or first recognition during pregnancy. The definition applies irrespective of whether or not insulin is used for treatment or the condition persists after pregnancy. It does not exclude the possibility that unrecognized glucose intolerance may have antedated the pregnancy.

Class A_1 gestational diabetes is diet controlled; Class A_2 gestational diabetes requires diet and pharmacological treatment (insulin or oral agent such as glyburide).

Consequences: Why bother to screen?

1 Maternal: subsequent type 2 diabetes mellitus, shortened life expectancy.
2 Fetal and neonatal:
  * excessive fetal growth and birth trauma; neonatal hypoglycemia, hypocalcemia, hyperbilirubinemia;
  * increased perinatal mortality associated with significant maternal hyperglycemia.

Screening and diagnosis

Detection

Most practitioners continue to screen all pregnant women for glucose intolerance since selective screening based on clinical attributes or past obstetric history has been shown to be inadequate. There may be a group of women at low enough risk that screening is not necessary (see below).

According to the Fourth International Workshop Conference on GDM, Screening Strategy, risk assessment for GDM should be ascertained at the first prenatal visit.

Low risk

Blood glucose testing is not routinely required if all of the following characteristics are present:
* Member of an ethnic group with a low prevalence of GDM
* No known diabetes in first-degree relatives
* Age younger than 25 years
* Weight normal before pregnancy
* No history of abnormal glucose metabolism
* No history of poor obstetric outcome.

Average risk

Perform blood glucose screening at 24–28 weeks using one of the following:

- Two-step procedure: 1-hour 50 g GCT (glucose challenge test) followed by a diagnostic OGTT (oral glucose tolerance test) in those meeting the threshold value in GCT (130–140 mg/dl).
- One-step procedure: diagnostic OGTT performed on all subjects.

High risk

- Perform blood glucose testing as soon as feasible, using the procedures described above.
- If GDM is not diagnosed, blood glucose testing should be repeated at 24–28 weeks or at any time a patient has symptoms or signs suggestive of hyperglycemia.

Adapted from Fourth International Workshop Conference on GDM, *Diabetes Care*, Volume 21, Supplement 2, August 1998.

With a GCT cutoff value of 140 mg/dL, sensitivity is 90%, and 15% of patients require a GTT. With a cutoff of 130 mg/dL, sensitivity is nearly 100%, but 25% of patients require a GTT.

A plasma glucose measurement 200 mg/dL or higher outside the context of a formal glucose challenge test, or a truly fasting plasma glucose 126 mg/dL or higher, suggests the diabetic state and warrants further investigation.

Diagnosis

100 g oral glucose load, administered in the morning after overnight fast for at least 8 hours but not more than 14 hours, and following at least 3 days of unrestricted diet (150 g carbohydrate or more) and usual physical activity.

Venous plasma glucose is measured fasting and at 1, 2 and 3 hours. Subject should remain seated and not smoke throughout the test.

Two or more of the following venous plasma concentrations must be met or exceeded for a positive diagnosis (Table 20.2).

Table 20.2 Venous plasma concentrations for positive diagnosis of diabetes mellitus

	NDDG (mg/dL)	Carpenter and Coustan* (mg/dL)
Fasting	105	95
1-hour	190	180
2-hour	165	155
3-hour	145	140

*Carpenter MW, Coustan DR. Criteria for screening tests for gestational diabetes. *Am J Obstet Gynecol* 1982;144:768–73.

Other diagnostic criteria

The Hyperglycemia and Adverse Pregnancy Outcome (HAPO) study suggested a continuous relationship between maternal glucose levels (including levels below those currently diagnostic of GDM) and perinatal outcomes. Based on the HAPO data, the IADPSG criteria were derived by consensus. The IADPSG approach utilizes universal 2-hour 75 gram OGTT with the diagnosis of GDM established if one value is abnormal. The IADPSG criteria are as follows: fasting, 92 mg/dl; one-hour, 180 mg/dl; two-hour, 153 mg/dl. This approach results in a 2–3 times increased frequency of GDM. Currently, the ADA endorses either the IADPSG approach or the two-step approach with a diagnostic three-hour OGTT. ACOG endorses only the three-hour 100-gram OGTT criteria.

Antepartum management
Program of care
Visits every 1–2 weeks until 36 weeks, then weekly.

Dietary recommendations in pregnancy
- Plan: 3 meals, bedtime snack.
- Diet: 2000 to 2200 kcal/day. Normal weight: 30 kcal/kg ideal prepregnancy body weight. Lean: 35 kcal/kg ideal prepregnancy body weight. Obese: 25 kcal/kg ideal prepregnancy body weight.
- Composition: carbohydrate 40–50% complex, high fiber; protein 20%; fat 30–40% (less than 10% saturated).
- Weight gain: 20 lb; 16 lb for very obese.

Note: Check morning urine for ketones if using caloric restriction in obese patients (1600–1800 kcal/day). Increase caloric intake if fasting ketonuria noted.

Exercise
Encourage regular exercise, 20–30 minutes brisk walking, 3–4 times/week.

Surveillance of maternal diabetes
1 Self-monitoring of capillary blood glucose to check fasting and 1- or 2-hour postprandial glucose levels daily to assess efficacy of diet.
2 If repetitive fasting plasma values are more than 95 mg/dL and/or 1-hour values are more than 140 mg/dL and/or 2-hour values are more than 120 mg/dL, insulin or glyburide therapy is recommended.
3 Starting insulin dose calculated based on patient's weight; 0.8 U/kg actual body weight per day in first trimester, 1.0 U/kg in second trimester, 1.2 U/kg in third trimester. Give two-thirds of total dose in fasting state: two-thirds as NPH, one-third as regular or insulin lispro; give one-third

of total dose as one-half regular or insulin lispro at dinner, one-half as NPH at bedtime.

4 Glyburide can be used as alternative to insulin, although it is usually not effective if fasting glucose exceeds 115 mg/dL. Glyburide, unlike insulin, does cross the placenta and patients should be informed of this although short-term safety is established. The usual starting dose is 2.5 mg at breakfast and 2.5 mg at dinner with doses as high as 20 mg/day employed.

Delivery

1 Women with well-controlled class A_1 gestational diabetes allow to go to 39 weeks of gestation.
2 If undelivered at 40 weeks, begin fetal assessment with twice-weekly NSTs. Women with prior stillbirth or those with hypertension should be followed with twice-weekly NSTs at 32 weeks.
3 Clinical estimation of fetal size and ultrasonographic indices should be used to detect excessive fetal growth. To reduce birth trauma, counsel regarding cesarean delivery if estimated fetal weight is at least 4500 g. For estimated weight 4000–4500 g, consider prior obstetric history, fetal growth indices, pelvic capacity and patient preference in selecting mode of delivery.
4 Class A_2 women should be followed with twice-weekly NSTs.
5 Suboptimally controlled GDM women may require delivery before 39 weeks.
6 Alert neonatal team as infant may require observation for hypoglycemia, hypocalcemia, and hyperbilirubinemia.

Postpartum care
Evaluation for persistent carbohydrate intolerance

1 Women can continue self-blood-glucose monitoring to evaluate glucose profile although class A_1 patients generally demonstrate normoglycemia.
2 At 6–12 weeks postpartum, oral GTT with 75 g glucose load, administered under conditions described for 100 g oral test. Venous plasma glucose is measured fasting and at 2 hours (Table 20.3).
3 If normal, evaluate at minimum of 3-year intervals with fasting glucose; encourage exercise and, if obese, weight loss.

Effects of oral contraceptives
Deterioration of carbohydrate intolerance not reported with low-dose pills.

Recurrence risk
Approximately 60%.

Table 20.3   Values for venous plasma glucose

Normal	Impaired glucose tolerance (mg/dL)	Diabetes mellitus
Fasting less than 100 mg/dL	100–125	126 mg/dL or higher
2 h less than 140 mg/dL	140–199	200 mg/dL or higher

Suggested reading

Type 1 and type 2 diabetes mellitus in pregnancy

DeWitt DE, Hirsch IB. Outpatient insulin therapy in type 1 and type 2 diabetes mellitus. *JAMA* 2003;289(17):2254–64.

Gabbe SG, Graves CR. Management of diabetes mellitus complicating pregnancy. *Obstet Gynecol* 2003;102:4:857–68.

Kitzmiller JL, Buchanan TA, Kjos S, Combs CA, Ratner RE. Pre-conception care of diabetes, congenital malformations, and spontaneous abortions. *Diabetes Care* 1996;19:514–40.

Landon MB, Catalano PM, Gabbe SG. Diabetes mellitus complicating pregnancy. In: Gabbe SG, Neibyl JR, Simpson JL (eds) *Obstetrics: Normal and Problem Pregnancies,* 6th edn. *Elsevier* 2012; pp. 887–921.

Landon MB, Gabbe, SG. Medical therapy. In: Reece EA, Coustan D, Gabbe SG (eds) *Diabetes Mellitus in Women.* Lippincott Williams & Wilkins, 2004.

Pregestational diabetes mellitus. ACOG Practice Bulletin No. 60. American College of Obstetricians and Gynecologists. *Obstet Gynecol* 2005;105:675–85.

Gestational diabetes mellitus

American Diabetes Association. Standards of Medical care in Diabetes- 2014 *Diabetes Care 2014;* 37(Suppl.1):S14–80.

Carpenter MW, Coustan DR. Criteria for screening tests for gestational diabetes. *Am J Obstet Gynecol* 1982;144:768–73.

Crowther CA, Hiller JE, Moss JR, McPhee AJ, *et al.* Australian Carbohydrate Intolerance Study in Pregnant Women (ACHOIS) Trial Group. *N Engl J Med* 2005;352(24):2477–86.

Gestational diabetes mellitus. Practice Bulletin No. 137. American College of Obstetricians and Gynecologists. *Obstet Gynecol* 2013;122:406–16.

HAPO Study Cooperative Research Group. Hyperglycemia and Adverse Pregnancy Outcome (HAPO) Study: association with neonatal anthropometrics. *Diabetes* 2009;58(2):453–9.

Metzger BE, Gabbe SG Persson B for the IADPSG Consensus Panel: recommendations on the diagnosis and classification of hyperglycemia in pregnancy. *Diabetes Care* 2010;33:676.

Landon MB, Spong CY, Thom E, Carpenter MW, *et al.* A Multicenter, Randomized Trial of Treatment for Mild Gestational Diabetes. *N Engl J Med* 2009;361;14:1339–1348.

Langer O, Conway DL, Berkus MD, Xenakis EMJ, Gonzales O. A comparison of glyburide and insulin in women with gestational diabetes mellitus. *N Engl J Med* 2000;343:1134–8.

PROTOCOL 21

Thyroid Disorders

Stephen F. Thung

Department of Obstetrics and Gynecology, The Ohio State University College of Medicine, Columbus, OH, USA

Overview

Thyroid disease during pregnancy is common, second only to diabetes amongst endocrine disorders. The overlap between common pregnancy complaints and physiologic changes and the signs and symptoms of both hyperthyroidism and hypothyroidism can make recognition of disease challenging. Proper identification and management prevents many of the sequela that affects these complicated pregnancies.

Maternal euthyroid status is critical for healthy maternal and fetal health and development. The fetal thyroid becomes active at 18–20 weeks of gestation and until this time the fetus is largely dependent upon placental transported maternal thyroid hormone for proper development.

Pregnancy induces tremendous thyroid physiologic changes from the nonpregnant state. Estrogens stimulate the rapid production of both thyroid binding globulins as well as total thyroid hormones (T3 and T4) to magnitudes significantly above the nonpregnant state. Despite this rapid increase in thyroid hormone, active free thyroid hormone levels (free T3 and free T4) do not change significantly from nonpregnant levels and pregnant women are not considered hyperthyroid. Thyroid-stimulating hormone (TSH) changes modestly during pregnancy, particularly in the first trimester when levels are commonly reduced below nonpregnant norms as a result of a physiologic rise of human chorionic gonadotropin (HCG), which is structurally similar to TSH. Trimester-specific norms have been described for TSH.

Diagnosis

Typically a TSH and free T4 are required to make the diagnosis for the vast majority of thyroid disorders (Table 21.1).

Protocols for High-Risk Pregnancies: An Evidence-Based Approach, Sixth Edition.
Edited by John T. Queenan, Catherine Y. Spong and Charles J. Lockwood.
© 2015 John Wiley & Sons, Ltd. Published 2015 by John Wiley & Sons, Ltd.

Table 21.1 Diagnosis of thyroid disorders

Condition	TSH	Free T4
Overt hypothyroidism	High	Low
Subclinical hypothyroidism	High	Normal range
Overt hyperthyroidism	Low (commonly undetectable)	High
Subclinical hyperthyroidism	Low	Normal range
Hypothyroxinemia	Normal range	Low

Additional studies

- *Free T3*: When there is a strong clinical suspicion for thyroid disease with an abnormal TSH and free T4 evaluation is unremarkable, testing a free T3 may be useful.
- *Thyroid-stimulating immunoglobulins (TSI)* are the pathologic antibodies found in Graves' disease-related hyperthyroidism that mediate the many signs and symptoms of the disorder. They can be used to confirm the diagnosis. Moreover, TSI cross the placenta (IgG) and on rare occasions stimulate clinically relevant fetal hyperthyroidism regardless of maternal thyroid state. Testing TSI is particularly useful in women who have had a diagnosis of Graves' disease and have had an ablative procedure in the past (surgery or radioactive iodine) and no longer have a significant risk for maternal hyperthyroidism. Euthyroid pregnant women with high TSI should have close fetal follow up, similar to mothers with active hyperthyroidism as the fetus remains at risk.
- *Antithyroid peroxidase antibodies (TPO)* are antibodies commonly associated with Hashimoto disease and hypothyroidism. TPO antibodies in euthyroid women have been associated with future thyroiditis risks as well as pregnancy loss. TPO testing may be indicated in women with recurrent pregnancy loss, as some studies demonstrate that low-dose thyroid hormone supplementation may reduce the risk of recurrent loss or prematurity in euthyroid women.

Hypothyroidism

Unrecognized overt hypothyroidism is uncommon during pregnancy due to a high prevalence of infertility. However, caring for pregnant women with a managed preexisting diagnosis is common. In the United States, Hashimoto thyroiditis is the most common etiology, an autoimmune disease that results in the destruction of thyroid gland. Surgical thyroidectomy or radioactive iodine ablation are other causes.

Worldwide, iodine deficiency remains the most common etiology for maternal hypothyroidism and is the leading cause of offspring mental retardation. Even in the United States, moderate iodine deficiency is becoming a growing concern as Americans consume less salt due to cardiovascular concern as well as larger proportions of daily salt intake lacking significant iodine supplementation such as processed foods and popular salt products (sea salt and kosher salts).

Implications for pregnancy

Overt hypothyroidism is clearly associated with adverse pregnancy outcomes when unmanaged. When managed judiciously, outcomes can be similar to uncomplicated low-risk gestations. Adverse pregnancy outcomes due to hypothyroidism can include:
- Spontaneous abortion and fetal demise
- Placental abruption
- Gestational hypertension and preeclampsia
- Idiopathic preterm delivery
- Offspring developmental delay

Subclinical hypothyroidism is commonly defined as a TSH above the 95% or 97.5% for pregnancy and a normal free T4. Given the name, it is asymptomatic. In the past, many experts suggested thyroid hormone supplementation due to a concern for delayed neurologic development, similar to that of overt hypothyroidism. However, a recent randomized trial has not demonstrated improved offspring outcomes with this strategy (Lazarus et al 2012). Screening for this condition is not indicated.

Hypothyroxinemia has not been clearly associated with adverse pregnancy outcomes and thyroid hormone supplementation is not required. Attention to diet and adequate iodine intake is prudent in these cases.

Thyroid cancer is rare during pregnancy. In general, most thyroid neoplasms are slow growing and in most cases surgery may be deferred until after delivery. That being said, current data suggest no significant differences in pregnancy outcome if thyroidectomy is performed in the second trimester. Attention to adequate thyroid supplementation is essential after thyroidectomy.

Treatment

Therapy for overt hypothyroidism is straightforward in most cases.
- Levothyroxine dosing for overt hypothyroidism is typically 100–125 micrograms daily but may be significantly higher in women who have had a thyroidectomy/ablation. For mild to moderate cases 1 mcg/kg/day

is appropriate as an initial dose, while severe cases may require 1.5 mcg/kg/day.

- Dosing typically increases in the first trimester, approximately 20–25%. Some experts empirically increase dosing once pregnancy is determined while others determine dosing changes based upon TSH and free T4 levels at a first prenatal visit. Both approaches are acceptable.
- Adequate levothyroxine supplementation should be assessed at baseline and every 4–6 weeks with a TSH and free T4 as dosing is titrated. TSH levels do not change significantly with more frequent testing intervals. Once a stable dose is realized, testing once per trimester is sufficient.
- Be aware that iron supplementation can interfere with thyroid hormone supplementation and dosing should be staggered, 4–6 hours before or after levothyroxine.
- TSH goals for levothyroxine titration are not agreed upon. I typically titrate levothyroxine dosing to keep TSH less than 2.5 mU/L.
- In the postpartum period levothyroxine dosing should be returned to prepregnancy levels. TSH and free T4 should be tested at the routine postpartum visit to assure a euthyroid state and rule out postpartum thyroiditis. There are no concerns with breastfeeding and levothyroxine therapy.

Hyperthyroidism

Antenatal management of hyperthyroidism is rare, affecting approximately 0.2% of pregnancies. Of these women, the overwhelming majority has pre-existing Graves' disease. Other etiologies include active thyroid adenomas and toxic nodular goiter, thyroiditis, and transient gestational thyrotoxicosis (HCG-induced).

Graves' disease is an autoimmune disorder that may involve many organ systems, including the thyroid. Thyroid-stimulating immunoglobulins mediate the disease state including triggering over-activity of the thyroid gland. These IgG autoantibodies cross the placenta to stimulate fetal disease in rare cases (1%). Even when the maternal thyroid gland is removed, circulating TSI may mediate fetal disease in a euthyroid mother.

Implications for pregnancy

The impact of overt hyperthyroidism during pregnancy is related to severity of the disease state. Mild disease can be tolerated while moderate and severe disease generally requires pharmacotherapy or thyroidectomy in recalcitrant cases. Women not optimally managed face risks of preeclampsia/gestational hypertension. In severe cases, particularly when found to be in thyroid storm, women are at significant risk for cardiac heart failure and death.

Thyroid storm is an acute medical emergency characterized by a hypermetabolic state that when unmanaged results in heart failure and death. Recognition and aggressive management in an intensive care setting is required to prevent death.

Fetal consequences include growth restriction and fetal/neonatal demise. Neonatal hyperthyroidism is found in 1–2% of Graves' disease pregnancies, mediated by TSI that cross the placenta. Findings include: fetal tachycardia, fetal goiter, cardiac heart failure/hydrops, accelerated bone maturity, and craniosynostosis. Goiters are enlarged thyroid glands, best seen by a specialist. On ultrasound, a homogenous echogenic anterior neck mass may be seen measuring more than 95th percentile on available nomograms.

Transient gestational thyrotoxicosis is generally a self-limited consequence of common alpha subunits of HCG and TSH. As such, HCG is a weak stimulator of thyroid hormone release and as HCG levels rise in the first trimester so does the potential for subclinical hyperthyroidism or mild overt hyperthyroidism. As HCG levels taper in the second trimester, so does the thyrotoxicosis. Typically, therapy is not required beyond reassurance.

Subclinical hyperthyroidism is well tolerated during pregnancy. In older women it may be associated with cardiac arrhythmias but no significant adverse outcomes have been identified during pregnancy. Treatment is not indicated for young pregnant women.

Management

Subclinical hyperthyroidism: No therapy is required; however follow up for development to overt hyperthyroidism may be prudent, particularly in the postpartum period.

Pharmacotherapy management of overt maternal hyperthyroidism alleviates maternal and fetal risks, but may result in unintentional fetal hypothyroidism due to placental transfer. As such, utilizing minimal dosing of pharmacologic agents is necessary to minimize fetal risk. Titrating therapy to achieve a euthyroid state bordering upon subclinical hyperthyroidism is ideal as it is well tolerated.

Antithyroid therapy. Two therapeutic options are available for treatment. Propylthiouracil (PTU) has been used more commonly during pregnancy due to concerns of small but increased risks of teratogenicity with methimazole (MMI) use in the first trimester. Unfortunately, PTU has been associated with fulminant hepatitis for all users (1/10,000) that may result in death or liver transplantation. As such, MMI is now the first-line hyperthyroidism therapy for nonpregnant users due to its safer side-effect profile and once daily dosing. This is the case for pregnancy, except in the first trimester. *Current recommendations are to use PTU in the preconception period and first trimester followed by MMI for the remainder of pregnancy to minimize both fetal and maternal risks.*

- *MMI* use has concerns including maternal hepatitis and *possible* concerns for fetal abnormalities such as aplasia cutis, choanal atresia, and tracheal-esophageal fistulas. Absolute risks are low and if a woman arrives to care well through the period of organogenesis, MMI therapy should be maintained, rather than changed to alternative agents. Initial dosing commonly ranges from 5–10 mg daily with upward titration to 10–30 mg daily.

- *PTU* side effects include risk of rash, hepatitis and liver failure (1/10,000) resulting in death or liver transplant, and agranulocytosis (first three months typically less than 1% risk). Typical starting dose should be determined by severity of disease, but I commonly will start with 50 mg three times daily and increase monthly to a typical 100–150 mg every 8 hours. Serial liver function tests are not thought to be useful due to rapid progression of hepatitis when it occurs.

- *Changing between PTU and MMI.* MMI is 20-fold to 25-fold more active per milligram than PTU. As such, someone requiring 450 mg (total daily dose) of PTU could be expected to require 15–20 mg of MMI daily. For both therapies, monthly thyroid function follow up is needed to actively titrate dosing. In more concerning cases, free T4 can be measured more frequently to guide increasing dosage. Dosing should be titrated close to subclinical hyperthyroid ranges to minimize fetal thyroid suppression. Requirements typically fall in the third trimester due to less active disease. Both therapies are acceptable for breastfeeding.

For *severe cases with symptoms*, propranolol 20 mg every 6–8 hours can be used, and I prefer this over other beta blockers such as atenolol which have been known to be associated with fetal growth restriction. This is particularly useful as antithyroid therapies are titrated upwards.

Fetal surveillance. Given the fetal risks, a detailed anatomical survey is indicated with serial ultrasound for growth, commonly done on a monthly basis. For women with a history of Graves' disease, fetal hyperthyroidism is a concern through TSI pathogenesis. In these cases, TSI can be measured to determine if there is fetal risk, however attention to the presence of fetal tachycardia and subsequent evaluation of the neck for goiter (homogenous echogenic enlargement on the anterior neck more than 95%) is typically sufficient.

In rare cases of treated hyperthyroidism when a fetal goiter is identified, determining whether the fetus is hyperthyroid or hypothyroid can be unclear. In these cases, utilizing cordocentesis to sample fetal blood and thyroid levels for therapy guidance has been described. These cases should be referred to a tertiary center that has experience with this management.

In *recalcitrant cases* that do not respond to pharmacotherapy, thyroidectomy can be performed. Surgical removal can be done safely, especially in the second trimester. Radioactive iodine is contraindicated as it is concentrated in the fetal thyroid.

Thyroid storm management:

- This is a medical emergency that requires immediate admission to a medical intensive care unit.
- Common symptoms include fever, agitation, delirium, tachycardia, and congestive heart failure.
- Therapy is no different than the nonpregnant state.
- Immediate IV access and hydration.
- PTU 600–800 mg PO/crushed in a nasogastric tube, followed by 150–200 mg every 4–6 hours.
- Iodide product to suppress T3 and T4 release from thyroid gland, options include:
  - Sodium Iodide 500–1000 mg IV (1 hour after PTU administration) every 8 hours (or)
  - Potassium Iodide (SSKI) 5 drops every 8 hours (or)
  - Lugol Solution 8 drops PO every 6 hours (or)
  - Lithium carbonate 300 mg every 6 hours (if allergic to the above)
- Dexamethasone 2 mg IV every 6 hours for 4 doses (blocks peripheral conversion of T4 to T3)
- Beta blockers if the patient is not hypotensive or in heart failure. Options include:
  - Propranolol 1 mg IV (slow) every 5 minutes for a total of 6 mg followed by 1–10 mg IV every 4 hours (or)
  - Propanolol 20–80 mg PO or nasogastric tube every 4–6 hours (or)
  - Esmolol drip, 250–500 µg/kg with continuous drip of 50–100 µg/kg/min.

Suggested reading

Alexander EK, Marqusee E, Lawrence J, *et al.* Timing and magnitude of increases in levothyroxine requirements during pregnancy in women with hypothyroidism. *N Engl J Med* 2004;351(3):241–9.

Bahn RS, Burch HS, Cooper DS, Garber JR, Greenlee CM, Klein IL, Laurberg P, McDougall IR, Rivkees SA, Ross D, Sosa JA, Stan MN. The Role of Propylthiouracil in the Management of Graves' Disease in Adults: report of a meeting jointly sponsored by the American Thyroid Association and the Food and Drug Administration. *Thyroid.* 2009;19(7):673.

Casey BM, Leveno KJ. Thyroid disease in pregnancy. *Obstet Gynecol* 2006;108(5):1283–92.

Casey BM, Dashe JS, Wells CE, *et al.* Subclinical hyperthyroidism and pregnancy outcomes. *Obstet Gynecol* 2006;107(2pt1):337–41.

Lazarus JH, Bestwick JP, Channon S, *et al.* Antenatal thyroid screening and childhood cognitive function. *N Engl J Med* 2012;366(6):493–501.

Morreale De Escobar G, Obregon MJ, Escobar Del Rey F. Role of thyroid hormone during early brain development. *Eur J Endocrinol* 2004;151(Suppl 3):U25–U37.

Sheffield JS, Cunningham FG. Thyrotoxicosis and heart failure that complicate pregnancy. *Am J Obstet Gynecol* 2004;190:211.

Subclinical Hypothyroidism in Pregnancy. ACOG Committee Opinion No. 381. American College of Obstetricians and Gynecologists. *Obstet Gynecol* 2007;110:959–60. (Reaffirmed 2012).

Thyroid disease in pregnancy. ACOG Practice Bulletin No. 37. American College of Obstetricians and Gynecologists. *Obstet Gynecol* 2002;100:387–396. (Reaffirmed 2013).

PROTOCOL 22

Acute and Chronic Hepatitis

Patrick Duff

Department of Obstetrics and Gynecology, University of Florida College of Medicine, Gainesville, FL, USA

Clinical significance

The principal forms of hepatitis that complicate pregnancy are hepatitis A, B, C, D, and E. Hepatitis G is a relatively benign clinical disorder that does not pose a serious risk to either the pregnant woman or her baby.

Hepatitis A is the second most common cause of hepatitis in the United States, but it is relatively uncommon in pregnancy. It is caused by an RNA virus that is transmitted by fecal–oral contact. Infections in children are usually asymptomatic; infections in adults are usually symptomatic. The disease is most prevalent in areas of poor sanitation and close living. Infection does not result in a chronic carrier state, and perinatal transmission essentially never occurs.

Hepatitis B is the most common form of viral hepatitis in obstetric patients. It is caused by a DNA virus that is transmitted parenterally and via sexual contact. Acute hepatitis B occurs in approximately 1 to 2 per 1000 pregnancies in the United States. The chronic carrier state is more frequent, occurring in 6 to 10 per 1000 pregnancies. In the United States, approximately 1.25 million persons are chronically infected. Worldwide, more than 400 million individuals are infected.

Hepatitis C is caused by an RNA virus that is transmitted parenterally, via sexual contact, and perinatally. In some patient populations, hepatitis C is actually as common as, if not more common than, hepatitis B. Chronic hepatitis C infection now is the number one indication for liver transplantation in the United States. Worldwide, almost 170 million people are infected with this virus.

Hepatitis D is an RNA virus that depends upon co-infection with hepatitis B for replication. The epidemiology of hepatitis D is essentially identical to that of hepatitis B. Hepatitis D may cause a chronic carrier state,

---

Protocols for High-Risk Pregnancies: An Evidence-Based Approach, Sixth Edition.
Edited by John T. Queenan, Catherine Y. Spong and Charles J. Lockwood.
© 2015 John Wiley & Sons, Ltd. Published 2015 by John Wiley & Sons, Ltd.

and perinatal transmission is possible if hepatitis B transmission occurs simultaneously.

Hepatitis E is caused by an RNA virus. The epidemiology of hepatitis E is similar to that of hepatitis A. The disease is quite rare in the United States but is endemic in developing countries of the world. In these countries, maternal infection with hepatitis E often has an alarmingly high mortality, in the range of 10 to 20%. A chronic carrier state does not exist, and perinatal transmission has only rarely been documented.

Pathophysiology and clinical manifestations

Hepatitis A has an incubation period of 15 to 50 days, and usually causes symptomatic infection in adults. The typical clinical manifestations include low-grade fever, malaise, poor appetite, right upper quadrant pain and tenderness, jaundice, and acholic stools. Because hepatitis A does not cause a chronic carrier state, perinatal transmission virtually never occurs. The disease poses a risk only if the mother develops fulminant hepatitis and liver failure. Fortunately, such a situation is extremely rare.

Hepatitis B may be transmitted by sharing contaminated drug paraphernalia and via sexual contact and blood transfusion. Infection also can be transmitted to healthcare workers as a result of occupational exposure through needle stick or splash injuries. After exposure to the virus, approximately 90% of patients mount an effective immunologic response to the virus and completely clear the infection. Less than 1% develop fulminant hepatitis and die. Approximately 10% of patients develop a chronic carrier state. These patients pose a major risk of transmission of infection to their sexual partner and their infant, and they are the patients most commonly encountered by obstetricians in clinical practice.

Hepatitis C may be transmitted parenterally, via sexual contact, perinatally and via occupational exposure. The disease usually is asymptomatic, but, unfortunately, it typically results in chronic infection that, ultimately, causes severe hepatic impairment. Fifteen to 30% of patients develop cirrhosis. Of those with cirrhosis, 1–3% each year will develop hepatocellular carcinoma.

Hepatitis D infection always occurs in association with hepatitis B infection. Patients may have two types of infection. Some have both acute hepatitis D and acute hepatitis B (*co-infection*). These individuals typically clear their viremia and have a favorable long-term prognosis. Other individuals have chronic hepatitis D infection superimposed upon chronic hepatitis B infection (*super-infection*). These patients are particularly likely to develop chronic liver disease.

Hepatitis E is transmitted almost entirely by fecal–oral contact. The incubation period averages 45 days, and patients typically have a symptomatic acute infection. The maternal mortality in endemic areas is high, primarily because of the associated poor nutrition, poor general health and lack of access to modern medical care within the population. Hepatitis E does not cause a chronic carrier state, and perinatal transmission is extremely rare.

Diagnosis

The best test to confirm the diagnosis of acute hepatitis A is identification of anti-hepatitis A-IgM antibody. Acutely infected patients also may have elevated liver transaminase enzymes and an elevated serum concentration of direct and indirect bilirubin. In severe cases, coagulation abnormalities may be present.

Hepatitis B virus has three distinct antigens: the surface antigen (HBsAg) which is found in the serum, the core antigen (HBcAg) which is found only in hepatocytes, and the e antigen (HBeAg) which also is found in the serum. Detection of the last antigen is indicative of an extremely high rate of viral replication. Patients with *acute* hepatitis B typically have a positive serologic test for the surface antigen and a positive IgM antibody directed against the core antigen. Patients with *chronic* hepatitis B infection are seropositive for the surface antigen and have positive IgG antibody directed against the core antigen. Some patients will also test positive for hepatitis B*e* antigen. The seroprevalence of hepatitis e antigen is particularly high in Asian women. Patients who are positive for both the surface antigen and e antigen have an extremely high risk of perinatal transmission of infection that approaches 90% in the absence of neonatal immunoprophylaxis. Table 22.1 summarizes the possible serologic profiles related to hepatitis B infection.

The initial screening test for hepatitis C should be an enzyme immunoassay (EIA). The confirmatory test is a recombinant immunoblot assay (RIBA). Seroconversion may not occur for up to 16 weeks following infection. In addition, these immunologic tests do not precisely distinguish between IgM and IgG antibodies. Patients who have hepatitis C infection

Table 22.1 Serologic Diagnosis of Hepatitis B Infection

Condition	HBs antigen	HBs antibody	HB c antibody
Immune – natural infection	Negative	Positive IgG	Positive IgG
Immune – vaccination	Negative	Positive IgG	Negative
Acute infection	Positive	Negative	Positive IgM
Chronic infection	Positive	Negative	Positive IgG

also should be tested for hepatitis C RNA, a test that is analogous to quantitation of the viral load in patients with HIV infection. Detection of hepatitis C RNA is indicative of a high rate of viral replication.

The diagnosis of hepatitis D can be confirmed by performing a liver biopsy and identifying the delta antigen in liver tissue. However, the most useful diagnostic test for confirmation of acute infection is detection of hepatitis D IgM antibody. The corresponding test for diagnosis of chronic hepatitis D infection is identification of anti-D-IgG.

The diagnosis of acute hepatitis E can be established by using electron microscopy to identify viral particles in the stool of infected patients and by identification of IgM antibody in the serum.

Treatment

Patients with acute hepatitis A require supportive therapy. Their nutrition should be optimized. Coagulation abnormalities, if present, should be corrected, and trauma to the upper abdomen should be avoided. Of great importance, household contacts should be vaccinated with hepatitis A vaccine.

Patients with acute hepatitis B require similar supportive care. Their household contacts and sexual partners should receive hepatitis B immune globulin, followed by the hepatitis B vaccine series. Infants delivered to mothers with hepatitis B infection should immediately receive the hepatitis B immune globulin and first dose of hepatitis B vaccine while still in the hospital. These children subsequently should receive the second and third doses of the vaccine at 1 and 6 months after delivery. There is no contraindication to breastfeeding in women who have chronic hepatitis B infection.

On a long-term basis, women with hepatitis B infection should be referred to a gastroenterologist for consideration of medical treatment. Seven drugs currently are licensed for the treatment of hepatitis B infection: interferon alfa, pegylated interferon alfa-2A, lamivudine, adefovir, entecavir, telbivudine, and tenofovir. The most commonly used therapy for chronic hepatitis B infection is long-acting pegylated interferon, which is injected once weekly. In patients who do not respond to interferon, the nucleoside and nucleotide analogs have been extremely effective. These agents have played a major role in reducing the need for liver transplantation in patients who have chronic hepatitis B infection. More than 80% of patients, even those who are HBeAg-positive, will have sustained virologic responses with extended courses of therapy.

Patients with hepatitis C, particularly those who have evidence of high viral replication and ongoing liver injury, are candidates for medical therapy. The first drug widely used for the treatment of hepatitis C was recombinant human interferon alfa. The second important advance in the therapy of hepatitis C was ribavirin, a nucleoside analog. The third major advance was the introduction of pegylated forms of interferon that allowed for once-weekly treatment. Subsequently, protease inhibitors such as telaprevir, simeprevir, and boceprevir, dramatically increased viral response rates. More recently, short courses of treatment (12 to 24 weeks) with new regimens that include direct-acting antiviral agents (DAAs) such as ledipasvir, sofosbuvir, ABT-450r, ombitasvir, and dasabuvir have achieved sustained virologic responses in up to 96% of patients with HCV genotype 1a or 1b. These new regimens, although very expensive (approximately $90,000 for a 12-week course), are much better tolerated than the older regimens that included interferon alpha. In truth, the new regimens offer the bright prospect of a microbiologic cure in patients who are able to afford the medications.

The treatment for hepatitis D parallels that described above for hepatitis B. The treatment of hepatitis E is similar to that described for hepatitis A.

Complications

The principal concern with hepatitis A infection in pregnancy is that the mother will develop fulminant hepatitis and liver failure. Fortunately, this complication is extremely rare. Hepatitis A does not cause a chronic carrier state. Perianal transmission virtually never occurs and, therefore, the infection does not pose a major risk to the baby.

Hepatitis B, particularly when associated with hepatitis D infection, may result in chronic liver disease such as chronic active hepatitis, chronic persistent hepatitis, and cirrhosis. Chronic disease also predisposes to the development of hepatocellular carcinoma. Pregnant women who are infected with hepatitis B pose a significant risk of transmission to their offspring. Most neonates become infected at the time of delivery as a result of exposure to contaminated blood and genital tract secretions. Patients who are seropositive for the surface antigen alone have at least a 20% risk of transmitting infection to their neonate. Women who are seropositive for both the surface antigen and e antigen have almost a 90% risk of perinatal transmission. Neonates who become infected as a result of perinatal transmission subsequently are at risk for all the complications associated with chronic hepatic disease.

The most important sequela of hepatitis C infection is severe chronic liver disease. Infection with hepatitis C virus remains the most important indication for liver transplantation in the United States. Perinatal transmission of hepatitis C is also an important concern. In pregnant women who have a low serum concentration of hepatitis C RNA and who do not have coexisting HIV infection, the risk of perinatal transmission of hepatitis C is less than 5%. If the patient's serum concentration of hepatitis C RNA is high and/or she has concurrent HIV infection, perinatal transmission may approach 25%.

Hepatitis D virus, when superimposed upon chronic hepatitis B infection, is a major risk factor for severe chronic liver disease. Like hepatitis A, hepatitis E does not usually cause a chronic carrier state. Assuming the patient survives the acute episode, the infection usually does not have long-term sequelae. In addition, perinatal transmission of hepatitis E is exceedingly rare.

Follow up

Patients with chronic hepatitis B (with or without co-infection with hepatitis D) and hepatitis C require long-term follow-up with a gastroenterologist. Many of them will be excellent candidates for the new treatment regimens outlined above. Patients with chronic hepatitis of any type should not receive any medications that may exacerbate hepatic injury. For example, oral contraceptives should be avoided if a patient has clear evidence of on-going hepatocellular disease. In some individuals, chronic infection progresses to such a serious disease that liver transplantation will be required.

Prevention

Hepatitis A can be prevented by administration of an inactivated vaccine. Two formulations of the vaccine now are available – Vaqta® and Havrix®. Both vaccines require an initial intramuscular injection, followed by a second dose 6 to 12 months later. The vaccine should be offered to the following individuals:
- International travelers
- Children in endemic areas
- Intravenous drug users
- Individuals who have occupational exposure to hepatitis A virus, e.g., workers in a primate laboratory
- Residents and staff of chronic care institutions
- Individuals with chronic liver disease
- Homosexual men
- Individuals with clotting factor disorders.

Immunoglobulin provides reasonably effective passive immunization for hepatitis A if it is given within 2 weeks of exposure. The standard intramuscular dose of immunoglobulin is 0.02 mg/kg. However, a recent report demonstrated that hepatitis A vaccine should be the preferred method of prophylaxis both for pre-exposure and post-exposure. The principal advantage of the vaccine, compared to immune globulin, is that it provides more long-lasting protection.

There are two important immunoprophylactic agents for prevention of hepatitis B infection. The first is hepatitis B immune globulin, which can be administered immediately after an exposure to provide acute protection against a high viral inoculum. The second immunoprophylactic agent is the hepatitis B vaccine. This vaccine is prepared by recombinant technology and poses no risk of transmission of another infection such as HIV. The agent is administered intramuscularly in three separate doses and is highly effective. In healthy immunocompetent adults, seroconversion rates approach 90% after the three-dose regimen.

Immunoprophylaxis of the neonate delivered of a hepatitis B-positive mother also is highly effective. In view of this high rate of effectiveness, there is no indication for cesarean delivery in women with hepatitis B infection. Interestingly, prevention of hepatitis B infection also prevents hepatitis D co-infection.

Passive and active immunization of the neonate with HBIG and HBV is approximately 90% effective in preventing perinatal transmission of hepatitis B. Presumably, some prophylaxis failures result from antenatal transmission of the virus from mother to baby. Recent evidence suggests that daily administration of oral lamivudine, 100 mg, from 28 weeks of gestation until delivery, or monthly administration of intramuscular HBIG, 200 international units, at 28, 32, and 36 weeks of gestation, may provide additional protection against infection of the infant.

Unfortunately, there is no hyperimmune globulin or vaccine for the prevention of hepatitis C infection. Appropriate preventive measures include adoption of universal precautions in the care of patients, intensive screening of blood donations and adherence to safe sexual practices. As a routine, cesarean delivery is not indicated in patients who have hepatitis C infection. However, in patients who are co-infected with HIV, caesarean delivery should be performed to decrease the risk of perinatal transmission of both infections. Breast feeding is permissible regardless of the mode of delivery.

There is no hyperglobulin or vaccine for prevention of hepatitis E infection.

Conclusion

The key features of hepatitis in pregnancy are summarized in Table 22.2.

Table 22.2 Principal features of hepatitis A, B, C, D, and E

Type of hepatitis	Mechanism of transmission	Diagnostic test	Carrier state	Perinatal transmission	Prevention and treatment
A	Fecal–oral	Detection of IgM antibody	No	No	Immunoglobulin and vaccine Supportive care
B	Parenteral/sexual	Detection of surface antigen	Yes	Yes	HBIG Hepatitis B vaccine Interferon Nucleoside/nucleotide analogs
C	Parenteral/sexual	Detection of antibody	Yes	Yes	Direct acting antiviral agents
D	Parenteral/sexual	Detection of antibody	Yes	Yes	Hepatitis B vaccine protects against hepatitis D
E	Fecal–oral	Detection of antibody	No	No	Supportive care

Suggested reading

Afdhal N, Reddy KR, Nelson DR, *et al.* Ledipasvir and sofosbuvir for previously treated HCV genotype 1 infection. *N Engl J Med* 2014;370:1483–93.

Chung RT, Baumert TF. Curing chronic hepatitis C–the arc of a medical triumph. *N Engl J Med* 2014;370:1576–8.

Dienstag JL. Hepatitis B virus infection. *N Engl J Med* 2008;359:1486–500.

Duff P. Hepatitis in pregnancy. *Semin Perinatol* 1998;22:277–83.

Feld JJ, Kowdley KV, Coakley E, *et al.* Treatment of HCV with ABT-450/r-ombitasvir and dasabuvir with ribavirin. *N Engl J Med* 2014;370:1594–603.

European Pediatric Hepatitis C Virus Network. A significant sex – but not elective cesarean section – effect on mother-to-child transmission of hepatitis C virus infection. *J Infect Dis* 2005;192:1872–9.

Gibb DM, Goodall, RI, Dunn DT, *et al.* Mother-to-child transmission of hepatitis C virus: evidence for preventable peripartum transmission. *Lancet* 2000;356:904–7.

Hoofagle JH. A step forward in therapy for hepatitis C. *N Engl J Med* 2009;360:1899–901.

Hoofnagle JH, Sherker AH. Therapy for hepatitis C–the costs of success. *N Engl J Med* 2014;370:1552–3.

Poland GA, Jacobson RM. Prevention of hepatitis B with the hepatitis B vaccine. *N Engl J Med* 2004;351:2832–8.

Victor JC, Monto AS, Surdina TY, *et al.* Hepatitis A vaccine versus immune globulin for postexposure prophylaxis. *N Engl J Med* 2007;357:1685–94.

Zaretti AR, Paccagnini S, Principi N, *et al.* Mother-to-infant transmission of hepatitis C virus. *Lancet* 1995;345:289–91.

Asthma

Michael Schatz

Department of Allergy, Kaiser-Permanente Medical Center, San Diego, CA, USA

Overview

Asthma currently affects approximately 8% of pregnant women, making it probably the most common potentially serious medical problem to complicate pregnancy. Although data have been conflicting, recent meta-analyses have suggested that maternal asthma increases the risk of perinatal mortality, preeclampsia, preterm birth and low-birth-weight infants. More severe asthma is associated with increased risks, while better-controlled asthma is associated with decreased risks.

Pathophysiology

Asthma is an inflammatory disease of the airways that is associated with reversible airway obstruction and airway hyper-reactivity to a variety of stimuli. Although the cause of asthma is unknown, a number of clinical triggering factors can be identified, including viral infections, allergens, exercise, sinusitis, reflux, weather changes and stress.

Airway obstruction in asthma can be produced by varying degrees of mucosal edema, bronchoconstriction, mucus plugging, and airway remodeling. In acute asthma, these changes can lead to ventilation perfusion imbalance and hypoxia. Although early acute asthma is typically associated with hyperventilation and hypocapnea, progressive acute asthma can cause respiratory failure with associated carbon dioxide retention and acidosis.

Diagnosis

Many patients with asthma during pregnancy will already have a physician diagnosis of asthma. A new diagnosis of asthma is usually suspected on the

Protocols for High-Risk Pregnancies: An Evidence-Based Approach, Sixth Edition.
Edited by John T. Queenan, Catherine Y. Spong and Charles J. Lockwood.
© 2015 John Wiley & Sons, Ltd. Published 2015 by John Wiley & Sons, Ltd.

basis of typical symptoms – wheezing, chest tightness, cough and associated shortness of breath – which tend to be episodic or at least fluctuating in intensity and are typically worse at night. Identification of the characteristic triggers further supports the diagnosis. Wheezing may be present on auscultation of the lungs, but the absence of wheezing on auscultation does not exclude the diagnosis. The diagnosis is ideally confirmed by spirometry, which shows a reduced forced expiratory volume $(FEV)_1$ with an increase in FEV_1 of 12% or more after an inhaled short-acting bronchodilator.

It is sometimes difficult to demonstrate reversible airway obstruction in patients with mild or intermittent asthma. Although methacholine challenge testing may be considered in nonpregnant patients with normal pulmonary function to confirm asthma, such testing is not recommended during pregnancy. Thus, therapeutic trials of asthma therapy should generally be used during pregnancy in patients with possible but unconfirmed asthma. Improvement with asthma therapy supports the diagnosis, which can then be confirmed postpartum with additional testing if necessary.

The most common differential diagnosis is dyspnea of pregnancy, which may occur in early pregnancy in approximately 70% of women. This dyspnea is differentiated from asthma by its lack of association with cough, wheezing or airway obstruction.

Another aspect of asthma diagnosis is an assessment of severity. Although more complicated severity schemes have been proposed, the most important determination is whether the patient has intermittent versus persistent asthma. This distinction has both prognostic and therapeutic significance during pregnancy. Patients with *intermittent asthma* have short episodes less than three times per week, nocturnal symptoms less than three times a month, and normal pulmonary function between episodes. Patients with more frequent symptoms or who require daily asthma medications are considered to have *persistent asthma*.

Asthma severity often changes during pregnancy; it can get either better or worse. Patients with more severe asthma prior to pregnancy are more likely to further worsen during pregnancy. Since gestational asthma course in an individual woman is unpredictable, women with asthma must be followed particularly closely during pregnancy so that any change in course can be matched with an appropriate change in therapy.

Management

General

Identifying and avoiding asthma triggers can lead to improved maternal well-being with less need for medications. In previously untested patients, in vitro (RAST, ELISA) tests should be performed to identify relevant allergens, such as mite, animal dander, mold spores and cockroach, for which specific environmental control instructions can be given. Smokers must be encouraged to discontinue smoking, and all patients should try to avoid exposure to environmental tobacco smoke and other potential irritants as much as possible. Effective allergen immunotherapy can be continued during pregnancy, but benefit–risk considerations do not generally favor beginning immunotherapy during pregnancy.

Asthma medicines are classified into two types: relievers and long-term controllers. Relievers provide quick relief of bronchospasm and include short-acting beta agonists (albuterol is preferred during pregnancy, 2–4 puffs every 4 h as needed) and the anticholinergic bronchodilator ipratropium (generally used as second-line therapy for acute asthma – see below). Long-tem control medications are described in Tables 23.1 and 23.2.

Chronic asthma

Patients with intermittent asthma do not need controller therapy. In patients with persistent asthma, controller therapy should be initiated and progressed in steps (Table 23.3) until adequate control is achieved. A classification of asthma control has been published (Table 23.4). Well-controlled asthma means symptoms or rescue therapy requirement less than three times per week, nocturnal symptoms less than three times per month, no activity limitation due to asthma, and, ideally, normal pulmonary function tests. For patients with "not well controlled" asthma (Table 23.4), one step up in therapy (Table 23.3) is recommended. For patients with "very poorly controlled" asthma, a two-step increase, a course of oral corticosteroids, or both should be considered. Before stepping up pharmacological therapy in women whose asthma is not well controlled, adverse environmental exposures, co-morbidities, adherence and inhaler technique should be considered as targets for therapy.

Inhaled corticosteroids are the mainstay of controller therapy during pregnancy. Because it has the most published reassuring human gestational safety data, budesonide is considered the inhaled corticosteroid of choice for asthma during pregnancy. It is important to note, though, that no data indicate that the other inhaled corticosteroid preparations are unsafe. Therefore, inhaled corticosteroids other than budesonide may be continued in patients who were well controlled by these agents prior to pregnancy, especially if it is thought that changing formulations may jeopardize asthma control. A long-acting beta agonist (salmeterol or formoterol) should be added in patients inadequately controlled on medium dose inhaled corticosteroids (Table 23.1). As described in Table 23.1,

Table 23.1 Long-term control medications for asthma during pregnancy

Medication	Mechanism of action	Dosage form	Adult dose	Use during pregnancy
Inhaled corticosteroids	Topical anti-inflammatory	See Table 23.2		First-line controller therapy
Systemic corticosteroids	Systemic anti-inflammatory		Short course "burst" to achieve control: 40–60 mg/day as single or 2 divided doses for 3–10 days	Burst therapy for severe acute symptoms Maintenance therapy for severe asthma uncontrolled by other means
Methylprednisolone		2, 4, 8, 16, 32 mg tablets		
Prednisolone		5 mg tablets, 5 mg/mL, 15 mg/mL		
Prednisone		1, 2.5, 5, 10, 20, 50 mg tablet 5 mg/mL, 5 mg/5 mL	7.5–60 mg daily in a single dose in a.m. every other day, as needed for control of severe asthma	
Long-acting beta agonists	beta agonist-mediated smooth muscle relaxation that lasts 12 hours			Add-on therapy in patients not controlled by low-medium dose inhaled corticosteroids
Salmeterol		DPI 50 microgram/blister	1 blister every 12 h	
Formoterol		DPI 12 microgram/single-use capsule	1 capsule every 12 h	
Leukotriene receptor antagonists	Blocks activity of leukotrienes (inflammatory mediators) by means of receptor antagonism			Alternative therapy for persistent asthma in patients who have shown good response prior to pregnancy
Montelukast		10 mg tablets	10 mg every HS	
Zafirlukast		10 or 20 mg tablets	20 mg twice daily	
Theophylline	Bronchodilator (? anti-inflammatory effects)	Liquids, sustained-release tablets, and capsules	400–800 mg/day to achieve serum concentration of 5–12 microgram/mL	Alternative therapy for persistent asthma during pregnancy
Inhaled combination medications	Inhaled corticosteroid and long-acting beta agonist in a single device			For patients not controlled on medium dose inhaled corticosteroids
Fluticasone and salmetero		DPI: 100 microgram/50 microgram, 250 microgram/50 microgram, or 500 microgram/50 microgram	1 inhalation twice daily	
Budesonide and formterol		MDI: 45 microgram/21 microgram, 115 microgram/21 microgram or 230 microgram/21 microgram	2 puffs twice daily	
Mometasone and formoterol		MDI 80 microgram/4.5 microgram or 160 microgram/4.5 microgram	2 inhalations twice	
		MDI 100 microgram/5 microgram or 200 microgram/5 microgram	2 inhalations bid	

Source: National Asthma Education and Prevention Program, 2005. Adapted with permission of Elsevier.

Table 23.2 Estimated comparative daily adult dosages for inhaled corticosteroids

Drug	Low daily dose (microgram)	Medium daily dose (microgram)	High daily dose (microgram)
Beclomethasone HFA 40 or 80 microgram/puff	80–240	241–480	>480
Budesonide DPI 90 or 180 microgram/inhalation	180–540	541–1080	>1080
Ciclesonide 80 or 160 microgram/actuation	160–320	321–640	>640
Flunisolide HFA HFA 80 microgram/puff	320	321–640	>640
Fluticasone HFA MDI: 44, 110, 220 microgram/puff	88–264	265–440	>440
DPI: 50, 100, or 250 microgram/inhalation	100–300	301–500	>500
Mometasone DPI 110 or 220 microgram /inhalation	110–220	221–440	>440

Source: National Asthma Education and Prevention Program, 2009 and Kelly, Ann Pharmacother. 2009;43:519–27.

Table 23.3 Recommendations for preferred step therapy for asthma during pregnancy

Step one	No controller
Step two	Low-dose inhaled corticosteroids
Step three	Medium-dose inhaled corticosteroids
Step four	Medium-dose inhaled corticosteroids plus long-acting beta agonist
Step five	High-dose inhaled corticosteroids plus long-acting beta agonist
Step six	High-dose inhaled corticosteroids plus long-acting beta agonist plus oral corticosteroids at lowest effective dose*

*Addition of montelukast or theophylline to combination inhaled corticosteroid/long-acting beta agonist therapy may be considered in order to try to prevent oral corticosteroid dependence. Source: National Asthma Education and Prevention Program, 2004 and 2007.

the following drugs are considered by the National Asthma Education and Prevention Program (NAEPP) to be alternative, but not preferred, treatments for persistent asthma during pregnancy: cromolyn, due to decreased efficacy compared to inhaled corticosteroids; theophylline, due primarily to increased side effects compared to alternatives; and leukotriene-receptor antagonists, due to the availability of less published human gestational data for these drugs. Although oral corticosteroids have been associated with possible increased risks during pregnancy (oral clefts, prematurity, lower birth weight), if needed during pregnancy, they should be used because these risks are less than the potential risks of severe uncontrolled asthma (which include maternal or fetal mortality).

Table 23.4 Classification of asthma control during pregnancy*

Variable	Well controlled asthma	Asthma not well controlled	Very poorly controlled asthma
Frequency of symptoms	2 or fewer days/week	More than 2 days/week	Throughout the day
Frequency of night-time awakening	2 or fewer times/month	1 to 3 times/week	4 or more times/week
Interference with normal activity	None	Some	Extreme
Use of short-acting beta agonist for symptom control	2 or fewer days/week	2 or more days/week	Several times per day
FEV₁ or peak flow	Greater than 80%[†]	60–80%[†]	Less than 60%[†]
Exacerbations requiring use of systemic corticosteroid (no.)	0–1 in past 12 months	2 or more in past 12 months	

*The level of control is based on the most severe category. The frequency and effect of symptoms should be assessed according to the patient's recall of the previous 2–4 weeks.
[†]Percentage of the predicted or personal best value.
Source: Schatz and Dombrowski, 2009. Reproduced with permission of Massachusetts Medical Society

Acute asthma

A major goal of chronic asthma management is the prevention of acute asthmatic episodes. When acute asthma does not respond to home therapy, expeditious acute management is necessary for both the health of the mother and that of the fetus.

Due to progesterone-induced hyperventilation, normal blood gases during pregnancy reveal a higher PO_2 (100–106 mmHg) and a lower PCO_2 (28–30 mmHg) than in the nonpregnant state. The changes in blood gases that occur secondary to acute asthma during pregnancy will be superimposed on the "normal" hyperventilation of pregnancy. Thus, a PCO_2 35 or greater or a PO_2 70 or lower associated with acute asthma will represent more severe compromise during pregnancy than will similar blood gases in the nongravid state.

The recommended pharmacological therapy of acute asthma during pregnancy is summarized in Table 23.5. Intensive fetal monitoring as well as maternal monitoring is essential. In addition to pharmacological therapy, supplemental oxygen (initially 3 to 4 L/min by nasal cannula) should be administered, adjusting FiO_2 to maintain at PO_2 70 or greater and/or O_2 saturation by pulse oximetry 95% or greater. Intravenous fluids (containing glucose if the patient is not hyperglycemic) should also be administered, initially at a rate of at least 100 mL/h.

Table 23.5 Pharmacological management of acute asthma during pregnancy

1 β_2-agonist bronchodilator (nebulized or metered-dose inhaler)
  • up to 3 doses in first 60–90 minutes
  • every 1–2 hours thereafter until adequate response
2 Nebulized ipratropium (may be repeated every 6 hours)
3 Systemic corticosteroids with initial therapy in patients on regular corticosteroids and in patients with severe exacerbations (peak expiratory flow rate less than 40% predicted or personal best) and for those with incomplete response to initial therapy
  • 40–80 mg/day in 1 or 2 divided doses until peak expiratory flow rate reaches 70% of predicted or personal best
  • may be given orally; IV for severe exacerbation
  • taper as patient improves
4 Consider intravenous magnesium sulfate (2 grams) for women with life-threatening exacerbations (peak expiratory flow rate less than 25% predicted or personal best) and for those whose exacerbations remain in the severe category after 1 hour of intensive conventional therapy

Systemic corticosteroids (40–80 mg/day in one or two divided doses) are recommended for patients who do not respond well (FEV_1 or peak expiratory flow rate [PEF] less than 70% predicted) to the first beta agonist treatment as well as for patients who have recently taken systemic steroids and for those who present with severe exacerbations (FEV_1 or PEF less than 40% of predicted). Patients with good responses to emergency therapy (FEV_1 or PEF 70% or greater predicted) can be discharged home, generally on a course of oral corticosteroids. Inhaled corticosteroids should also be continued or initiated upon discharge until review at medical follow-up. Hospitalization should be considered for patients with an incomplete response (FEV_1 or PEF 40% or greater but 70% or less predicted). Admission to an intensive care unit should be considered for patients with persistent FEV_1 or PEF 40% or less predicted, PCO_2 42 or greater or sensorium changes. Intubation and mechanical ventilation may be required for patients whose condition deteriorates or fails to improve associated with decreasing PO_2, increasing PCO_2, progressive respiratory acidosis, declining mental status or increasing fatigue.

Follow up

Careful follow-up by physicians experienced in managing asthma is an essential aspect of optimal gestational asthma management. Asthmatic women requiring regular medication should be evaluated at least monthly. In addition to symptomatic and auscultatory assessment, objective measures of respiratory status (optimally spirometry, minimally PEF) should be obtained on every clinic visit. In addition, patients with more severe or labile asthma should be considered for home PEF monitoring. All pregnant patients should have a written action plan for increased symptoms and facilitated access to their physician for uncontrolled symptoms.

Conclusion

Asthma is a common medical problem during pregnancy. Optimal diagnosis and management of asthma during pregnancy should maximize maternal and fetal health.

Suggested reading

Asthma in pregnancy. ACOG Practice Bulletin No. 90. American College of Obstetricians and Gynecologists. *Obstet Gynecol* 2008;111:457–64. (Reaffirmed 2012).

Elsayegh D, Shapiro J. Management of the obstetric patient with status asthmaticus. *J Int Care Med* 2008;23:396–402.

Gluck JC, Gluck PA. The effect of pregnancy on the course of asthma. *Immunol All Clin N Am* 2006;26:63–80.

Murphy VE, Namazy JA, Powell H, *et al.* A meta-analysis of adverse perinatal outcomes in women with asthma. *BJOG* 2011;118:1314–1323.

Murphy VE, Gibson PG. Asthma in pregnancy. *Clin Chest Med* 2011;32:93–110.

Namazy JA, Murphy VE, Powell H, *et al.* Effects of asthma severity, exacerbations, and oral corticosteroids on perinatal outcomes. *Eur Resp J* 2013;41:1082–90.

National Asthma Education and Prevention Program. Expert Panel Report 3: Guidelines for the diagnosis and management of asthma. SummaryReport. *J Allergy Clin Immunol* 2007;120:S93–138.

National Asthma Education and Prevention Program. Expert Panel Report Managing Asthma During Pregnancy: Recommendations for Pharmacologic Treatment – Update 2004. *J Allergy Clin Immunol* 2005;115:34–46.

Racusin DA, Fox KA, Ramin SM. Severe acute asthma. *Semin Perinatol* 2013;37:234–45.

Schatz M, Dombrowski MP. Asthma in pregnancy. *N Engl J Med* 2009;360:1862–9.

Tamasi L, Horvath I, Bohacs A, *et al.* Asthma in pregnancy—Immunological changes and clinical management. *Res Med* 2011;105:159–64.

PROTOCOL 24

Epilepsy

Men-Jean Lee
Department of Obstetrics & Gynecology, Icahn School of Medicine at Mount Sinai,
New York, NY, USA

Overview

Women of childbearing age with epilepsy should be offered preconception and early pregnancy consultation with a neurologist and perinatologist to evaluate their need for antiepileptic drugs (AED), determine the minimum number of agents needed and dosage(s) required to prevent seizures, and discuss the teratogenic potential of the drugs. In addition, folate supplementation is recommended prior to conception to potentially decrease risk for fetal neural tube defects. To optimize pregnancy outcomes, the patient should be treated with the lowest effective dosage and, if possible, a single AED prior to attempting pregnancy; however, the frequency of seizures tends to increase during pregnancy so careful monitoring of AED levels in the blood is recommended to minimize seizure activity.

Pathophysiology

Epilepsy complicates approximately 0.3–0.5% of pregnancies. Between 14% and 32% of these patients will experience an increase in seizure frequency during pregnancy, which is most often attributable to a reduction in the plasma concentration of anticonvulsant drugs. In addition, pregnancy hormone levels, emotional stress, and sleep deprivation also lower neuronal seizure thresholds. In general, the reasons for changes in plasma AED levels include increased plasma volume, electrolyte changes, physiological respiratory alkalosis, and reduced plasma protein binding. Additionally, factors known to affect the pharmacokinetics of AED in pregnancy include: (1) decreased motility of the gastrointestinal tract may change the bioavailability of orally administered dosage forms; (2) increases in glomerular filtration rate and creatinine clearance during

Protocols for High-Risk Pregnancies: An Evidence-Based Approach, Sixth Edition.
Edited by John T. Queenan, Catherine Y. Spong and Charles J. Lockwood.
© 2015 John Wiley & Sons, Ltd. Published 2015 by John Wiley & Sons, Ltd.

pregnancy influence the renal clearance rates of many drugs; and (3) hormonal changes increase hepatic enzyme systems responsible for the metabolism and clearance of many AEDs.

Whatever the underlying cause of the increase in seizure frequency during pregnancy, the potential for seizure-induced fetal damage secondary to hypoxia, and the added maternal risk of seizures (e.g., aspiration pneumonia) necessitate close observation and careful management by a neurologist and perinatologist. Women who continue to have seizures during pregnancy tend to be at increased risk for preterm birth and fetuses with growth restriction compared to women with epilepsy who have no seizures.

Teratogenicity of anticonvulsants

There is considerable controversy concerning the teratogenicity of anticonvulsant drugs. The overall rate of congenital abnormalities in association with maternal intake of AEDs is 5–6%. This is twice the expected rate of 2.5–3.0% in the general unaffected population. In addition, children of mothers with epilepsy, even when untreated with AEDs, tend to have slightly more minor anomalies than do children of women without epilepsy.

Trimethadione has been shown to result in spontaneous abortions and fetal malformations in over 80% pregnancies. Its use is, therefore, contraindicated during pregnancy and it probably should not be given to women of childbearing age. Valproic acid is also considered a highly teratogenic AED that should be avoided during pregnancy, if at all possible. Valproate monotherapy during the first trimester of pregnancy contributes to the development of major congenital malformations (MCMs) in the offspring of women using this medication. Valproate as a part of polytherapy in the first trimester of pregnancy probably contributes to the development of MCMs when compared to polytherapy that does not include valproate. There appears to be a relationship between the dose of valproate and the risk of development of MCMs in the offspring of women with epilepsy. In addition to structural defects, valproate use during pregnancy is associated with the development of fetal valproate syndrome (similar to fetal alcohol syndrome), which includes developmental delay and neurobehavioral issues. The cognitive and behavioral impairments have been attributed to prolonged intrauterine exposure of the developing fetus to valproate even after embryogenesis has been completed. Therefore, valproic acid is one AED that should be discontinued even after the first trimester if an alternative effective AED can be used. Carbamazepine does not appear to substantially increase the risk of MCMs when used as monotherapy. Data from a number of pregnancy registries suggest that lamotrigine, levetiracetam, oxcarbazepine, topiramate, and gabapentin are not significantly associated with an increased risk of MCMs in pregnancy. However, topiramate and zonizamide use in pregnancy is associated with lower birth-weight newborns than lamotrigine.

The incidence of MCMs increases with increasing number of anticonvulsant medications used to control seizures. As noted, if possible, only one AED should be used during pregnancy and the lowest effective dose of each AED is recommended. Exposure to polytherapy and valproate during pregnancy are associated with significantly reduced verbal intelligence in the offspring. Carbamazepine monotherapy with maternal serum levels within the recommended range does not impair intelligence in prenatally exposed offspring. It should be remembered that 95% of infants born to mothers receiving AED treatment will be normal.

Serum levels

Pregnancy appears to cause an increase in clearance and a significant decrease in the levels of lamotrigine, carbamazepine, and phenytoin. Sufficient data are not available to provide evidence for a change in clearance or levels during pregnancy for valproate. In general, the unbound concentration of the AED is the pharmacologically active level of the medication that should be monitored during pregnancy.

Breast feeding

Primidone probably enters breast milk in potentially clinically important amounts, whereas valproate, phenytoin, and carbamazepine probably do not. Lamotrigine may penetrate into breast milk in clinically important amounts. There is insufficient evidence to determine if indirect exposure to maternally ingested AEDs has symptomatic effects on the newborns. In general, nursing mothers receiving ethosuximide, phenobarbital, primidone, or lamotrigine should be advised to closely monitor the infant for sedation, poor suckling, and lethargy. Phenytoin, carbamazepine, and valproate are probably safe to take if the woman chooses to breastfeed. These AEDs are all moderately to highly protein-bound, and are not transferred in high concentrations in breast milk.

Management

The treatment of the pregnant epileptic patient should ideally begin preconceptionally. At this time, her seizure status should be assessed to ascertain whether or not she truly needs an anticonvulsant drug. If she has been seizure-free for a long interval (at least 9 months) on minimal doses of anticonvulsant drugs and has a negative electroencephalogram (EEG), it may be reasonable to attempt anticonvulsant withdrawal before conception. Women who report seizure activity within 2 years of pregnancy are significantly more likely to experience antenatal, intrapartum, and postpartum seizures when compared with women whose last seizure occurred more than 2 years before pregnancy. Given the potential teratogenic risks of AED exposure in early pregnancy, discontinuation or decreasing the dosage of AED in those women who have not had a seizure in the past 2 years under the direct supervision of a neurologist can be considered prior to pregnancy.

Risk for relapse increases when the history includes clonic–tonic grand mal convulsions, prolonged seizures, failure of AED treatment, or seizure control achieved with a combination of two or three drugs. One should, therefore, hesitate in withdrawing AED treatment from women who are planning pregnancy if their history includes the above risks for relapse. The current recommendation is that AEDs, if withdrawn, should be withdrawn at least 6 months prior to pregnancy. When possible, monotherapy should be used rather than polytherapy. After monotherapy is established, the lowest plasma AED level that prevents seizures should be determined.

Counseling pregnant women with epilepsy later in pregnancy is also important. Women who are late registrants to prenatal care or do not realize that they are pregnant until after the first trimester of pregnancy often self-discontinue AEDs without realizing that embryogenesis has already been completed and the risk of seizures during pregnancy outweighs any further risk for developing any new anomalies. Women with intractable seizures or drug-resistant epilepsy should be referred to an epilepsy center and evaluated for noncompliance with medications and to rule out structural intracranial pathology. Women with treatable seizures should be counseled to continue taking the lowest effective dose of AED to control seizure activity. A single seizure is unlikely to induce birth defects; however five or more seizures during pregnancy have been associated with impaired cognitive development of the offspring.

Several observations can serve as guidelines for management throughout pregnancy:

1 Steady-state plasma concentrations of most anticonvulsants decrease as pregnancy progresses.
2 These changes may be associated with breakthrough seizures, requiring an increase in anticonvulsant medications.
3 Patients appear to have a threshold concentration of drug below which seizure control is lost. In other words, some patients may be adequately

controlled by drug concentrations below the quoted therapeutic range.

4 The use of divided doses or slow-release preparations results in lower peak levels and may reduce the risk of malformations.

5 For valproate, the use of a single daily dose is not advisable because the adverse effects are believed to be the result of high peak serum level.

6 Total serum AED levels and, if possible, free AED fractions should be measured at regular intervals throughout pregnancy, particularly for lamotrigine, phenytoin, and carbamazepine.

Treatment

Preconceptional

1 Ascertain the patient's need for anticonvulsant medications.

2 Determine the fewest agents (ideally monotherapy) and lowest effective level of anticonvulsant medication at which the patient is seizure-free.

3 The use of divided doses or slow-release preparations results in lower peak levels and may reduce the risk of malformations.

4 Discuss the risks of anticonvulsant medications to the fetus.

5 Recommend folate supplementation (1 mg/day) beginning before conception.

Antenatal

1 Maintain the concentration of anticonvulsant medication(s) at the level(s) required by the patient.

2 Obtain plasma anticonvulsant levels every 3 to 4 weeks, or if a seizure occurs, if potential drug interaction is suspected, or if signs of toxicity develop.

3 Raise doses if necessary to maintain effective anticonvulsant activity. Dosage increments may need to be small (e.g., the use of 30 mg rather than 100 mg phenytoin capsules).

4 Assess drug toxicity clinically after an appropriate interval based on the estimated time to reach a steady state.

5 If seizure control is not maintained and the anticonvulsant dose has been increased until toxic effects are apparent (Table 24.1), add additional anticonvulsant medication.

6 Prescribe supplements containing at least 0.4 mg folic acid to all patients on anticonvulsant medication and follow their complete blood counts (CBCs), since folic acid deficiency anemia is frequent in this group of patients.

7 Offer prenatal diagnosis to patients receiving AEDs (Level 2 sonogram, MSAFP, and fetal echocardiogram).

Table 24.1 Frequently prescribed anticonvulsants

For grand mal and focal psychomotor seizures	Adult daily dosage (mg)	Therapeutic level (micrograms/mL)	Toxicity
Carbamazepine (Tegretol)	800–1200	4–16	Ataxia, drowsiness, nystagmus, agitation
Phenytoin (Dilantin)	300–400	10–20	Ataxia, slurred speech, vertigo, nystagmus, seizures
Phenobarbital (Luminal, Solfoton)	90–120	15–40	Ataxia, drowsiness
Primidone (Mysoline)*	750–1500	5–15	Ataxia, vertigo, nystagmus
Lamotrigine (Lamictal)	300–600	1–20	Life-threatening rash, vertigo, ataxia, blurred vision
Topiramate (Topamax)	100–600	10–20	Vertigo, drowsiness, ataxia, slurred speech, diplopia
Oxacarbazipine (Trileptal)	600–3600	10–40	Diplopia, dizziness, headache
Levetiracetam (Keppra)	1000–3000	1–20	Vertigo, fatigue, irritability
Gabapentin (Neurontin)	900–3600	4–20	Drowsiness, fatigue, ataxia, nausea, shortness of breath

*Primidone is metabolized to phenobarbital, and combined use of phenobarbital and primidone should be avoided.

8 Consider Vitamin K, 10 mg/day orally after 36 weeks of pregnancy until delivery to prevent neonatal hemorrhage.

9 Epilepsy is not usually considered an indication for early delivery.

First seizure during pregnancy

For the patient who develops new onset seizures during pregnancy, eclamptic seizures must be ruled out. A detailed neurological history and examination are essential. Diagnostic studies, including electroencephalography, magnetic resonance imaging, serum electrolytes and metabolic studies including serum calcium level, urine protein, and fasting and postprandial blood glucose determinations, should be performed on all patients. A lumbar puncture following computed tomography or magnetic resonance imaging may be indicated to rule out intracranial bleed or mass. Based on these studies and evidence of other neurological signs or symptoms, angiographic studies may be helpful.

Postpartum

1 Administer 1 mg of vitamin K intramuscularly to all newborns of patients receiving AEDs.

2 Examine the newborn carefully for signs of fetal teratogenic effects.

3 Reduction of anticonvulsant medication may be required in the postpartum period. Check the patient every 2 or 3 weeks after delivery.

Suggested reading

Delgado-Escueta AV, Janz D. Consensus guidelines: preconception counseling, management, and care of the pregnant woman with epilepsy. *Neurology* 1992;42:149–60.

DeToledo J. Pregnancy in epilepsy: issues of concern. *Int Rev Neurobiol* 2009;83:169–80.

Ditte M-N, Anders H. Newer-generation antiepileptic drugs and the risk of major birth defects *JAMA* 2011, 305(19).

Hernández-Díaz S, Smith CR, Shen A, *et al.* Comparative safety of antiepileptic drugs during pregnancy. *Neurology* 2012;78;1692–1699.

Hernández-Díaz S, Mittendorf R, Smith CR, Hauser WA, Yerby M, Holmes LB; North American Antiepileptic Drug Pregnancy Registry. Association between topiramate and zonisamide use during pregnancy and low birth weight. *Obstet Gynecol* 2014;123(1): 21–8.

Management issues for women with epilepsy – focus on pregnancy (an evidence-based review): Report of the Quality Standards Subcommittee and the Therapeutics and Technology Assessment Subcommittee of the American Academy of Neurology and the American Epilepsy Society. I. Obstetrical complications and change in seizure frequency. *Epilepsia* 2009;50(5):1229–36. II. Teratogenesis and perinatal outcomes. *Epilepsia* 2009;50(5):1237–46. III. Vitamin K, folic acid, blood levels, and breast-feeding. *Epilepsia* 2009;50(5):1247–55.

Meador KJ, *et al.* Cognitive function at 3 years of age after fetal exposure to antiepileptic-drugs. *N Eng J Med* 2009;360(16):1597–605.

Meadow R. Anticonvulsant in pregnancy. *Arch Dis Child* 1991, 66: 62–5.

Pennell PB. Antiepileptic drug pharmacokinetics during pregnancy and lactation. *Neurology* 2003, 61: S35–S42.

Richmond JR, *et al.* Epilepsy and pregnancy: an obstetric perspective. *Am J Obstet Gynecol* 2004;190:371–9.

Shorvon SD, *et al.* The management of epilepsy during pregnancy: progress is painfully slow. *Epilepsia* 2009;50(5):973–4.

St. Louis EK. Monitoring Antiepileptic Drugs: A Level-Headed Approach. *Current Neuropharm.* 2009;7:115–119.

Tomson T, *et al.* Antiepileptic drug treatment in pregnancy: Changes in drug disposition and their clinical implications. *Epilepsia* 2013;54(3):405–414.

Walker SP, *et al.* The management of epilepsy in pregnancy. *Br J Obstet Gynaecol* 2009; 116:758–67.

Yerby MS. Management issues for women with epilepsy. *Neurology* 2003;61:S23–S26.

Chronic Hypertension

Baha M. Sibai

Department of Obstetrics and Gynaecology and Reproductive Sciences, The University of Texas Medical School at Houston, Houston, TX, USA

According to data derived from the National Health and Nutrition Examination Survey, 1988–1991, the prevalence of chronic hypertension among women of childbearing age increases from 0.6–2.0% for women 18–29 years old to 4.6–22.3% for women 30–39 years old. The lower rates are for white women and higher rates are for African Americans. Because of the current trend of childbearing at an older age, it is expected that the incidence of chronic hypertension in pregnancy will continue to rise. Recent data from the ACOG Hypertension in Pregnancy Task force suggest that chronic hypertension will complicate 5% of all pregnancies. This indicates that at least 200,000 pregnant women (5% of 4 million pregnancies) with chronic hypertension will be seen in the United States each year.

Definition and diagnosis

In pregnant women, chronic hypertension is defined as elevated blood pressure that is present and documented before pregnancy. In women whose prepregnancy blood pressure is unknown, the diagnosis is assumed to be present based on the presence of sustained hypertension before 20 weeks of gestation, defined as either systolic blood pressure of at least 140 mmHg or diastolic blood pressure of at least 90 mmHg on at least two occasions measured at least 4 hours apart.

Women with chronic hypertension are at increased risk of superimposed preeclampsia. The Task Force recommended that superimposed preeclampsia be stratified into two groups to guide management.

1 Superimposed preeclampsia defined as:
  • A sudden increase in blood pressure (BP) that was previously well controlled or escalation of antihypertensive medications to control BP or

Protocols for High-Risk Pregnancies: An Evidence-Based Approach, Sixth Edition. Edited by John T. Queenan, Catherine Y. Spong and Charles J. Lockwood.

- New-onset proteinuria (300 mg or more/24-hour collection or a protein:creatinine ratio of 0.3 or more) or sudden increase in proteinuria in a woman with known proteinuria before or early in pregnancy.
2 The diagnosis of superimposed preeclampsia with severe features should be made in the presence of any of the following:
  - Severe-range BP (160 mmHg or higher systolic or 110 mmHg or higher diastolic) despite escalation of antihypertensive therapy
  - Persistent cerebral (headaches) or visual disturbances
  - Significant increase in liver enzymes (two times the upper limit of normal concentration for a particular laboratory)
  - Thrombocytopenia (platelet count less than 100,000/microliter)
  - New-onset and worsening renal insufficiency
  - Pulmonary edema.

Etiology and classification

The etiology as well as the severity of chronic hypertension is an important consideration in the management of pregnancy. Chronic hypertension is subdivided into primary (essential) and secondary. Primary hypertension is by far the most common cause of chronic hypertension seen during pregnancy (90%). In 10% of the cases, chronic hypertension is secondary to one or more underlying disorders such as renal disease (glomerulonephritis, interstitial nephritis, polycystic kidneys, renal artery stenosis), collagen vascular disease (lupus, scleroderma), endocrine disorders (diabetes mellitus with vascular involvement, pheochromocytoma, thyrotoxicosis, Cushing disease, hyperaldosteronism), or coarctation of the aorta.

Chronic hypertension during pregnancy can be subclassified as either mild or severe, depending on the systolic and diastolic BP readings. Systolic and diastolic (Korotkoff phase V) blood pressures of at least 160 mmHg and/or 105 mmHg, respectively, constitute severe hypertension requiring antihypertensive therapy.

For management and counseling purposes, chronic hypertension in pregnancy is also categorized as either low-risk or high-risk as described in Fig. 25.1. The patient is considered to be at low risk when she has mild essential hypertension without any organ involvement.

Maternal–perinatal risks

Pregnancies complicated by chronic hypertension are at increased risk for superimposed preeclampsia and abruptio placentae, fetal growth restriction, and preterm delivery, and adverse maternal outcomes. The reported

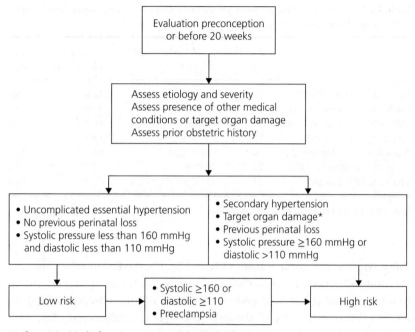

*Left ventricular dysfunction, rentinopathy, dyslipidemia, maternal age above 40 years, microvascular disease, stroke.

Figure 25.1   Initial evaluation of women with chronic hypertension.

rates of superimposed preeclampsia in the literature in mild hypertension range from 10% to 25% (Table 25.1). The rate of preeclampsia in women with severe chronic hypertension approaches 50%. Sibai and associates studied the rate of superimposed preeclampsia among 763 women with chronic hypertension followed prospectively at several medical centers in the United States. The overall rate of superimposed preeclampsia was 25%. The rate was not affected by maternal age, race, or presence of proteinuria early in pregnancy. However, the rate was significantly greater in women who had hypertension for at least 4 years (31% vs 22%), in those who had had preeclampsia during a previous pregnancy (32% vs 23%), and in those whose diastolic blood pressure was 100–110 mmHg when compared with those whose diastolic blood pressure was below 100 mmHg at baseline (42% vs 24%).

The reported rate of abruptio placentae in women with mild chronic hypertension has ranged from 0.5 to 1.5% (Table 25.1). The rate in those with severe or high-risk hypertension may be 5–10%. In a recent multicenter study that included 763 women with chronic hypertension, the overall rate of abruptio placentae was reported at 1.5% and the rate was significantly higher in those who developed superimposed preeclampsia than in

Table 25.1 Rates of adverse pregnancy outcome in observational studies describing mild chronic hypertension in pregnancy

	Preeclampsia (%)	Abruptio placentae (%)	Delivery at <37 weeks (%)	SGA (%)
Sibai et al. 1983 (n = 211)	10	1.4	12.0	8.0
Rey & Couturier 1994 (n = 337)	21	0.7	34.4	15.5
McCowan et al. 1996 (n = 142)	14	NR	16	11.0
Sibai et al. 1998 (n = 763)	25	1.5	33.3	11.1
Giannubilo et al. 2006 (n = 233)	28	0.5	NR	16.5
Chappell et al. 2008 (n = 822)	22	NR	22.7	27.2
Sibai et al. 2009 (n = 369)	17	2.4	29.3	15.0

SGA, small for gestational age; NR, not reported.

those without this complication (3% vs 1%, $P < 0.04$). However, the rate was not influenced by maternal age, race, or duration of hypertension. In addition, the results of a systematic review of nine observational studies revealed that the rate of abruptio placentae is doubled (OR, 2.1; 95% CI, 1.1–3.9) in women with chronic hypertension compared with either normotensive or general obstetric population.

Fetal and neonatal complications are also increased in women with chronic hypertension. The risk of perinatal mortality is increased 3–4 times compared with the general obstetric population. The rates of premature deliveries and small-for-gestational-age (SGA) infants are also increased in women with chronic hypertension (Table 25.1).

Chappell et al. studied 822 women with chronic hypertension that were part of patients enrolled in a randomized trial to evaluate the benefits of antioxidants (vitamin C and vitamin E) for the prevention of preeclampsia (no benefit was found). The incidence of preeclampsia was 22%. The incidence of preeclampsia was significantly higher in those with systolic blood pressure higher than 130 mmHg and/or those with diastolic blood pressure higher than 80 mmHg at the time of enrollment as compared to the other groups. The rate of SGA was 48% in those with superimposed preeclampsia and 21% in those without. In addition, the rate of preterm delivery at 37 weeks was 51% in those with superimposed preeclampsia as compared to 15% in those without preeclampsia.

Treatment

Most women with chronic hypertension during pregnancy have mild essential uncomplicated hypertension and are at minimal risk for cardiovascular complications within the short time frame of pregnancy. Several retrospective and prospective studies have been conducted to determine whether antihypertensive therapy in these women would improve pregnancy outcome. An overall summary of reviewed studies in the Task Force Report revealed that, regardless of the antihypertensive therapy used, maternal cardiovascular and renal complications were minimal or absent. Based on the available data, there is no compelling evidence that short-term antihypertensive therapy is beneficial for the pregnant woman with low-risk hypertension except for a reduction in the rate of exacerbation of hypertension.

Antihypertensive therapy is necessary in women with severe hypertension to reduce the acute risk of stroke, congestive heart failure or renal failure. In addition, control of severe hypertension may also permit pregnancy prolongation and possibly improve perinatal outcome. However, there is no evidence that control of severe hypertension reduces the rates of either superimposed preeclampsia or abruptio placentae.

There are many retrospective and prospective studies examining the potential fetal–neonatal benefits of pharmacological therapy in women with mild essential uncomplicated hypertension (low-risk). Some compared treatment with no treatment or with a placebo, others compared two different antihypertensive drugs, and others used a combination of drugs. Only four of these studies were randomized trials that included women enrolled prior to 20 weeks of gestation. Only two trials had a moderate sample size to evaluate the risks of superimposed preeclampsia and abruptio placentae. Therefore, treatment of mild chronic hypertension remains controversial.

Suggested management

The primary objective in the management of pregnancies complicated with chronic hypertension is to reduce maternal risks and achieve optimal perinatal survival. This objective can be achieved by formulating a rational approach that includes preconception evaluation and counseling, early antenatal care, timely antepartum visits to monitor both maternal and fetal well-being, timely delivery with intensive intrapartum monitoring, and proper postpartum management.

Evaluation and classification

Management of patients with chronic hypertension should ideally begin prior to pregnancy, whereby evaluation and workup are undertaken to assess the etiology, the severity, as well as the presence of other medical illnesses, and to rule out the presence of target organ damage of longstanding hypertension. An in-depth history should delineate in particular the duration of hypertension, the use of antihypertensive medications, their type, and the response to these medications. Also, attention should be given to the presence of cardiac or renal disease, diabetes, thyroid disease, and a history of cerebrovascular accident, or congestive heart failure. A detailed obstetric history should include maternal, as well as neonatal, outcome of previous pregnancies with stresses on history of development of abruptio placentae, superimposed preeclampsia, preterm delivery, SGA infants and intrauterine fetal death.

Laboratory evaluation is obtained to assess the function of different organ systems that are likely to be affected by chronic hypertension, and as a baseline for future assessments. These should include the following for all patients: urine analysis, urine culture and sensitivity, 24-hour urine evaluations for protein, electrolytes, complete blood count and glucose tolerance test.

Low-risk hypertension

Women with low-risk chronic hypertension without superimposed pre-eclampsia usually have a pregnancy outcome similar to that in the general obstetric population. In addition, discontinuation of antihypertensive therapy early in pregnancy does not affect the rates of preeclampsia, abruptio placentae or preterm delivery in these women. My policy is to discontinue antihypertensive treatment at the first prenatal visit because the majority of these women will have good pregnancy outcome without such therapy. Although these women do not require pharmacological therapy, a careful management is still essential (Fig. 25.2). At the time of initial and subsequent visits, the patient is educated about nutritional requirements, weight gain and sodium intake (maximum of 2.4 g of sodium per day). During each subsequent visit, they are observed very closely for early signs of preeclampsia and fetal growth restriction.

The development of severe hypertension (systolic BP 160 mmHg or higher or diastolic BP 105 mmHg or higher), preeclampsia or abnormal fetal growth requires urgent fetal testing with non-stress test or biophysical profile. Women who have superimposed preeclampsia with severe features, and those with documented severe fetal growth restriction (less than 5th percentile) require hospitalization and delivery at 34 weeks of gestation or earlier as indicated. Those who have superimposed preeclampsia only should receive frequent monitoring and deliver at 37 weeks or earlier if indicated. In the absence of these complications, the pregnancy may be continued till 38–39 weeks of gestation.

High-risk hypertension

Women with high-risk chronic hypertension are at increased risk for adverse maternal and perinatal complications. Women with significant renal insufficiency (serum creatinine 1.4 mg/dL or higher), diabetes

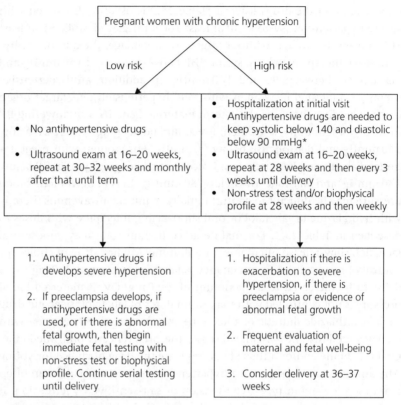

Pregnant women with chronic hypertension

Low risk   High risk

- No antihypertensive drugs

- Ultrasound exam at 16–20 weeks, repeat at 30–32 weeks and monthly after that until term

- Hospitalization at initial visit
- Antihypertensive drugs are needed to keep systolic below 140 and diastolic below 90 mmHg*
- Ultrasound exam at 16–20 weeks, repeat at 28 weeks and then every 3 weeks until delivery
- Non-stress test and/or biophysical profile at 28 weeks and then weekly

1. Antihypertensive drugs if develops severe hypertension

2. If preeclampsia develops, if antihypertensive drugs are used, or if there is abnormal fetal growth, then begin immediate fetal testing with non-stress test or biophysical profile. Continue serial testing until delivery

1. Hospitalization if there is exacerbation to severe hypertension, if there is preeclampsia or evidence of abnormal fetal growth

2. Frequent evaluation of maternal and fetal well-being

3. Consider delivery at 36–37 weeks

*For women with target organ damage

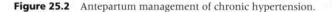

Figure 25.2 Antepartum management of chronic hypertension.

mellitus with vascular involvement (class R/F), severe collagen vascular disease, cardiomyopathy or coarctation of the aorta should receive thorough counseling regarding the adverse effects of pregnancy before conception. These women should be advised that pregnancy may exacerbate their condition with the potential for congestive heart failure, acute renal failure requiring dialysis, and even death. In addition, perinatal loss and neonatal complications are markedly increased in these women. All such women should be managed by or in consultation with a subspecialist in maternal-fetal medicine, as well as in association with other medical specialists as needed.

Women with high-risk hypertension may require hospitalization at the time of first prenatal visit for evaluation of cardiovascular and renal status and for regulation of antihypertensive medications, as well as other prescribed medications (Fig. 25.2). Women receiving atenolol, ACE inhibitors or angiotensin II receptor antagonists should have these medications discontinued under close observation. Antihypertensive therapy with one or more of the drugs listed in Table 25.2 is used in all women with severe hypertension (systolic BP at least 160 mmHg or diastolic BP at least 105 mmHg). In women without target organ damage, the aim of antihypertensive therapy is to keep systolic BP between 140 and 150 mmHg and diastolic BP between 90 and 100 mmHg. In addition, antihypertensive therapy is indicated in women with mild hypertension plus target organ damage because there are short-term maternal benefits from lowering BP in such women. In these women, I recommend keeping systolic BP below 140 mmHg and diastolic BP below 90 mmHg. For women with pregestational diabetes and hypertension, I recommend keeping systolic BP below 130 mmHg and diastolic BP below 80 mmHg. In some women, blood pressure may be difficult to control initially requiring intravenous therapy with hydralazine or labetalol or oral short-acting nifedipine with doses as described in Table 25.2. For maintenance therapy, one may choose oral labetalol, slow-release nifedipine, or a diuretic. My first drug of choice for control of hypertension in pregnancy is labetalol starting at 200 mg twice daily, to be increased to a maximum of 2400 mg/day. If maternal blood pressure is not controlled with maximum doses of labetalol, a second drug such as a thiazide diuretic or nifedipine may be added. For women with diabetes mellitus and vascular disease, the preference is oral nifedipine. Oral nifedipine and/or a thiazide diuretic are the drug of choice for young African American women with hypertension because these women often manifest a low-renin type hypertension or salt-sensitive hypertension. If maternal blood pressure is adequately controlled with these medications, the patient can continue with the same drug after delivery. Alternatively, the patient can be started on their prepregnancy medications.

Early and frequent prenatal visits are the key for successful pregnancy outcome in women with high-risk chronic hypertension. These women

Table 25.2   Drugs used to treat hypertension in pregnancy

Drug	Starting dose	Maximum dose
Acute treatment of severe hypertension		
Hydralazine	5–10 mg IV every 20 min	25 mg*
Labetalol[†]	20–40 mg IV every 10–15 min	300 mg*
Nifedipine	10–20 mg oral every 20–30 min	50 mg*
Long-term treatment of hypertension		
Labetalol	100 mg bid	2400 mg/day
Nifedipine	10 mg bid	120 mg/day
Thiazide diuretic	12.5 mg bid	50 mg/day

*If desired blood pressure levels are not achieved, switch to another drug.
[†]Avoid labetalol in women with asthma or congestive heart failure.

need close observation throughout pregnancy and may require serial evaluation of renal function, and complete blood count with metabolic profile at least once every trimester. Further laboratory testing can be performed depending on the clinical progress of the pregnancy. Fetal evaluation should be carried out as recommended in Fig. 25.2.

The development of uncontrolled severe hypertension, superimposed preeclampsia or evidence of fetal growth restriction requires maternal hospitalization for more frequent evaluation of maternal and fetal well-being. The development of any of these complications at or beyond 34 weeks of gestation should be considered an indication for delivery. In all other women, consider delivery at 36–37 weeks of gestation. In the postpartum period, these women are at increased risk for development of exacerbation of hypertension and pulmonary edema. Therefore, it is important to monitor BP, and intake-output very carefully. In addition, it is advisable to avoid using nonsteroidal anti-inflammatory agents for pain control.

Summary

Chronic hypertension in pregnancy is associated with increased rates of adverse maternal and fetal outcomes, both acute and long term. These adverse outcomes are particularly seen in women with uncontrolled severe hypertension, in those with target organ damage, and those who are noncompliant with prenatal visits. In addition, adverse outcomes are substantially increased in women who develop superimposed preeclampsia or abruptio placentae. Women with chronic hypertension should be evaluated either prior to conception or at time of first prenatal visit. Depending on this evaluation, they can be divided into categories of either high-risk or low-risk chronic hypertension. High-risk women should receive aggressive antihypertensive therapy, lifestyle changes and frequent evaluations of maternal and fetal well-being.

Acknowledgment

The author would like to acknowledge the contributions of Hind N. Moussa, MD to this protocol.

Suggested reading

American College of Obstetricians and Gynecologists Task Force on Hypertension in Pregnancy. Hypertension in pregnancy. Washington, DC: American College of Obstetricians and Gynecologists; 2013.

Burt VL, Whetton P, Rochella EJ, Brown C, Cutler JA, Higgins M, *et al.* Prevalence of hypertension in the US adult population: results from the third national health and nutrition examination survey, 1988–1991. *Hypertension* 1995;23:305–13.

Chappell LC, Enye S, Seed P, Driley AL, *et al.* Adverse perinatal outcomes and risk factors for preeclampsia in women with chronic hypertension: a prospective study. *Hypertension* 2008;51:1002–9.

Giannubilo SR, Dell Uomo B, Tranquilli AL. Perinatal outcomes, blood pressure patterns and risk assessment of superimposed preeclampsia in mild chronic hypertensive pregnancy. *Eur J Obstet Gynecol Reprod Biol* 2006;126:63–7.

McCowan LM, Buist RG, North RA, Gamble G. Perinatal morbidity in chronic hypertension. *Br J Obstet Gynaecol* 1996;103:123–9.

Powrie RO. A 30-year-old woman with chronic hypertension trying to conceive: clinical cross roads. *JAMA* 2007;298:1548–59.

Rey E, Couturier A. The prognosis of pregnancy in women with chronic hypertension. *Am J Obstet Gynecol* 1994;171:410–16.

Sibai BM. Chronic hypertension in pregnancy. *Obstet Gynecol* 2002;100:369–77.

Sibai BM, Abdella TN, Anderson GD. Pregnancy outcome in 211 patients with mild chronic hypertension. *Obstet Gynecol* 1983;61:571–6.

Sibai BM, Anderson GD. Pregnancy outcome of intensive therapy in severe hypertension in first trimester. *Obstet Gynecol* 1986;67:517–22.

Sibai BM, Lindheimer M, Hauth J, Caritis S, Van Dorsten P, Klebanoff M, *et al.* Risk factors for preeclampsia, abruptio placentae, and adverse neonatal outcomes among women with chronic hypertension. *N Engl J Med* 1998;339:667–71.

Sibai BM, Koch M, Freire S, *et al.* The impact of a history of previous preeclampsia on the risk of superimposed preeclampsia and adverse pregnancy outcome in patients with chronic hypertension. *Am J Obstet Gynecol* 2009;201:752.

PROTOCOL 26

Cytomegalovirus, Genital Herpes, Rubella, Syphilis, and Toxoplasmosis

Brenna L. Hughes

Department of Obstetrics and Gynecology, Warren Alpert Medical School of Brown University/Women & Infants Hospital, Providence, RI, USA

Cytomegalovirus

Congenital cytomegalovirus (CMV) infection is among the most prevalent congenital infection and the most common infectious cause of childhood deafness. It typically occurs via transplacental passage of virus from a mother with primary infection, reinfection or reactivation of latent disease. Maternal primary CMV infection results in 30–40% of infants with congenital infection, while less than 1% of infants born to mothers with recurrent CMV infection will have perinatal infection. Overall, it is estimated that approximately 0.5–1% of all newborns are CMV-infected in the United States.

Women with primary CMV infection are usually asymptomatic, but about 10% of women can have an infectious mononucleosis-like disease (but with a negative heterophile antibody test). Primary infection during any trimester can lead to intrauterine infection and the risk of transmission increases with increasing gestational age, but infection in the first half of pregnancy carries the highest risk for adverse neonatal outcome. Between 85% and 90% of congenitally infected infants are born clinically asymptomatic; but up to 10–15% of these asymptomatic infants will later have abnormal development, most commonly unilateral or bilateral hearing impairment. Infants who are symptomatic at birth can present with thrombocytopenia, hepatosplenomegaly, chorioretinitis, deafness, microcephaly, cerebral calcification, mental retardation or early death, often due to disseminated intravascular coagulation, myocardial dysfunction, or hepatic failure.

Protocols for High-Risk Pregnancies: An Evidence-Based Approach, Sixth Edition.
Edited by John T. Queenan, Catherine Y. Spong and Charles J. Lockwood.
© 2015 John Wiley & Sons, Ltd. Published 2015 by John Wiley & Sons, Ltd.

Postnatal CMV infection of the infant can occur from exposure to genital tract virus or through breast milk; however, it does not lead to visceral or neurological sequelae.

Diagnosis

The great majority of CMV infections in women are asymptomatic and can be identified only by prospective antibody testing. After primary CMV infection, virus replication may persist for many months and can be reactivated months or years later, with intermittent CMV shedding from the cervix and other sites. The diagnosis of primary infection can be made with serial titers and evidence of seroconversion from IgG-negative to IgG-positive serology. Because most women with the infection are asymptomatic, the clinical utility of serial titers is somewhat limited since they would need to be performed in asymptomatic women in order to capture 90% of infections. Women who have antibody (IgG) to CMV before being pregnant can be assured that it is very unlikely that subsequent children will have sequelae due to congenital CMV infection.

The presence of IgM-specific CMV antibody is associated with an increased chance of infection, but only approximately 10% are indicative of true infection. For this reason, CMV IgG avidity testing may be of value in assessing a patient's likelihood of recent infection. Low IgG avidity suggests that primary infection has occurred within the prior 3–4 months. Fetal diagnosis can be achieved with the use of amniocentesis. Unlike the case of aneuploidy testing, though, amniocentesis has imperfect sensitivity and specificity, with increasing sensitivity later in gestation and at least 6 weeks from the time of maternal infection.

Management

If a pregnant woman develops primary infection with CMV, there is a 30–40% chance her child will be infected and thus, approximately a 6–7% chance her child will have some damage due to this infection. Therapeutic abortion may be considered when a diagnosis of fetal infection is made. Abnormal ultrasound findings, such as microcephaly, ascites, intra-cranial or intra-peritoneal calcifications, or echogenic bowel may be present. Amniocentesis can be used to aid in making the diagnosis when infection is suspected either on the basis of maternal serology or ultrasound findings.

Some studies have suggested that there may be role for anti-CMV-specific hyperimmune globulin as prophylaxis to reduce the risk of fetal infection after maternal infection and as treatment to prevent fetal sequelae after in utero infection. However, a small prospective randomized study has not shown this practice to be efficacious. Larger studies are needed before this strategy can be considered.

Genital herpes simplex virus

Herpes infection is a common cause of minor maternal symptoms and a rare cause of devastating neonatal infection. Congenital in utero infection is distinctly rare. However, neonatal infection is associated with high mortality and occurs in approximately 1 per 3000–5000 births.

The majority of neonatal herpes cases are born to women who have subclinical genital viral shedding at delivery and who often have no history of disease, making transmission prevention difficult. The risk of transmission from asymptomatic shedding in a woman with recurrent HSV is much lower, approximately 1 in 10,000 deliveries. The duration of rupture of membranes, the use of fetal scalp electrodes, and the mode of delivery also influence neonatal transmission. Two-thirds of neonatal HSV infection is due to HSV-2 and the remaining one-third is due to HSV-1 infection. Both HSV-1 and HSV-2 cause clinical maternal and neonatal disease. Most orolabial lesions are secondary to HSV-1, and either virus may cause genital lesions.

Diagnosis

The diagnosis of HSV infection is often made clinically, either in the setting of maternal or neonatal disease. Isolation of virus by cell culture is the most sensitive test widely available. PCR is highly sensitive but not as widely available. Antibodies begin to develop within 2–3 weeks of infection. Serological tests now available are based on antibodies formed to type-specific G-glycoproteins. These tests allow specific typing for HSV-1 and HSV-2 and are useful for counseling when diagnosis is in question.

Management
Antepartum management

Late pregnancy primary HSV has the highest likelihood for neonatal transmission. Though some experts recommend screening, at this time universal screening of all pregnant women with type-specific serology is not recommended. Delivery during a primary infection should be avoided if possible.

An active lesion in the antepartum period should be cultured to confirm the clinical diagnosis. If this is an initial episode, type-specific serology should be performed to determine if this is a primary or nonprimary infection. Systemic antivirals may be used to attenuate signs and symptoms of HSV, especially if this is a primary infection. However, these will not eradicate latent virus.

Antiviral suppression therapy with acyclovir or valacyclovir in the latter part of pregnancy (36 weeks until delivery) has been shown to decrease the rate of clinical HSV recurrences at delivery and the rate of asymptomatic shedding at delivery.

Intrapartum management

A woman with a history of HSV should be asked about prodromal symptoms and recent HSV lesions. A careful vulvar, vaginal and cervical examination should be performed at the time of admission for labor and delivery. Suspicious lesions should be cultured. Currently, cesarean delivery is indicated if the woman has an active lesion or prodromal symptoms. However, a cesarean delivery does not eliminate the risk. Ten to fifteen percent of infants with HSV are born to women who have had a cesarean delivery. If a lesion is present distant from the vulva, vagina or cervix, the risk of neonatal transmission is lower. The nongenital lesions may be covered with an occlusive dressing and a vaginal delivery allowed. Cesarean delivery should not be performed in a woman solely for a history of HSV.

The management of the woman presenting with an active HSV lesion and ruptured membranes is controversial. At term, cesarean delivery should be offered regardless of how long the membranes have been ruptured. In the setting of preterm PROM, especially remote from term, expectant management should be considered; as the risk of prematurity complications may outweigh the benefit of immediate delivery.

Rubella

Rubella virus infection is acquired via the upper respiratory tract through inhalation. Infection during the first 5 months of pregnancy can result in severe fetal damage or death. Fortunately, congenital rubella has been eradicated in the United States for a number of years. The mother with rubella may have no symptoms (30%) or a mild 3-day rash with posterior auricular adenopathy.

The infant, however, may experience severe congenital heart damage, cataracts, deafness, damage to major blood vessels, microcephaly, mental retardation or other abnormalities. In addition there may be severe disease during the newborn period, including thrombocytopenia, bleeding, hepatosplenomegaly, pneumonitis, or myocarditis. The risk of major fetal damage varies with the time of maternal infection: 80–90% in the first 3 months of pregnancy; 10% in the fourth month; and 6% in the fifth month, often as isolated hearing impairment. There is probably no risk after the fifth month.

Diagnosis

Routine prenatal care includes testing for evidence of rubella immunity. Aside from this, serologic testing of pregnant women is rarely indicated in the United States given the rarity of rubella and is generally not helpful in the presence of abnormal ultrasound findings. After true exposure, a woman will develop infection in 2–3 weeks, and antibody shortly thereafter. To document the infection, serial serology is necessary with evidence of seroconversion from IgG negative to IgG positive. IgM becomes positive shortly after the onset of rash and remains positive for about 4 weeks.

Management
Routine use of immune globulin (IG) for post-exposure prophylaxis in pregnant susceptible women is not recommended. IG has been shown to suppress symptoms; however, it does not prevent viremia. Congenital rubella infections have occurred despite immediate post-exposure use of IG.

The primary approach to the prevention of rubella is immunization. Vaccine for measles, mumps, and rubella (MMR) should be given to all children between 12 and 15 months of age and repeated at school age. Since all pregnant women are routinely tested for antibody to rubella, lack of immunity can be documented during pregnancy. Postpartum vaccination can be conducted for nonimmune women. Pregnant women should not receive the live virus vaccine. Nonpregnant vaccine recipients should be instructed not to become pregnant for 3 months. These reservations are based on the hypothetic possibility that the vaccine virus might damage the developing fetus early in pregnancy. However, data from the Centers for Disease Control (CDC) for over 800 susceptible pregnant women who inadvertently received the rubella vaccine during early pregnancy showed no evidence of rubella-related fetal damage.

Syphilis

Syphilis remains a major public health problem, with increasing prevalence in the United States following a significant decline in the latter part of the 1900s. The increase in prevalence is predominantly among the population of men who have sex with men, but the rate among women has increased as well. Congenital syphilis occurs in 7–10 per 100,000 live births. The most common clinical findings in congenital syphilis are hepatosplenomegaly, osteochondritis or periostitis, jaundice or hyperbilirubinemia, petechiae, purpura, lymphadenopathy and ascites or hydrops.

Diagnosis
The majority of pregnant women with syphilis are asymptomatic, and the diagnosis is frequently made by serological testing, which is recommended as part of routine prenatal care. Of infected fetuses, 40–50% will die in utero. The most common cause of fetal death is placental infection and

overwhelming fetal infection. *Treponema pallidum* can be identified in infected amniotic fluid using PCR testing; however, prenatal diagnosis is not recommended prior to maternal treatment.

Management

Patients with early syphilis (primary, secondary, and early latent syphilis of less than 1 year's duration) should receive a single intramuscular dose of 2.4 million units of benzathine penicillin G. After treatment of early disease, more than 60% of women will have the Jarisch-Herxheimer reaction. Pregnant patients should be monitored for fever, decreased fetal activity and signs of preterm labor.

For pregnant women with late latent syphilis of more than 1 year's duration or of unknown duration, or with cardiovascular syphilis, benzathine penicillin G, 2.4 million units intramuscularly, should be given weekly for three doses (7.2 million units total). Serological tests should be repeated at the previously recommended times during the third trimester and at delivery. It is expected that there will be a fourfold drop in serological test titers over a 6- to 12-month period in women treated for early syphilis. However, it is not unusual for pregnant women to have insufficient time to be evaluated for serological evidence of cure of their syphilis by delivery.

Treatment before 20 weeks is highly effective in preventing congenital syphilis, barring reinfection. Treatment failures occur in 1–2% of patients because of advanced, irreversible fetal infection. These failures are seen more frequently with maternal high-titer early latent syphilis, secondary syphilis or treatment after 30 weeks of gestation. In adults, HIV infection may affect the clinical presentation of syphilis, the serologies, and the response to recommended therapy.

Treatment after 20 weeks should be preceded by ultrasonography to look for evidence of fetal infection. In the case of an abnormal sonogram (hydrops, ascites, skin edema, hepatomegaly), antepartum fetal heart rate testing is useful prior to treatment. Spontaneous late decelerations and nonreactive fetal heart rate patterns have been associated with an infected fetus. When sonographic abnormalities are found and antepartum testing is abnormal, a neonatologist and maternal–fetal medicine specialist should be consulted.

The pregnant woman with syphilis who is allergic to penicillin presents a therapeutic challenge. Because of reported treatment failures, resistance concerns and the lack of clinical data in pregnancy, azithromycin is not recommended for routine use in pregnant patients. Referral for penicillin desensitization for the pregnant patient with a true allergy to penicillin is recommended. Desensitization can be accomplished either orally or intravenously.

Toxoplasmosis

Congenital toxoplasmosis is less uncommon in the United States than many other countries, with an estimated incidence of 500–5000 cases annually. The sequelae of congenital toxoplasmosis may be severe and include fetal death, blindness, deafness and mental retardation. At birth, infected children may have a maculopapular rash, hepatosplenomegaly, seizures or hydrocephalus. In the setting of maternal infection, the risk of having an affected child is approximately 2% in the first trimester, nearly 10% around 28 weeks, and about 4% at term. At this time, antepartum screening, optimal methods for prenatal diagnosis of congenital toxoplasmosis, and treatment are controversial.

Diagnosis

When maternal infection is present, the most common clinical sign is bilateral, nontender lymphadenopathy that often involves the posterior cervical nodes. Additional symptoms include generalized fatigue, myalgias, fevers and headaches.

Serological tests for IgG and IgM antibodies may be obtained in patients who have suggestive symptoms. IgG antibodies generally appear within 1–2 weeks of infection, and peak between 6 and 8 weeks following infection. IgM antibodies appear within the first week of infection and then usually decline over several months. IgM antibodies may persist for years, and their presence is not necessarily indicative of an active or recent infection. At reference laboratories, a combination of tests, including IgG avidity testing, is helpful in determining a recent or distant infection depending on the clinical risk. One such laboratory is the Palo Alto Medical Foundation Research Institute's Toxoplasma Serology Laboratory. PCR testing of the amniotic fluid is the most accurate method for diagnosing fetal infection. This is generally performed in the second trimester or at least 4 weeks after an acute maternal infection. There are multiple sonographic abnormalities that may be seen with congenital toxoplasmosis; however, these are only suggestive of fetal infection. Some of these abnormalities include the following:

- ventricular dilation
- intracranial calcifications
- increased placental thickness

- hepatomegaly and/or intrahepatic calcifications
- fetal ascites
- pericardial or pleural effusions.

Treatment

The rationale for treatment of women with *Toxoplasma* infection during pregnancy is that it has been shown to reduce the incidence of severe sequelae and that a shorter interval between diagnosis and treatment is associated with a lower incidence of sequelae. Randomized trials in this area are currently lacking.

Once maternal infection is confirmed, treatment should be started with spiramycin. This antibiotic is similar to erythromycin and concentrates in the placenta. This drug is not available commercially in the United States; however, it can be obtained with the permission of the U.S. Food and Drug Administration. If there is evidence of fetal infection, as diagnosed by amniocentesis and PCR, additional treatment is given. If the PCR is negative for fetal infection, spiramycin is generally continued until delivery.

When fetal infection is confirmed, treatment is changed in favor of medications that cross the placenta and penetrate the fetal brain and cerebrospinal fluid. This includes both pyrimethamine and sulfadiazine. Pyrimethamine and sulfadiazine are both folic acid antagonists that work synergistically against the *T. gondii* parasite. These are generally administered after the second trimester and with supplementation with folinic acid.

Suggested reading

Cytomegalovirus

Stagno S, *et al.* Primary cytomegalovirus infection in pregnancy. Incidence, transmission to fetus, and clinical outcome. *JAMA* 1986;256(14):1904–8.

Fowler KB, *et al.* The outcome of congenital cytomegalovirus infection in relation to maternal antibody status. *N Engl J Med* 1992;326(10):663–7.

Cannon MJ, Davis KF. Washing our hands of the congenital cytomegalovirus disease epidemic. *BMC Public Health* 2005;5:70.

Revello MG, Lazzarotto T, Guerra B, Spinillo A, Ferrazzi E, Kustermann A, Guaschino S, Vergani P, Todros T, Frusca T, Arossa A, Furione M, Rognoni V, Rizzo N, Gabrielli L, Klersy C, Gerna G, CHIP Study Group. A randomized trial of hyperimmune globulin to prevent congenital cytomegalovirus. *N Engl J Med* 2014 Apr 3;370(14):1316–26.

Genital herpes simplex virus

American College of Obstetricians and Gynecologists. ACOG Practice Bulletin #82, June 2007. Management of herpes in pregnancy. *Obstet Gynecol* 2007;109:1489–98.

Hollier LM, Wendel GD. Third trimester antiviral prophylaxis for preventing maternal genital herpes simplex virus (HSV) recurrences and neonatal infection. *Cochrane Database Syst Rev* 2008 Jan 23;1:CD004946.

Rubella

Best JM. Rubella. *Semin Fetal Neonatal Med* 2007;12:182–92.

Haas DM, Flowers CA, Congdon CL. Rubella, rubeola, and mumps in pregnant women: susceptibilities and strategies for testing and vaccinating. *Obstet Gynecol* 2005;106: 295–300.

Syphilis

Centers for Disease Control and Prevention, Workowski KA, Berman SM. Sexually transmitted diseases treatment guidelines, 2006. *MMWR Recomm Rep* 2006;55(RR-11):1–94.

Wendel GD Jr, Sheffield JS, Hollier LM, Hill JB, Ramsey PS, Sánchez PJ. Treatment of syphilis in pregnancy and prevention of congenital syphilis. *Am J Obstet Gynecol* 2003;189:1178–83.

Toxoplasmosis

Montoya JG, Remington JS. Management of Toxoplasma gondii infection during pregnancy. *Clin Infect Dis* 2008;47:554–66.

SYROCOT (Systematic Review on Congenital Toxoplasmosis) study group, Thiébaut R, Leproust S, Chêne G, Gilbert R. Effectiveness of prenatal treatment for congenital toxoplasmosis: a meta-analysis of individual patients' data. *Lancet* 2007;369:115–22.

PROTOCOL 27

Influenza, West Nile Virus, Varicella-Zoster, and Tuberculosis

Jeanne S. Sheffield
Division of Maternal-Fetal Medicine, University of Texas Southwestern Medical Center, Dallas, TX, USA

Influenza

Influenza infection, while clinically recognized for centuries, remains a significant contributor to morbidity and mortality from febrile respiratory illness. Occurring annually, this viral infection affects all age groups and causes anywhere from 3000 to 50,000 deaths per year in the United States depending on the length and severity of the season. While children and adults aged 65 and older are at highest risk for serious complications and death, other high-risk groups have been identified, including pregnant women.

Early studies from the 1918 and 1957 influenza pandemics reported higher risks of complications such as abortion, stillbirth, low birth weight, congenital anomalies, and maternal mortality rates (as high as 30%) in pregnant women compared to the general population. However, studies over the last three decades including data obtained during the recent 2009–2010 influenza A/H_1N_1 pandemic have noted that while these complications remain higher than the nonpregnant reproductive age population, contemporary medical care and antiviral agents have decreased the overall complication rate. Complications such as stillbirth, first trimester abortion, and preterm delivery appear to correlate with maternal disease severity.

Pathophysiology

Influenza is an orthomyxovirus with three antigenic types – A, B, and C. Only influenza A and B cause clinically significant disease. Influenza A is further subtyped using two surface glycoproteins, hemagglutinin (H) and neuraminidase (N). Hemagglutinin is a viral attachment protein and mediates viral entry. The neuraminidase enzyme facilitates viral spread. The annual antigenic variation noted worldwide is secondary to either antigenic drift or shift. Antigenic drift occurs when mutations accumulate in the N or H antigen gene. It is a slow, often subtle process and the mutations directly affect vaccine efficacy. Antigenic shift, seen only in influenza A, involves replacement of the current H or N antigen with a new subtype. This shift to a novel antigen subtype is responsible for the intermittent worldwide influenza pandemics.

The emergence of the novel influenza A virus subtype A/H_1N_1 in 2008/2009 has been associated with significant febrile illness worldwide – the World Health Organization declared a pandemic on June 11, 2009. Since that time, several other influenza subtypes have been reported worldwide, including the highly pathogenic Avian influenza A H_5N_1 and H_7N_9 viruses, and the Swine influenza variant viruses (e.g. H_3N_2 variant) causing sporadic human infections. These strains normally do not infect humans; however, the number of human infections in recent years has risen to include rare human-to-human transmission. The international health agencies are monitoring these cases closely and vaccine trials are underway.

The influenza virus is spread through respiratory droplets and direct contact with recently contaminated articles. The incubation period ranges from 1 to 4 days. Adults often shed virus the day before symptoms develop until 5 days after symptom onset. Though many cases of influenza are asymptomatic, adults often present with a sudden onset of fever and rigors, diffuse myalgias, malaise, headache, and a nonproductive cough. Sore throat, rhinitis, abdominal pain, nausea and vomiting may also be present. Tachycardia and tachypnea are common, especially in pregnant women. Though most symptoms resolve within a few days, the cough and malaise may persist for greater than 2 weeks. Viremia is infrequent and vertical transmission is rare.

Diagnosis

During the influenza "season," the diagnosis is usually made using clinical features. Diagnostic tests are best performed within 72 hours of onset of illness, as viral shedding is greatest at this time. Viral culture of throat washings and nasopharyngeal secretions allow subtyping of the virus, important for epidemiologic evaluation and vaccine development. Serology, PCR, and immunofluorescent testing are also available. Finally, rapid antigen tests, though lower sensitivity than the viral culture, are readily available and allow rapid viral detection of nasopharyngeal secretions.

Treatment

The decision to hospitalize a pregnant woman with influenza depends on the severity of symptoms and associated complications. The patient should be evaluated for evidence of pneumonia and other complications as the clinical findings dictate. If influenza is suspected, initiate droplet and contact isolation procedures along with strict hand hygiene.

Two classes of antiviral medications are currently marketed for use during influenza outbreaks. Amantadine and ramantadine are adamantanes with activity against influenza A only. Their use in pregnancy has been reported with no adverse outcomes to date. However, due to the rapid rise in resistance to the adamantanes in the last decade, this class is currently not recommended for treatment of influenza. The second class of antiviral medications, the neuraminidase inhibitors, includes zanamivir, oseltamivir, and peramivir, all highly effective for influenza A and B. Secondary to yearly variations in resistance patterns, the Centers for Disease Control & Prevention publish treatment guidelines every year based on the influenza subtypes and antiviral sensitivity patterns (www.cdc.gov). Optimally, treatment should begin within 48 hours of symptom onset.

Complications

Immunologic changes that occur during pregnancy (e.g., the shift to Th2 immunity with the associated decrease in cell-mediated immunity) may alter the response to infection and increase the severity of influenza. Physiologic changes in pregnancy such as an elevated diaphragm, increased oxygen consumption, and decreased functional residual capacity may worsen the pulmonary complications of influenza (i.e., pneumonia). Secondary bacterial infections, particularly pneumonia, are not uncommon. Myocarditis has also been reported. Death, though rare, usually complicates influenza in patients with underlying chronic disease. There is no evidence that influenza A or B cause congenital malformations and congenital infection is negligible.

Prevention

Vaccination is the primary method to prevent influenza and its severe complications. Each year, a new vaccine formulation consisting of two influenza A subtypes and one or two influenza B viruses is determined based on typing of current virus worldwide. The efficacy of the vaccine is variable depending on how well the vaccine antigens correlate with the virus circulating in a specific community. Pregnant women respond to vaccination with increases in antibody titers similar to the nonpregnant women. Only the inactivated influenza vaccine is recommended in pregnancy and it should be given to all pregnant women and can be used in any trimester. Secondary prevention strategies such as hand hygiene, respiratory, and contact isolation should be implemented.

West Nile Virus

West Nile Virus, originally isolated in 1937 in Uganda and endemic in Africa, Asia, and the Middle East, was first reported in North America in 1999. By 2003, there were 9858 reported cases with 2864 cases of neuroinvasive disease. Subsequent years have witnessed a decrease in numbers, though in 2012 some 5674 cases were reported, the largest number since 2003. There were 286 deaths, 95% associated with neuroinvasive disease. Most patients are asymptomatic or have mild symptoms – less than 1% develops neuroinvasive disease.

Pathophysiology

West Nile Virus is an anthropod-borne RNA flavivirus, a member of the Japanese encephalitis virus antigenic complex. It is maintained in nature through biologic transmission involving bird reservoirs and mosquitoes, with humans an incidental host via a bite of an infected mosquito. Human transmission occurs mainly in the late summer months and there is no documented animal-to-human (except mosquitoes) or human-to-human transmission. The incubation period is 2 to 14 days.

Diagnosis

Most human West Nile Virus infections are subclinical – only one in five develop a mild febrile illness with symptoms lasting 3 to 6 days. Pregnant women with symptoms may present with fever, headache, fatigue, rare truncal skin rash, lymphadenopathy, and eye pain. Central nervous system involvement or neuroinvasive disease is diagnosed in less than 1% of adult cases. The diagnosis of West Nile Virus is based on clinical symptoms and serology. West Nile Virus serum IgM and IgG and cerebrospinal fluid IgM are used for laboratory confirmation, though cross-reaction to other flaviruses has been reported. Polymerase chain reaction (PCR) testing is limited secondary to transient and low viremia. Amniotic fluid, chorionic villi, fetal serum or products of conception can be tested for evidence of fetal West Nile Virus infection though the sensitivity and specificity are not known.

Treatment

There is no known effective antiviral treatment – management is supportive based on the severity of the disease. Clinical trials are ongoing.

Complications

Patients with neuroinvasive disease often have long-term sequelae including fatigue, memory loss, difficulty walking, muscle weakness, and depression. Fetal infection has been reported complicating pregnancy. A CDC West Nile Virus Pregnancy Registry found a small rate of neonatal infection (3/72 liveborn infants) though it could not be established conclusively that the infection was acquired congenitally. Transmission through breast milk has been reported though rare.

Prevention

The primary strategy for preventing exposure in pregnancy is the use of mosquito repellent containing *N,N*-diethyl-*m*-toluamide (DEET). Avoid outdoor activity around stagnant water and wear protective clothing from dusk to dawn. A vaccine is not currently available.

Varicella-Zoster

Varicella-zoster virus (VZV) is a double-stranded DNA herpes virus acquired predominantly during childhood – in the United States, 95% of adults have serologic evidence of immunity. Primary infection with VZV manifests as varicella (chickenpox). Herpes zoster (shingles) is an eruption that results from reactivation of latent VZV infection from the dorsal root ganglia.

Pathophysiology

Humans are the only source of infection with VZV. The virus is highly contagious and transmission occurs primarily through direct contact with an infected individual, although airborne spread from respiratory tract secretions has been reported. The incubation period is 10–21 days and a susceptible woman has a 60–95% risk of becoming infected with exposure. The patients are contagious from 1 to 2 days prior to the onset of rash until the lesions are crusted.

Diagnosis

Varicella is usually diagnosed clinically. A 1- to 2-day prodrome of fever, malaise, myalgias, and headache is followed by a rash on the head and trunk which then spreads to the extremities and abdomen. The rash occurs in "crops" of maculopapular lesions that rapidly form vesicles. It is intensely pruritic and slowly crust over several days. Herpes zoster presents as painful skin lesions over sensory nerve root distributions (dermatomes).

   Laboratory diagnosis is occasionally helpful. The virus may be isolated by scraping the vesicles and performing a tissue culture, Tzank smear or direct fluorescent antibody testing. Nucleic acid amplification tests are available and are very sensitive and specific. Serologic testing is commonly available – the enzyme-linked immunosorbent assay (ELISA) is the most popular though useful mainly to confirm prior infection.

Treatment

Pregnant women with uncomplicated varicella who are immunocompetent require only supportive care. Acyclovir (500 mg/m^2 or 10–15 mg/kg every 8 hours) is reserved for pregnant women with complicated varicella infection (e.g., varicella pneumonia) or who are immunocompromised.

Complications

Primary varicella infection in adults has higher complication rates than in children and is most pronounced in pregnant women. The increased morbidity is primarily respiratory in nature. Pneumonitis is diagnosed in 5–14% of pregnant women with varicella, especially in smokers and women with ≥100 skin lesions; mortality has decreased to less than 2%. VZV encephalitis and other neurologic complications are rare. Bacterial super-infection can lead to cellulitis, abscess formation, or rarely necrotizing fasciitis.

Congenital varicella syndrome among infants born to mothers with varicella occurs in approximately 2% when infection occurs before 20 weeks of gestation. Children exposed to VZV in utero during the second 20 weeks of pregnancy can develop inapparent varicella and subsequent zoster early in life without having had extrauterine varicella. Fetal infection after maternal varicella during the first or early second trimester of pregnancy occasionally results in varicella embryopathy, characterized by cutaneous scars, denuded skin, limb hypoplasia, muscle atrophy, and rudimentary digits. Other more frequent abnormalities are microcephaly, intracranial calcifications, cortical atrophy, cataracts, chorioretinitis, microphthalmia, and psychomotor retardation. Fetal exposure just before or during delivery results in neonatal VZV infection in 25–50% of cases. The case fatality rate approaches 30%, as there is no protective transplacental passage of maternal VZV-specific IgG. Varicella zoster immune globulin (VariZIG) should be given to neonates whose mothers developed varicella 5 days before and up to 2 days post delivery.

Prevention

Pregnant women exposed to VZV who deny prior infection should have a VZV IgG titer performed – 70% of individuals with no history of VZV are actually immune. Seronegative women should be given VariZIG. It is most effective when given early but may be given up to 10 days post-exposure. A live virus vaccine (Varivax©) is available in the United States but is not recommended for pregnant women.

Tuberculosis

While tuberculosis (TB) remains a serious health problem worldwide, TB has been steadily declining in the United States, to a lowest recorded rate in 2012 of 3.2 cases per 100,000 persons. The TB rate in foreign-born persons was 10 times greater than that of U.S.-born persons, with almost three-fifths of all TB cases in the United States occurring in immigrants. It is estimated that one-third of the world's population is infected with TB. The majority of cases in the United States are latent tuberculosis infection (LTI).

Pathophysiology

TB is a chronic bacterial infection caused mainly by *Mycobacterium tuberculosis* or *M. bovis*, which is transmitted by respiratory droplet and spread from person to person via air. Transmission of TB is dependent on the number and/or viability of bacilli in expelled air, susceptible host factors, environment/shared air, and duration and/or frequency of exposure. In over 90% of patients, infection is dormant for long periods and remains localized to the respiratory tract.

Primary TB infection can be asymptomatic, can produce a primary complex, or result in typical chronic pulmonary TB without a demonstrable primary complex. Early pulmonary TB is usually asymptomatic, and does not produce symptoms until the bacillary population has reached a certain size. When symptoms occur they range from nonspecific constitutional symptoms such as anorexia, fatigue, weight loss, chills, afternoon fever, and when this subsides, night sweats. A productive cough is usually present, and hemoptysis can occur. In some women, extrapulmonary disease may occur – the greatest risk is in the immunocompromised patient. Pregnancy does not appear to increase the risk for developing active TB.

Children born to women with active TB have an increased risk of morbidity and mortality in the neonatal period, with an increase in prematurity, perinatal death, and low birth weight. However, when adequate therapy is initiated, TB appears to have no adverse effect on the pregnancy. Most perinatal infections occur when a mother with active TB handles her infant, and the risk of the child contracting TB from a mother with active disease during the first year of life may be as high as 50%. Transplacental passage of TB is extremely rare.

Diagnosis

The Centers for Disease Control & Prevention recommend testing of pregnant women in high-risk groups (Table 27.1). Most pregnant women diagnosed with TB are asymptomatic and are only detected secondary to screening. There are currently two main screening methods, purified protein derivative (PPD) skin testing and interferon-gamma release assays (IGRAs). The PPD skin test is performed using an intradermal injection to produce a 6 to 10 mm wheal. The skin reaction is read at 48 to 72 hours by measuring the induration. Interpretation of the results depends on patient risk factors (Fig. 27.1). The IGRAs, Quantiferon TB Gold and T-Spot, can

Table 27.1 High-risk groups for latent tuberculosis

HIV-infected
Known recent contact with TB-infected person
Healthcare workers
Foreign-born (high-prevalence areas)
Alcohol and/or illicit drug use
Resident of a long-term care facility, prison or shelter
Organ transplant recipient

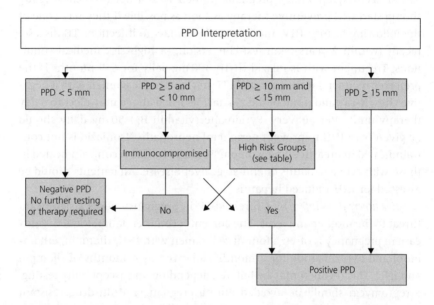

Figure 27.1 Interpretation of purified protein derivative (PPD) skin testing.

also be used to screen for latent TB and are useful in patients who have received BCG vaccination.

The definitive diagnosis of TB is based on identifying *M. tuberculosis* by culture or acid-fast stain of the sputum. First morning sputum specimens obtained on three consecutive days are usually the best source for detecting TB and should be undertaken in those with symptoms of active TB and those with a positive PPD and abnormal chest X-ray.

Treatment

A positive PPD only means that the patient has been previously exposed to TB and that there are latent organisms present. Less than 10% of patients with a positive PPD and an intact immune system will progress to active disease. However, targeted tuberculin skin testing for LTI is a strategic component of TB control to identify persons at high risk for developing TB who would benefit by treatment of LTI, if detected. Persons with increased risk for developing active TB include those who have recent infection with *M. tuberculosis* and those who have clinical conditions that are associated with an increased risk for progression of LTI to active TB, such as HIV infection, injection drug use, chest radiograph evidence or prior TB or chronic illness.

Latent infection: Individuals with LTI who are at high risk for progression to TB disease should be given high priority for treatment of LTI regardless of age. Asymptomatic pregnant women with a negative chest X-ray should start INH preventive therapy as soon as possible if they have one of the following factors: HIV infection; close contact to infectious TB disease; recent (within 2 years) skin test conversion; or high-risk medical conditions. Treatment with Isoniazid (INH) 300 mg daily for 6–9 months is the preferred regimen for treatment of LTI. Asymptomatic women with a negative chest X-ray and none of the risk factors listed above may elect to delay therapy until after delivery. Pyridoxine (vitamin B_6) 50 mg daily should be given with INH to prevent peripheral neuropathy. Isoniazid is not contraindicated in breastfeeding women. Isoniazid for LTI is contraindicated in those with active hepatitis or end-stage liver disease. All patients should be assessed for INH-induced hepatitis.

Active tuberculosis infection: Untreated TB in pregnancy poses a significant threat to the mother and fetus. The current recommendation for active disease in pregnancy is often a four drug regimen with INH, rifampin, ethambutol and pyrazinamide for 2 months, followed by 4 months of rifampin and INH. This regimen may be tailored depending on susceptibility testing. Streptomycin should be avoided during pregnancy. Multi-drug-resistant tuberculosis (MDR TB) is defined as resistance to at least INH and rifampin. Extensively drug-resistant tuberculosis (XDR TB) is resistant to at least INH, rifampin, fluoroquinolones and at least one of the injectable second-line drugs. Fortunately these remain rare in the United States – compliance with appropriate medication regimens remains one of the most important steps to prevent the development of drug resistance.

Complications

Congenital and neonatal TB are fortunately uncommon. They present with hepatosplenomegaly, fever, respiratory disease and lymphadenopathy. Neonatal infection is unlikely if the mother is adequately treated. Isolation of the uninfected newborn until the mother has a negative sputum culture is recommended.

Suggested reading

American College of Obstetricians and Gynecologists. Influenza vaccination during pregnancy. Committee Opinion No. 468. American College of Obstetricians and Gynecologists. *Obstet Gynecol* 2010;116:1006–7.

Centers for Disease Control and Prevention. Maternal and infant outcomes among severely ill pregnant and postpartum women with 2009 pandemic influenza A (H1N1) – United States, April 2009–August 2010. *MMWR* 2011;60(35):1193.

Centers for Disease Control and Prevention. (2013a). Final 2012 West Nile virus update. Available at: http://www.cdc.gov/ncidod/dvbid/westnile. Accessed May 21, 2014.

Centers for Disease Control and Prevention. Prevention and control of seasonal influenza with vaccines: recommendations of the Advisory Committee on Immunization Practices – United States, 2013–2014. *MMWR* 2013b;62(7):1.

Centers for Disease Control and Prevention. Updated recommendations for use of VariZIG-United States, 2013. *MMWR* 2013c;62(28):574.

Harger JH, Ernest JM, Thurnau GR, *et al.* Frequency of Congenital Varicella Syndrome in a Prospective Cohort of 347 Pregnant Women. *Obstet Gynecol* 2002;100(2):260–5.

http://www.cdc.gov/TB/publications/guidelines/default.htm. Accessed May 21, 2014.

http://www.cdc.gov/TB/statistics/default.htm. Accessed May 21, 2014.

Jamieson DJ, Honein MA, Rasmussen SA, Williams JL, *et al.* H1N1 2009 influenza virus infection during pregnancy in the USA. *Lancet* 2009;374:451–58.

Lamont RF, Sobel JD, Carrington D, *et al.* Varicella-zoster virus (chickenpox) infection in pregnancy. *BJOG* 2011;118:1155.

O'Leary DR, Kuhn S, Kniss KL, Hinckley AF, Pape WJ, Kightlinger LK, Beecham BD, Miller TK, Neitzel DF, Michaels SR, Campbell GL, Rasmussen SA, Hayes EB. Birth Outcomes Following West Nile Virus Infection of Pregnant Women, United States, 2003–2004. *Pediatrics* 2006;117(3):e537–45.

Rasmussen SA, Jamieson DJ, Uyeki TM. Effects of influenza on pregnant women and infants. *Am J Obstet Gynecol* 2012;207(3 Suppl):S3.

PROTOCOL 28

Malaria

Richard M.K. Adanu

Population Family and Reproductive Health Department, University of Ghana School of Public Health, Accra, Ghana, Africa

Malaria is a parasitic infestation caused by the protozoa *Plasmodium*, which is transmitted through the bite of the female Anopheles mosquito. The four species of *Plasmodium* responsible for malaria are *P. falciparum, P. vivax, P. ovale*, and *P. malariae*. *P. falciparum* is, however, responsible for most of the cases of malaria worldwide. It has been reported that, worldwide, there are about 350–500 cases of malaria annually with 1 to 3 million deaths. Malaria in pregnancy is responsible for 5–12% of all low birth weight (LBW) babies and for 35% of all preventable LBW deliveries resulting in 75,000 to 200,000 infant deaths per year. Over 90% of malaria cases occur in sub-Saharan Africa.

Clinical significance

Pregnancy results in a reduction in cell-mediated immunity. This decreased immunity makes pregnant women more susceptible to malaria than nonpregnant women. Among pregnant women, it has shown that primigravida are at increased risk from malaria than are multigravid women. Even in places that are holoendemic for malaria, where people have an acquired immunity to malaria, pregnant women tend to have more severe episodes of malaria and are more likely to die from the complications of malaria than other adults. The presentation and effects of malaria are more severe and result in higher case fatality when the sufferer, being from an area where the disease is not common, does not have any acquired immunity. Immunocompromised people such as those suffering from human immunodeficiency virus (HIV) infection also tend to suffer from more severe malaria with a higher mortality rate.

Anemia in pregnancy is estimated to occur in about 56% of all pregnancies in low-income countries. Figures for Africa give a prevalence

Protocols for High-Risk Pregnancies: An Evidence-Based Approach, Sixth Edition.
Edited by John T. Queenan, Catherine Y. Spong and Charles J. Lockwood.
© 2015 John Wiley & Sons, Ltd. Published 2015 by John Wiley & Sons, Ltd.

ranging from 35% in Southern Africa to 56% in West Africa. Untreated anemia leads to several complications in pregnancy and anemia-related causes play a major role in maternal mortality. Malaria in pregnancy is a major cause of anemia and this is one of the routes through which malaria causes maternal death.

Pathophysiology

Malaria starts with the bite of an infected female Anopheles mosquito. These mosquitoes usually bite between dusk and dawn. When a person is bitten by an infected mosquito, the sporozoite of the *Plasmodium* parasite is introduced into the bloodstream. In the bloodstream, the sporozoites move into the hepatocytes, where they mature and develop into the hepatic schizonts. This process takes between 7 and 30 days. These schizonts then burst within the hepatocytes resulting in the release of merozoites into the circulation. The merozoites enter the red blood cells and go through another stage of development to become trophozoites within the red blood cells. The trophozoites in the red blood cells develop into erythrocytic stage schizonts which later rupture and release merozoites into the blood stream. This erythrocytic stage of the life cycle is repeated several times resulting in the destruction of the red blood cells. Some of the trophozites later develop into the sexual form of the *Plasmodium* parasite known as gametocytes. These gametocytes are taken up by the female Anopheles mosquito when it bites an infected person. In the gut of the female Anopheles mosquito, the gametocytes develop into gametes, which then fuse and develop into sporozoites. The sporozoites migrate to the salivary glands of the mosquito from where they are transmitted to an uninfected person to re-start the life cycle of the parasite.

Clinical features

Infestation with *P. falciparum* initially causes a nonspecific flu-like reaction. This presents as a fever, headaches, and general malaise. Among people in holoendemic areas with acquired immunity, this stage of the disease might pass unnoticed. It is more severe in people without acquired immunity and in the immunocompromised resulting in mild jaundice and hepatosplenomegaly.

Malaria is characterized by febrile paroxysms, which occur with the periodic release of merozoites from the red blood cells. The febrile episodes last for between 6 and 10 hours and are characterized by three stages. There is first a cold stage, which causes intense shivering. This is followed by the development of a high-grade fever, which later breaks and brings on the sweating stage. After the resolution of these stages, symptoms subside for a time and then recur within 36 to 48 hours.

The repeated destruction of red blood cells during the erythrocytic stage of the life cycle results in anemia. The destruction of the red blood cells is also responsible for the jaundice that occurs during the disease. This is from the breakdown of the heme portion of the hemoglobin. There is also splenomegaly as the spleen works to remove the destroyed red blood cells from the circulation.

These clinical features are most severe in pregnant women without acquired immunity. Pregnant women with acquired immunity could be either less symptomatic or asymptomatic despite having *P. falciparum* infestation.

Pregnancy-associated malaria results in placental malaria, which occurs even when the pregnant woman is asymptomatic. In placental malaria, the *Plasmodium*-infected red blood cells accumulate in the intervillous spaces of the placenta leading to damage of the trophoblastic basement membrane. The infected red blood cells bind to receptors in the placenta and so affect oxygen and nutrient transport across the placenta. Placental malaria is responsible for the effects of malaria seen on the fetus. Placental malaria is more severe in primigravid women. Immunity to placental malaria has been shown to develop over successive pregnancies.

Diagnosis

Diagnosis of malaria in pregnancy is made by a combination of the clinical features and laboratory investigations. In holoendemic areas, there is a tendency to overdiagnose malaria because of over-reliance on symptomatology and because it is known that the complete clinical picture is rare among those with acquired immunity.

Suspicion of malaria should be followed by performing a thick or thin peripheral blood film for microscopic examination. The thick blood film is used for low parasitemias and the thin blood film for high parasitemias. The level of parasitemia as well as the species of *Plasmodium* present can be determined by microscopic examination. Microscopy is the gold standard for routine laboratory diagnosis of malaria and is very reliable when performed by a laboratory technologist with experience in malaria diagnosis.

In places where medical laboratories do not usually deal with malaria, polymerase chain reaction (PCR) procedures are more accurate for making the diagnosis even though the PCR-based diagnostic testing is more expensive and takes longer to arrive at a diagnosis. Where laboratory facilities and microscopy expertise are limited, rapid diagnostic tests, which are able to determine the presence of plasmodial antigens, can be used for diagnosis.

Treatment

The treatment of malaria in pregnancy is determined by the stage of pregnancy at which the disease is diagnosed (see Fig. 28.1).

The recommended treatment for malaria diagnosed in the first trimester is a combination of quinine and clindamycin. Quinine alone can be used if clindamycin in unavailable or unaffordable.

Malaria in the second and third trimesters is treated using artemisin-based combination therapy (ACT). The recommended forms of ACT are artemether-lumefantrine, artesunate plus amodiaquine, artesunate plus mefloquine, and atesunate plus sulfadoxine-pyremethamine.

The use of ACT in the first trimester is not recommended because of limited availability of data on its effects. It is, however, recommended that

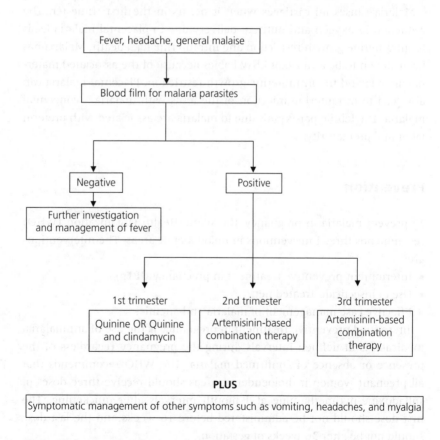

Figure 28.1 Flow chart for treatment of malaria in pregnancy.

in cases where ACT is the only available treatment it can be used in early pregnancy. In holoendemic areas, ACT is recommended as the standard preferred treatment in order to improve efficacy and limit drug resistance.

Anti-emetics and analgesics which are recommended for use in pregnancy are employed to manage severe vomiting, headaches and myalgia associated with malaria in pregnancy.

Complications

Malaria has effects on both the mother as well as the fetus. Malaria can result in severe anemia leading to cardiac failure. Malaria has been known to result in acute renal failure as a result of infected red blood cells causing endothelial damage and resultant reduced blood flow to the kidneys. It also causes hypoglycemia and could lead to central nervous complications of cerebral malaria characterized by seizures and loss of consciousness. These complications of malaria could result in maternal mortality.

Malaria causes miscarriages when it occurs in the first trimester. The reduction in oxygen and nutrient delivery due to placental malaria leads to intrauterine growth restriction and intrauterine fetal death. Malaria has been shown to be a cause of LBW babies because of the associated maternal anemia and the intrauterine growth restriction. Placental malaria can also lead to intrauterine infection of the fetus with malaria – congenital malaria. The febrile paroxysms due to malaria are associated with preterm labor and prematurity.

Prevention

To prevent malaria in pregnancy, the World Health Organization (WHO) recommends three interventions in holoendemic areas. The interventions are:
- Intermittent preventive treatment in pregnancy (IPTp)
- Use of insecticide-treated nets
- Effective case management of malaria and anemia.

Intermitted preventive treatment in pregnancy is the use of antimalarial medications at defined intervals during the pregnancy regardless of the presence or absence of confirmed malaria. The WHO recommends that all pregnant women in holoendemic areas should receive three doses of sulfadoxine-pyrimethamine at 1-month intervals after quickening. The first dose should not be administered before 16 weeks and the last dose should not be after 36 weeks of gestation.

It is recommended that pregnant women in holoendemic areas sleep under insecticide-treated bed-nets in order to reduce the frequency of mosquito bites during pregnancy.

Effective diagnosis and treatment of malaria helps prevent the occurrence of maternal and fetal complications of malaria.

Conclusion

Malaria in pregnancy is a leading cause of maternal morbidity and mortality with as many as 10,000 maternal deaths in sub-Saharan Africa being reported as due to malaria-related anemia. It is very important for both obstetricians and pregnant women to be aware of the disease so that proven methods of malaria prevention can be employed, there will be early reporting when symptoms of malaria are noticed, and recommended effective therapy is employed when the diagnosis is established.

Suggested Reading

Bardaji A, Sigauque B, Bruni L, Romagosa C, Sanz S, Mabunda S, *et al.* Clinical malaria in African pregnant women. *Malar J* 2008;7:27.

Brooks MI, Singh N, Hamer DH. Control measures for malaria in pregnancy in India. *Indian J Med Res* 2008 Sep;128(3):246–53.

Kabanywanyi AM, Macarthur JR, Stolk WA, Habbema JD, Mshinda H, Bloland PB, *et al.* Malaria in pregnant women in an area with sustained high coverage of insecticide-treated bed nets. *Malar J* 2008;7:133.

Lagerberg RE. Malaria in pregnancy: a literature review. *J Midwifery Womens Health* 2008 May;53(3):209–15.

Savage EJ, Msyamboza K, Gies S, D'Alessandro U, Brabin BJ. Maternal anaemia as an indicator for monitoring malaria control in pregnancy in sub-Saharan Africa. *BJOG* 2007 Oct;114(10):1222–31.

World Health Organization. Role of Laboratory Diagnosis to Support Malaria Disease Management – Report of a WHO Consultation. World Health Organization, Geneva; 2006a.

World Health Organization. The Use of Malaria Rapid Diagnostic Tests. 2nd ed. Geneva: World Health Organization; 2006b.

World Health Organization. Malaria in pregnancy. Guidelines for measuring key monitoring and evaluation indicators. Geneva: World Health Organization; 2007.

World Health Organization. Guidelines for the Treatment of Malaria. Geneva: World Health Organization; 2010.

World Health Organization. WHO policy brief for the implementation of intermittent preventive treatment of malaria in pregnancy using sulfadoxine-pyrimethamine (ITPp-SP). Geneva: World Health Organization; 2013.

PROTOCOL 29

Human Immunodeficiency Virus Infection

Jane Hitti
Department of Obstetrics and Gynecology, University of Washington, Seattle, WA, USA

Clinical significance

The past 20 years have brought tremendous advances in the prevention of human immunodeficiency virus (HIV) transmission from mother to infant. In the context of potent antiretroviral therapy (ART), excellent viral suppression (less than 1000 copies/µL) and absence of breastfeeding, perinatal transmission risk is approximately 1%. The increasing availability of potent ART in resource-limited settings, along with innovations such as prolonged maternal or infant antiretroviral prophylaxis during breast-feeding, promises the potential for similarly low perinatal transmission rates across the globe. However, in our enthusiasm to prevent pediatric HIV infection, obstetric providers also have an obligation to understand the impact of ART in pregnancy on women's health.

Pathophysiology

As a single-stranded ribonucleic acid (RNA) retrovirus, HIV has the ability to become incorporated into cellular deoxyribonucleic acid (DNA). It preferentially infects cells with the CD4 antigen, particularly T-helper lymphocytes (CD4 cells) and macrophages. At least two cell surface co-receptor molecules, CXCR4 and CCR5, help HIV to enter the host cell. Viral RNA is reverse-transcribed into proviral DNA, using the viral enzyme reverse transcriptase. The provirus enters the cell nucleus and integrates into the host cell genome using viral integrase, and will remain embedded in the host DNA for the lifetime of the cell, potentially creating a latent reservoir for HIV infection even during ART. When the host cell is stimulated to divide

---

Protocols for High-Risk Pregnancies: An Evidence-Based Approach, Sixth Edition.
Edited by John T. Queenan, Catherine Y. Spong and Charles J. Lockwood.

or in the context of other signals, proviral DNA is transcribed into viral RNA, eventually leading to the assembly of new virions; the viral enzyme protease assists with this process. The mature virions then bud from the host cell. Virions have a plasma half-life of about 6 hours. The high volume of HIV replication and high frequency of transcription errors by HIV reverse transcriptase and other enzymes result in many mutations, increasing the chance of producing strains resistant to host immunity and ART.

At the time of initial infection, there may be no symptoms or an acute mononucleosis-like syndrome, sometimes accompanied by aseptic meningitis, may develop. There is an immediate, dramatic viremia (up to a billion viral particles turned over per day) and a rapid immune response with similar levels of T-cell turnover. After the initial viremia, the level of virus returns to a set point at values that vary widely but average 30,000–100,000 copies/mL. In untreated chronic HIV infection about 10^8 to 10^9 virions are created and removed daily, accompanied by a similarly rapid turnover of host CD4 cells. The frenetic pace of viral replication and host-cell destruction create a proinflammatory environment that contributes to some of the clinical symptoms of HIV infection. The level of virus in the plasma at the time a set point is established correlates with long-term survival, in the absence of ART. The higher the set point, the more quickly the CD4 count decreases to a level that seriously impairs immunity (less than 200 cells/mL) and results in the opportunistic infections (e.g., *Pneumocystis carinii* pneumonia and central nervous system toxoplasmosis) and neoplasias (e.g., Kaposi sarcoma) that define acquired immunodeficiency syndrome (AIDS). A CD4 count drop below 200 cells/µL also makes the diagnosis of AIDS.

Diagnosis

- Recommend HIV serologic testing (ELISA and confirmatory Western blot) to all prenatal patients as part of standard prenatal care, using the opt-out model (see Fig. 29.1). Consider repeat testing in the third trimester if from a high prevalence area or engaged in risky behaviors.
  - Women with a positive ELISA and negative Western blot do not have HIV infection.
  - Women with an indeterminate Western blot may be in the process of HIV seroconversion. Repeat the Western blot and obtain a quantitative HIV RNA PCR. Seek expert consultation for interpretation of results.
- Offer a rapid HIV serologic test for women who present intrapartum with no documented prenatal HIV testing. These tests have high sensitivity but must be confirmed by standard serologic testing. Treatment to prevent transmission can begin prior to the confirmatory test.

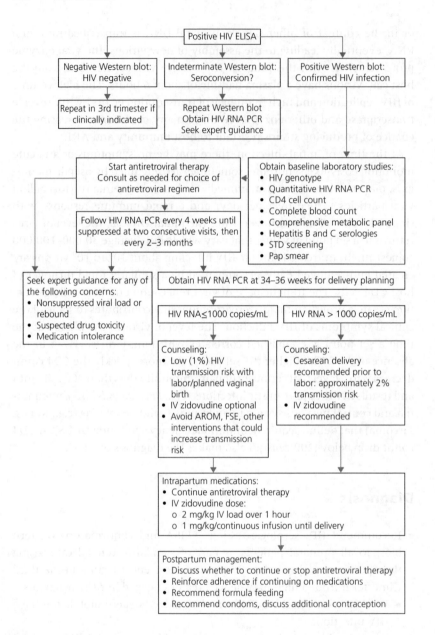

Figure 29.1   Algorithm for diagnosis and management of HIV in pregnancy.

- Obtain the following baseline laboratory studies for women with positive HIV serology:
  - HIV genotype, to assess for viral mutations and potential drug resistance
  - Quantitative HIV RNA by PCR, or viral load

- CD4 cell count, to assess immune status
- Complete blood count and comprehensive metabolic panel
- Hepatitis B and C serology, and viral loads if applicable
- Comprehensive STD screening, if not already completed (syphilis, chlamydia, gonorrhea)
- Pap smear, if not already completed.

Treatment

Standard ART requires the combination of at least three effective antiretroviral medications with the goal of complete viral suppression. Current recommended first-line regimens generally include two nucleoside reverse transcriptase inhibitors (NRTI) in combination with a third agent, which may be a non-nucleoside reverse transcriptase inhibitor (NNRTI), integrase inhibitor or protease inhibitor (PI). Co-formulations that combine two or three ART agents are now available, allowing for once-daily pill options for some patients. Specific medication choices should be made on the basis of HIV genotype if known, maternal co-morbidities, available data regarding maternal and fetal safety, expected adverse effect profile and other factors; expert consultation is recommended. The importance of excellent adherence must be emphasized, so as to avoid development of drug resistance.

In addition, women with CD4 cell counts below 200 cells/mL should receive *Pneumocystis carinii* prophylaxis (PCP) with an agent such as trimethoprim-sulfamethoxazole (TMP-SMZ). Women with CD4 cell counts below 100 cells/mL should receive prophylaxis against other opportunistic infections such as toxoplasmosis and *Mycobacterium avium* complex.

Available data and treatment options for HIV in pregnancy continue to expand rapidly. The Department of Health and Human Services Perinatal HIV Guidelines Working Group maintains a comprehensive, frequently updated summary of treatment recommendations at the following website: www.aidsinfo.nih.gov/contentfiles/perinatalGL.pdf.

Follow up

After initiation of ART, HIV viral load should be followed every 4 weeks until not detectable for at least two consecutive measurements. For women with a suppressed viral load, monitoring should occur every 2–3 months. A viral load should be obtained at 34–36 weeks to assist with delivery planning. Toxicity monitoring including complete blood count and comprehensive metabolic panel should occur, at a minimum, 4 weeks after initiation of ART and every 2–3 months thereafter. CD4 counts can be followed as clinically indicated.

Failure to suppress viral load, or rebound after suppression, may indicate poor adherence to medication and/or the development of viral resistance. The viral load should be repeated and another HIV genotype obtained. The patient should be asked in detail about skipped medication doses and any barriers to adherence. Expert consultation is suggested with regard to medication switches for virologic failure, toxicity or tolerability concerns.

Intrapartum management

- Planned labor and vaginal delivery is appropriate for women with viral suppression. Labor management should avoid amniotomy, fetal scalp electrode, and other invasive procedures.
- Planned cesarean delivery prior to labor will reduce perinatal HIV transmission for women with viral load greater than 1000 copies/μL. Per ACOG guidelines, cesarean delivery to prevent HIV transmission may be scheduled at 38 weeks without amniocentesis for fetal lung maturity testing.
- Intravenous zidovudine has long been recommended as intrapartum prophylaxis during active labor, or prior to a scheduled cesarean delivery. Recent guidelines have called into question the necessity of using IV zidovudine for women with a suppressed viral load; IV zidovudine is still recommended for women with detectable virus. The dose is 2 mg/kg IV load over 1 hour, followed by 1 mg/kg/hour continuous infusion until delivery.

Postpartum management

- The decision to continue or stop ART after delivery requires careful counseling. In general, women with a nadir CD4 count less than 500 cells/mL should continue ART for their own health. The health benefit for continuing medications for women with higher CD4 counts has not been well established, and is under active investigation.
- Women who do continue ART should be counseled about the challenges of maintaining excellent adherence in the early postpartum period, and should be helped to develop strategies to stay adherent to their regimen.
- Breastfeeding is not recommended unless there are no safe alternatives. In resource-limited settings with no safe water supply, exclusive breastfeeding is recommended over mixed feeding.

Prevention

Condom use is universally recommended to prevent STD acquisition as well as HIV transmission. There is a theoretical risk of super-infection with another HIV virus, so condoms are recommended even among partners who are both HIV-infected. A second method of contraception should be offered in addition to condoms for women who do not want another pregnancy in the near future. There are no contraindications to the use of intrauterine devices, emergency contraception and most hormonal contraception for HIV-infected women.

Conclusion

This protocol provides a brief summary of a complex topic. The choice of regimen and the starting point for initiating therapy should be tailored to the individual patient's needs and should be decided upon in collaboration with an HIV expert who will assume the ongoing care of the patient in the postpartum period. That same expert should be called upon to provide guidance in those cases in which adequate response to a first course of therapy is not obtained or the need for prophylaxis or treatment of opportunistic infections arises. Obstetricians have made a remarkable contribution to the rapid advances in the field of HIV, including improved survival and reduced rates of mother-to-child transmission. However, challenges remain and the price of progress has been complexity. By assisting women to learn their serostatus, to get optimal therapy and to be adherent to treatment, obstetricians will continue to earn their reputation as the principal advocates for the health of all pregnant women.

Suggested reading

American College of Obstetricians and Gynecologists. Scheduled Cesarean delivery and the prevention of vertical transmission of HIV infection. ACOG Committee Opinion 234. Washington, DC: ACOG; 2000. . (Reaffirmed 2010).

Connor EM, Sperling RS, Gelber R, *et al.* Reduction of maternal-infant transmission of human immunodeficiency virus type 1 with zidovudine treatment. *N Engl J Med* 1994;331(18):1173–80.

Garcia PM, Kalish LA, Pitt J, *et al.* Maternal levels of plasma human immunodeficiency virus type 1 RNA and the risk of perinatal transmission. *N Engl J Med* 1999;341(6): 394–402.

International Perinatal HIV Group. The mode of delivery and the risk of vertical transmission of human immunodeficiency virus type 1: a meta-analysis of 15 prospective cohort studies. *N Engl J Med* 1999;340(13):977–87.

Ioannidis JPA, Abrams EJ, Ammann A, *et al.* Perinatal transmission of human immun-odeficiency virus type 1 by pregnant women with RNA virus loads <1000 copies/mL. *J Infect Dis* 2001;183(4):539–45.

Panel on Treatment of HIV-Infected Pregnant Women and Prevention of Perinatal Trans-mission. Recommendations for Use of Antiretroviral Drugs in Pregnant HIV-1-Infected Women for Maternal Health *and* Interventions to Reduce Perinatal HIV Transmis-sion in the United States. Available at http://aidsinfo.nih.gov/contentfiles/lvguidelines /PerinatalGL.pdf. Accessed August 4, 2014.

Prenatal and Perinatal Human Immunodeficiency Virus Testing: Expanded Recommen-dations. ACOG Committee Opinion No. 418. American College of Obstetricians and Gynecologists. *Obstet Gynecol* 2008;112:739–42. (Reaffirmed 2011).

Tai JH, Udoji MA, Barkanic G, Byrne DW, Rebeiro PF, *et al.* Pregnancy and HIV disease progression during the era of highly active antiretroviral therapy. *J Infect Dis* 2007;196: 1044–52.

Wade NA, Birkhead GS, Warren BL, *et al.* Abbreviated regimens of zidovudine prophy-laxis and perinatal transmission of the human immunodeficiency virus. *N Engl J Med* 1998;339(20):1409–14.

World Health Organization. Hormonal contraceptive methods for women at high risk of HIV and living with HIV: 2014 guidance statement. WHO reference number: WHO/RHR/14.24. Available at http://apps.who.int/iris/bitstream/10665/128537/1 /WHO_RHR_14.24_eng.pdf?ua=1. Accessed August 4, 2014.

Parvovirus B19 Infection

Maureen P. Malee
University of Illinois McKinley Health Center, Urbana, IL, USA

Overview

The spectrum of clinical manifestations caused by parvovirus B19 infection, a single-stranded DNA virus, is unlikely completely described. In the normal host, B19 infection can be manifest as an asymptomatic or subclinical infection, erythema infectiosum (EI) or fifth disease, or as an arthropathy. In patients with thalassemia or sickle cell disease, B19 infection can cause a severe transient red cell aplasia (transient aplastic crisis; TAC). In the immunocompromised population, B19 infection can persist and manifest as chronic anemia. In the fetus, B19 infection is associated with anemia, nonimmune hydrops and death.

Pathophysiology

The rash of EI and B19 arthralgias are thought to be secondary to an immunological phenomenon. The hematological manifestations of B19 infection result from selective infection and lysis of erythroid precursor cells with interruption of normal red blood cell production. In the otherwise healthy but infected host, this infection produces a limited and clinically unapparent red cell aplasia. However, in the patient with chronic red cell destruction, dependent upon the ability to increase red blood cell production, B19 infection may lead to aplastic crisis.

The pathogenesis of fetal and congenital disease is fairly well understood. Infection of the fetus occurs through transplacental passage of the virus. The red cell aplasia is particularly devastating for the fetus, given the dramatic increase in red cell mass necessary to promote accelerated growth, as well as the shortened life span of the fetal red cell. Transient pleural or pericardial effusions may reflect direct pleural or myocardial inflammation. The pathogenic mechanism of hydrops is associated with severe

Protocols for High-Risk Pregnancies: An Evidence-Based Approach, Sixth Edition.
Edited by John T. Queenan, Catherine Y. Spong and Charles J. Lockwood.
© 2015 John Wiley & Sons, Ltd. Published 2015 by John Wiley & Sons, Ltd.

fetal anemia, which may result in tissue hypoxia and increased capillary permeability, as well as increased cardiac output and increased umbilical venous pressure. High output cardiac failure results is associated with increased hydrostatic pressure and decreased venous return, and as a result of ascites and/or organomegaly, leads to further cardiac decompensation. Compromised hepatic function and placental hydrops likely play a role as well.

Epidemiology

B19 is presumably transmitted person-to-person through direct contact with respiratory secretions, vertically from mother to fetus, and via transfusion with contaminated blood products or needles.

Cases of EI occur sporadically and as part of school outbreaks. The peak incidence of B19 infection occurs among school-aged children, with reported attack rates amongst susceptible students between 34% and 72%. Patients with EI are likely most contagious before the onset of the rash, and may remain contagious for a few days after appearance of the rash. During school outbreaks, reported attack rates amongst employees vary from 12% to 84%, with the highest rates in elementary school teachers, reflecting exposure to greater numbers of children or a greater likelihood of contacting respiratory secretions of younger children. When serological criteria are used, the frequency of asymptomatic infection was greater than 50% in most studies. Healthcare workers are another susceptible population, with over 30% demonstrating seroconversion following exposure to children with TAC.

Diagnosis

Seroprevalence
The seroprevalence of specific IgG antibodies increases with age, and is below 5% in those less than 5 years of age. The greatest increase in seroprevalence occurs between 5 and 20 years of age, increasing from 5% to 40%. Seroprevalence then increases more slowly, exceeding 75% by 50 years of age.

Specific IgM antibodies can be detected 10 days after inoculation, and IgG is detectable 2–3 days thereafter. Rash/arthropathy may develop about 18 days after inoculation. IgM antibodies persist typically for months, and IgG antibodies persist for years. Antibodies are detected by enzyme-linked immunoabsorbent assay (ELISA) or radioimmunoassay (RIA) and viral DNA by polymerase chain reaction.

An individual is susceptible in the absence of documented IgM and IgG. The presence of only IgG denotes an immune individual, who may have been infected as recently as 4 months previously. The presence of only IgM denotes a very recent infection, whereas the presence of both IgM and IgG is typical of a patient with recent (typically 7 days to 4 months) exposure.

Fifth disease

The most frequently recognized manifestation of B19 infection is the rash illness, EI. The most distinctive feature of EI, or slapped cheek disease, is an erythematous maculopapular rash that affects the cheeks and typically spares the remainder of the face. The trunk and extremities are also affected, and the rash may be pruritic. The rash occurs coincidentally with the production of specific antibodies, suggesting that it is an immune-mediated phenomenon.

Arthralgias, sometimes accompanied by inflammatory changes in affected joints, are a manifestation of acute B19 infection and can accompany EI, particularly in adults. Arthropathy, most often affecting wrists, hands and knees, can also be the sole manifestation of B19 infection. As with the rash, onset of arthropathy is accompanied by a rise in anti-B19 antibodies, suggesting an immunological phenomenon.

Fifth disease and pregnancy

Sequelae
Many pregnant women are susceptible to B19 infection, as the reported seroprevalence in reproductive-aged and pregnant women is between 35% and 55%. The infection rate during pregnancy is estimated at 1.1%. Transplacental transmission of B19 to the fetus may be common after maternal infection, but the frequency with which infection occurs is uncertain, and whether efficiency of transmission varies with gestational age is unknown. Many infants infected in utero are asymptomatic at birth.

Adverse pregnancy outcomes following B19 infection include nonimmune hydrops and fetal death. It is difficult to say with certainty the proportion of all deaths attributable to B19 infection. At present, it appears that the primary mechanism leading to fetal death is anemia and hydrops, in those gestations before 20 weeks, with demise usually in the second trimester. The crude fetal death rate is less than 10%. In the United States, it is likely that less than 1% of all demises result from B19 infection. Although infection with B19 may be a common cause of nonimmune hydrops especially during community outbreaks of EI, it does not follow that intrauterine

B19 infection frequently causes hydrops. The most common outcome is normal seronegative newborns, followed by liveborn seropositive babies and finally hydrops in less than 1%. Although there are case reports which support a link between B19 infection and congenital malformations, the relationship is not supported by epidemiological studies.

Management

Our knowledge of optimal management of B19 infection in pregnancy lags behind our understanding of the potential adverse consequences. As a result, there are considerable resources devoted to the pregnancy with this diagnosis, even though there are little data demonstrating efficacy of any particular therapeutic approach or intervention.

In the event that a pregnant patient presents with complaints potentially consistent with B19 infection, such as arthralgias, exposure to someone with EI, hydropic changes or a death on ultrasonography, for example, maternal blood should be sent for determination of anti-B19 IgM and IgG antibodies to determine immunity or risk. In the event of a school outbreak of EI, the decision to limit presumptive exposure of a pregnant schoolteacher should be individualized, as the risk of that teacher becoming infected and suffering a fetal demise is less than 1.5%. Intrauterine B19 infection can be determined by polymerase chain reaction DNA detection of viral B19 in amniotic fluid or fetal blood. An amniocentesis is the method of choice for fetal diagnosis, as cordocentesis carries a 1% loss rate.

There are no studies to identify the optimal management of a pregnant patient with an acute B19 infection. As the spectrum of fetal response is no effect versus hydrops versus demise, and the only treatment for hydropic changes is transfusion, which cannot be accomplished easily before 20 weeks, many question the utility of serial surveillance before 20 weeks. Serial ultrasonography is often advocated when infection is thought to have occurred before 20 weeks, as the peak in fetal morbidity and mortality is 4–6 weeks post-exposure, and as late as 3 months following onset of symptoms. However, the yield of such intensive observation is low. Serial determinations of fetal middle cerebral artery (MCA) Doppler velocimetry for detection of anemia has utility in the management of a B19-infected fetus, as increasing anemia may precede hydropic changes. If the MCA Doppler peak systolic velocity (PSV) (done after 18 weeks of gestation) is greater than 1.5 MOMs for gestational age, a periumbilical blood sampling (PUBs) can be offered to determine the fetal hematocrit, and would be the suggested plan for the overtly hydropic fetus. If anemia is detected, a transfusion to replace half of the RBC volume is accomplished during the same procedure, and the remainder in the next 48 hours. This strategy can be followed until the fetus recovers from the infection. However, this intervention is not without its own inherent risk of fetal morbidity and mortality (1% fetal loss). Two retrospective series demonstrate that transfusion confers a survival advantage to fetuses with B19-associated hydrops. There are no B19 vaccines for B19 immunization available at this time, and the role of hyperimmune serum globulin in the prevention or modification of B19 infection is unclear.

Summary

Intrauterine B19 infection is a cause of fetal anemia, hydrops and death, but unlikely of congenital anomalies. The best strategy for surveillance of the infected pregnant patient is unclear, as are strategies to decrease infection rate and untoward outcomes.

Suggested Reading

American College of Obstetricians and Gynecologists. Perinatal viral and parasitic infections. ACOG Practice Bulletin No. 20. ACOG: Washington, DC; 2000.

Centers for Disease Control. Risks associated with human parvovirus B19 infection. *MMWR* 1989;38:81–8.

Cosmi E, Mari G, Chiaie LD, Detti L, *et al.* Noninvasive diagnosis by Doppler ultrasonography of fetal anemia resulting from parvovirus infection. *Am J Obstet Gynecol* 2002;187:1290–3.

Divakaran TG, Waugh J, Clark TJ, Khan KS, Whittle MJ, Kilby MD. Noninvasive techniques to detect fetal anemia due to red blood cell alloimmunization: a systematic review. *Obstet Gynecol* 2001;98:509–17.

Goldenberg RL, Thompson C. The infectious origins of stillbirth. *Am J Obstet Gynecol* 2003;189:861–73.

Harger JH, Adler SP, Koch WC, Harger GF. Prospective evaluation of 618 pregnant women exposed to parvovirus B19: risks and symptoms. *Obstet Gynecol* 1998;91:413–20.

Hernandez-Andrade E, Scheier M, Dezerega V, Carmo A, Nicolaides KH. Fetal middle cerebral artery peak systolic velocity in the investigation of nonimmune hydrops. *Ultrasound Obstet Gynecol* 2004;23:442–5.

Kinney J, Anderson L, Farrar J, *et al.* Risk of adverse outcomes of pregnancy after human parvovirus B19 infection. *J Infect Dis* 1988;157:663.

Miller E, Fairley CK, Cohen BJ, Seng C. Immediate and long-term outcome of human parvovirus B19 infection in pregnancy. *Br J Obstet Gynecol* 1998;105:174–8.

Parilla BV, Tamura RK, Ginsberg NA. Association of parvovirus infection with isolated fetal effusions. *Am J Perinatol* 1997;14:357.

Pickering LK, Reves RR. Occupational risks for chil-care providers and teachers. *JAMA* 1990;263:2096.

Tolfvenstam T, Papadogiannakis N, Norbeck O, Petersson K, Broliden K. Frequency of human parvovirus B19 infection in intrauterine fetal death. *Lancet* 2001;357:1494–7.

Torok TJ. Human Parvovirus B19. In: Remington JS, Klein JO, editors. Infectious Diseases of the Fetus and Newborn Infant. Philadelphia: Saunders; 2001. p 770–811.

PROTOCOL 31

Group B Streptococcus

Mara J. Dinsmoor[1,2]

[1] Department of Obstetrics and Gynecology, NorthShore University Health System HealthSystem, Evanston, IL, USA
[2] Department of Obstetrics and Gynecology, Pritzker School of Medicine, University of Chicago, Chicago, IL, USA

Clinical significance

Between 10% and 30% of pregnant women are colonized with group B streptococcus (GBS), formally known as *Streptococcus agalactiae*. Colonization may result in symptomatic infection in some women, most commonly manifested as chorioamnionitis, postpartum endometritis, or urinary tract infections. Intrapartum and postpartum bacteremia may also occur in the face of maternal infection. Neonates may be colonized and develop symptomatic infections by transmission from the mother or by contact transmission in the nursery. These neonatal infections, including localized infections, meningitis, or septicemia, carry a high risk of sequelae, and are potentially fatal.

Pathophysiology

Carriage of GBS may be intermittent, and risk factors for maternal GBS colonization are imprecise, although African–American women and non-smokers appear to be at higher risk. However, risk factors for transmission to, and subsequent infection of, the neonate are well characterized. They include prematurity (less than 37 weeks of gestation), prolonged membrane rupture (18 hours or more), and fever in labor (100.5 °F or higher). The increased risk with prematurity is thought to be a result of incomplete GBS antibody transfer across the immature placenta. The latter two risk factors are likely related to prolonged contact with the organism and increased colony counts in the presence of acute maternal infection. Having a prior infected neonate is also a risk factor for having subsequent infected babies. Overall, the risk of neonatal colonization following delivery to a colonized

Protocols for High-Risk Pregnancies: An Evidence-Based Approach, Sixth Edition.
Edited by John T. Queenan, Catherine Y. Spong and Charles J. Lockwood.
© 2015 John Wiley & Sons, Ltd. Published 2015 by John Wiley & Sons, Ltd.

Table 31.1 Rate of early-onset neonatal group B streptococcus sepsis in the presence of maternal colonization and/or risk factors (prematurity, prolonged membrane rupture, fever in labor

Maternal colonization	Risk factor(s)	Rate per 1000 births
Present	Present	40.8
Present	Absent	5.1
Absent	Present	0.9
Absent	Absent	0.3

Source: Adapted from Boyer and Gotoff, 1985.

mother, in the absence of treatment, is approximately 50%. Up to 2% of these infants will develop symptomatic disease, so that the overall risk of neonatal disease following delivery to a colonized mother is less than 10 per 1000 exposed births, and is as low as 1–2 per 1000 in term neonates (Table 31.1).

There are five major serotypes of GBS (Ia, Ib, II, III, and V), and all appear capable of causing both maternal and neonatal disease. Serotype III is found in most cases of neonatal late-onset disease. Babies born to mothers who do not have antibodies to types II and III GBS appear to be at increased risk for developing GBS disease. Because of its predominance in neonatal infections, efforts at creating an effective vaccine have focused on serotype III.

Diagnosis

The most accurate mode of diagnosis of GBS is by culture. Although GBS will grow on ordinary blood agar, use of selective media will increase the detection of GBS by about 50%. For this reason, it is currently recommended that all GBS cultures be performed on sheep blood agar following incubation in selective broth medium. Examples include Todd-Hewitt broth supplemented with antibiotics and the commercially available medium, Trans-Vag broth, supplemented with 5% defibrinated sheep blood or LIM broth.

Most GBS cultures are done in the setting of late pregnancy (35–37 weeks), in an attempt to identify colonized women, so that they may be offered intrapartum antibiotic prophylaxis (IPAP). The highest yield is obtained when the culture is obtained from the distal vagina and the rectum, not anal orifice. Swabbing only the cervix or vaginal fornix will fail to detect approximately 50% of colonized women. To guide intrapartum therapy, antibiotic susceptibility testing should be performed on all isolates from penicillin-allergic women. GBS is also frequently isolated from amniotic fluid cultures obtained during the evaluation of patients with suspected subclinical or clinical intraamniotic infection.

In the postpartum period, GBS is commonly found in endometrial cultures from patients with postpartum endometritis. Some patients with uterine infections with GBS will also have bacteremia with the same organism. GBS rarely causes endocarditis in immunocompetent patients, but there have been case reports of endocarditis due to GBS.

Although a number of rapid tests for the detection of GBS have been evaluated, none have proven adequately sensitive for clinical use. A polymerase chain reaction (PCR)-based test has been developed, but is not widely available and is prohibitively expensive even in those institutions with PCR technology available.

The Centers for Disease Control and Prevention (CDC) currently recommend obtaining vaginal/rectal cultures in pregnant women between 35 and 37 weeks of gestation. These recommendations have been endorsed by the American Congress of Obstetricians and Gynecologists, the American Academy of Pediatrics, the American College of Nurse-Midwives, and the American Academy of Family Physicians.

Treatment

The recommended treatment regimens for intrapartum GBS prophylaxis are outlined in Table 31.2.

The treatment of clinically evident GBS infection depends somewhat on the clinical context in which it is identified. Appropriate antibiotic choices include penicillin, ampicillin, and first-generation cephalosporins. Because there has been increasing resistance of GBS strains to clindamycin

Table 31.2 Recommended regimens for intrapartum antibiotic prophylaxis*

Recommended	Penicillin G: 5 million units IV followed by 2.5–3.0 million units IV every 4 hours
Alternative	Ampicillin: 2 g IV followed by 1 g IV every 4 hours
Penicillin allergy: not high risk for anaphylaxis	Cefazolin: 2 g IV followed by 1 g IV every 8 hours
Penicillin allergy: high risk for anaphylaxis†	Clindamycin: 900 mg IV every 8 hours
Penicillin allergy: GBS resistant to clindamycin or erythromycin, or sensitivities unknown	Vancomycin: 1 g IV every 12 hours

*All antibiotics to be discontinued following delivery, in the absence of the clinical diagnosis of maternal infection.
†History of immediate hypersensitivity or history of anaphylaxis, angioedema, respiratory distress or urticaria following administration of a penicillin or cephalosporin.
Source: Adapted from Centers for Disease Control and Prevention, 2010.

and erythromycin, treatment of the penicillin-allergic patient should be based, if at all possible, on the results of sensitivity testing of the isolate. Up to 20% of GBS strains may be resistant to either clindamycin or erythromycin. The practitioner should also be mindful of the poor placental transfer of erythromycin when choosing this drug to treat any maternal infection that may potentially be transmitted to the fetus *in utero*. In addition, resistance to erythromycin is often associated with resistance to clindamycin as well. Vancomycin is another appropriate antibiotic choice for the penicillin-allergic patient, although concerns regarding the selection of vancomycin-resistant enterococcus and maternal side effects should temper its use.

Mothers who are colonized with GBS in the late third trimester should be offered IPAP, with penicillin being the preferred agent (Fig. 31.1). Patients with unknown GBS colonization status who are less than 37 weeks of gestation should also be offered IPAP. All mothers who have previously delivered a baby infected with invasive GBS disease should be offered IPAP, and the antepartum GBS culture may be eliminated.

Preterm labor

A GBS culture should be performed at the time of admission for preterm labor, and GBS prophylaxis begun (Fig. 31.2). If the preterm labor is arrested, or the culture is negative, the prophylactic antibiotics should be discontinued. If preterm labor recurs within 5 weeks of a negative culture, GBS prophylaxis is not necessary. If the initial culture was positive, GBS prophylaxis should be administered, regardless of the gestational age at which delivery occurs. If labor occurs 5 or more weeks later, and the patient is still preterm, GBS prophylaxis should be re-administered while awaiting the results of a repeat GBS culture. Patients with a negative culture at the time of preterm labor should be rescreened at 35–37 weeks if still pregnant, and treatment based on the most recent results.

Preterm premature rupture of the membranes

A GBS culture should be performed at the time of admission with preterm premature rupture of the membranes (PPROM) (Fig. 31.3). In most cases, the antibiotics administered to prolong the latency period will provide adequate coverage for GBS. If the culture is positive or the results are not yet known at the time of labor, GBS prophylaxis should be provided. If the culture is negative and labor occurs less than 5 weeks later, no further GBS prophylaxis is required. If 5 or more weeks have elapsed since the culture was obtained, either another culture should be performed, or if in labor, the patient should be managed based on the presence or absence of risk factors – i.e., given GBS prophylaxis for prolonged membrane rupture.

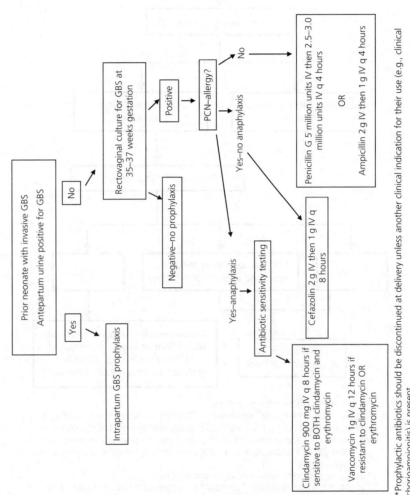

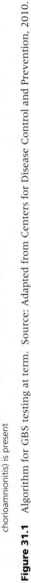

*Prophylactic antibiotics should be discontinued at delivery unless another clinical indication for their use (e.g., clinical chorioamnionitis) is present

Figure 31.1   Algorithm for GBS testing at term.   Source: Adapted from Centers for Disease Control and Prevention, 2010.

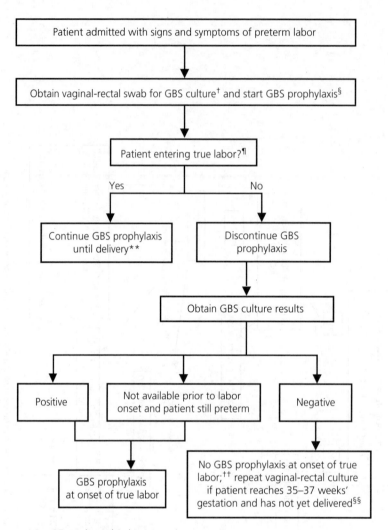

* At <37 weeks and 0 days' gestation.
† If patient has undergone vaginal-rectal GBS culture within the preceding 5
  weeks, the results of that culture should guide management. GBS-colonized
  women should receive intrapartum antibiotic prophylaxis. No antibiotics are
  indicated for GBS prophylaxis if a vaginal-rectal screen within 5 weeks was
  negative.
§ See Figure 8 for recommended antibiotic regimens.
¶ Patient should be regularly assessed for progression to true labor; if the
  patient is considered not to be in true labor, discontinue GBS prophylaxis.
** If GBS culture results become available prior to delivery and are negative,
  then discontinue GBS prophylaxis.
†† Unless subsequent GBS culture prior to delivery is positive.
§§ A negative GBS screen is considered valid for 5 weeks. If a patient with a history
  of PTL is re-admitted with signs and symptoms of PTL and had a negative GBS
  screen >5 weeks prior, she should be rescreened and managed according to
  this algorithm at that time.

Figure 31.2 Algorithm for GBS screening and prophylaxis in the setting of preterm
labor. Source: Adapted from Centers for Disease Control and Prevention, 2010.

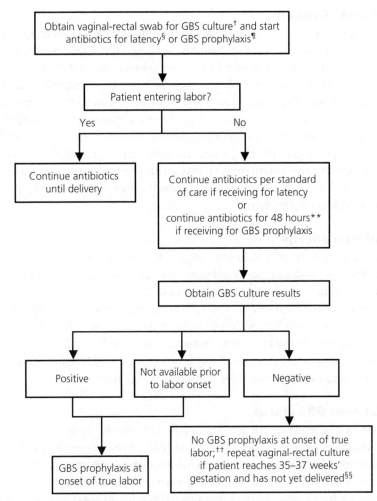

* At <37 weeks and 0 days' gestation.
† If patient has undergone vaginal-rectal GBS culture within the preceding 5 weeks, the results of that culture should guide management. GBS-colonized women should receive intrapartum antibiotic prophylaxis. No antibiotics are indicated for GBS prophylaxis if a vaginal-rectal screen within 5 weeks was negative.
§ Antibiotics given for latency in the setting of pPROM that include ampicillin 2 g intravenously (IV) once, followed by 1 g IV every 6 hours for at least 48 hours are adequate for GBS prophylaxis. If other regimens are used, GBS prophylaxis should be initiated in addition.
¶ See Figure 8 for recommended antibiotic regimens.
** GBS prophylaxis should be discontinued at 48 hours for women with pPROM who are not in labor. If results from a GBS screen performed on admission become available during the 48-hour period and are negative, GBS prophylaxis should be discontinued at that time.
†† Unless subsequent GBS culture prior to delivery is positive.
§§ A negative GBS screen is considered valid for 5 weeks. If a patient with pPROM is entering labor and had a negative GBS screen >5 weeks prior, she should be rescreened and managed according to this algorithm at that time.

Figure 31.3 Algorithm for GBS screening and prophylaxis in the setting of preterm premature rupture of the membranes. Source: Adapted from Centers for Disease Control and Prevention, 2010.

Cesarean Delivery

Although IPAP is not indicated in women undergoing planned cesarean delivery prior to labor or membrane rupture, the CDC recommends obtaining antepartum cultures from these patients so that IPAP may be offered in the event of membrane rupture prior to scheduled cesarean delivery. Cesarean delivery should not be delayed, however, to complete 4 hours of IPAP. Given that it is also recommended that women undergoing cesarean delivery be given perioperative antibiotic prophylaxis, usually a cephalosporin given prior to skin incision, many practitioners choose not to perform the antepartum culture, with the understanding that the administration of perioperative prophylactic antibiotics also serves to reduce GBS in the newborn.

Penicillin allergy

In those patients with a significant allergy to penicillin or a cephalosporin (anaphylaxis, angioedema, respiratory distress, urticaria), antibiotic sensitivity testing should be performed on all GBS isolates. If the isolate is sensitive to **both** clindamycin and erythromycin, the preferred IPAP regimen is clindamycin (900 mg IV q 8 hours). If not susceptible to clindamycin and erythromycin, the preferred regimen is vancomycin (1 g IV a 12 hours). If the severity of the penicillin allergy is unknown, consideration should be given to referring the patient for penicillin-allergy testing.

Unknown GBS status

In laboring patients *at term* for whom antepartum GBS culture results are not available, patients should be offered IPAP in the presence of risk factors for invasive GBS disease, i.e. prolonged membrane rupture (18 hours or more) or fever in labor. Ideally, women with a fever in labor should be treated for clinical chorioamnionitis, with a broad-spectrum antibiotic regimen that includes coverage for GBS.

Prevention

Although the CDC algorithms outlined above have reduced the incidence of early onset neonatal GBS sepsis by 50–80%, there are persistent cases that still occur. Some are a result of a false-negative maternal antepartum culture, while others are a result of "protocol violations" – i.e., the failure to administer appropriate or adequate antibiotic prophylaxis. Lastly, some babies will develop GBS sepsis despite appropriate and timely intrapartum antibiotic treatment. Although prevention of GBS sepsis appears to be effective, whether or not the overall incidence of early-onset neonatal sepsis is decreasing is somewhat controversial. Some institutions are reporting increases in neonatal infections with gram-negative organisms, particularly *Escherichia coli*, and particularly in low birth-weight babies. Although vaccine trials have been promising, no vaccine is currently available.

Conclusion

GBS is commonly isolated in maternal and neonatal infections, and can potentially lead to mortality and serious morbidity. However, since 1994, when the initial draft of the CDC guidelines for the prevention of GBS disease was released, the incidence of neonatal early-onset GBS sepsis has been declining. Although not well studied, maternal GBS disease may also be reduced by prenatal screening and intrapartum treatment. The long-term effects of such widespread antibiotic use remain unclear, however.

Suggested reading

Boyer KM, Gotoff SP. Strategies for chemoprophylaxis of GBS early-onset infections. *Antibiot Chemother* 1985;35:267–80.

Boyer KM, Gotoff SP. Prevention of early-onset neonatal group B streptococcal disease with selective intrapartum chemoprophylaxis. *N Engl J Med* 1986;314:1665–9.

Centers for Disease Control and Prevention. Prevention of perinatal group B streptococcal disease. *MMWR Recomm Rep* 2010;59:1–32.

Centers for Disease Control and Prevention. Perinatal Group B streptococcal disease after universal screening recommendations. *MMWR* 2007;46:701–5.

Honest H, Sharma S, Khan K. Rapid tests for group B streptococcus colonization in laboring women: a systematic review. *Pediatrics* 2006;117:1055–66.

Schrag SJ, Zell ER, Lynfield R, *et al.* A population-based comparison of strategies to prevent early-onset group B streptococcal disease in neonates. *N Engl J Med* 2002;347: 233–9.

Stoll BJ, Hansen N, Fanaroff AA, *et al.* Changes in pathogens causing early-onset sepsis in very-low-birth-weight infants. *N Engl J Med* 2002;347:240–7.

Van Dyke MK, Phares CR, Lynfield R, *et al.* Evaluation of universal screening for group B streptococcus. *N Engl J Med* 2009;360:2626–36.

Yancey MK, Schuchat A, Brown LK, Ventura VL, Markenson GR. The accuracy of late antenatal screening cultures in predicting genital group B streptococcal colonization at delivery. *Obstet Gynecol* 1996;88:811–5.

Acute Abdominal Pain Due to Nonobstetric Causes

Fred M. Howard

Department of Obstetrics and Gynecology, University of Rochester School of Medicine and Dentistry, Rochester, NY, USA

Overview

The pregnant woman with acute abdominal pain is a challenging clinical dilemma and her evaluation and treatment demand great care and judgment. Common pregnancy symptoms such as nausea, vomiting, and urinary frequency are similar to those of many nonobstetric illnesses that cause acute abdominal pain. The etiology of acute abdominal pain in pregnancy can be separated into obstetric and nonobstetric causes; only nonobstetric causes will be discussed in this protocol. The most common etiologies for nonobstetric causes of acute abdominal pain in the pregnant patient are appendicitis, cholecystitis, cystitis, pyelonephritis, hepatitis, pancreatitis, and degenerating uterine leiomyomata. Management is more complex, as interventions may adversely affect the pregnancy and concerns about harming the fetus may delay treatment. Clinical acumen to identify patients who need immediate interventions is essential.

Pathophysiology

Maternal physiologic and anatomic changes may modify symptoms and clinical responses from those seen in nonpregnant patients. The physical examination of the abdomen and pelvis are altered by pregnancy. By 12 weeks of gestation the uterine fundus rises from the pelvis and becomes an abdominal organ, as do the adnexal structures. The intestines and omentum are displaced superiorly and laterally with the appendix more likely to be closer to the gallbladder than to the McBurney point by late pregnancy (Fig. 32.1). Routine laboratory measures may also be altered in pregnancy.

Protocols for High-Risk Pregnancies: An Evidence-Based Approach, Sixth Edition.
Edited by John T. Queenan, Catherine Y. Spong and Charles J. Lockwood.
© 2015 John Wiley & Sons, Ltd. Published 2015 by John Wiley & Sons, Ltd.

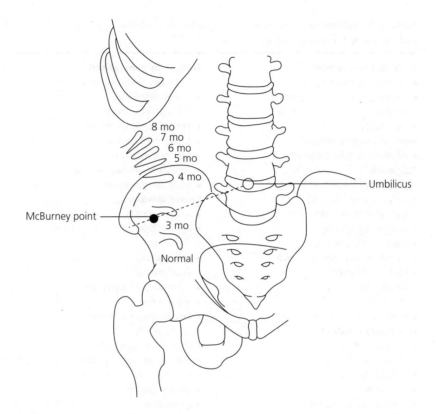

Figure 32.1 Location and orientation of the appendix in pregnancy.

For instance, the leukocyte count varies considerably during normal pregnancy with elevations up to 12,000 to 16,000/mL, levels that overlap with intraabdominal inflammatory conditions, such as appendicitis.

Diagnosis and treatment

History and physical examination
A systematic and detailed history and physical examination are essential and should guide the rest of the evaluation. Having the most common diagnoses in mind during evaluation is essential to formulating a differential diagnosis, yet the clinician must remain sufficiently open-minded and unhurried to avoid missing important information. Acute abdominal crises should be recognized expediently. They may present with pain as the sole symptom but often will also involve vomiting, muscular rigidity, abdominal distention or shock. In early pregnancy, excluding the possibility of ectopic pregnancy is often the first priority.

Table 32.1 Differential diagnosis of acute nonobstetric abdominopelvic pain by location (*the more common causes are in italics*)

Right upper quadrant
- *Cholecystitis/cholelithiasis*
- Diaphragmatic pleuritis/abscess
- *Hepatitis*
- *Pancreatitis*
- Pneumonia/pneumonitis
- *Appendicitis* (later gestation)

Epigastric
- *Cholecystitis/cholelithiasis*
- Early acute *appendicitis*
- Early small bowel obstruction
- *Gastroenteritis*/gastric ulcer
- *Gastroesophageal reflux*
- Mesenteric thrombosis/ischemia
- Myocardial infarction
- *Pancreatitis*
- Pericarditis
- Ruptured aortic aneurysm

Left upper quadrant
- *Gastroenteritis/gastric ulcer*
- Myocardial infarction
- *Pancreatitis*
- Pericarditis
- Pneumonia/pneumonitis
- Splenic rupture/abscess/infarction

Periumbilical
- All early-stage visceral diseases
- Abdominal trauma
- Abdominal wall hernias
- Bowel obstruction

Diffuse or generalized
- All late-stage visceral diseases
- Bowel obstruction
- Diabetic ketoacidosis
- Irritable bowel syndrome
- Mesenteric ischemia
- Metabolic disorders
- Peritonitis/perforated viscera
- Muscular strain/sprain

Lower quadrants
- *Adnexal torsion*
- *Appendicitis* (right lower quadrant)
- *Constipation*
- Diverticulitis
- Endometriosis
- Inflammatory bowel disease
- Inguinal hernia
- Irritable bowel syndrome
- *Leiomyomata*
- *Ovarian cyst/ruptured cyst*
- *Pelvic inflammatory disease*
- *Pyelonephritis*
- *Urinary calculi*

Suprapubic
- *Cystitis/urethritis*
- Obstruction of the urinary bladder
- *Urinary calculi*

Location is crucial to potential diagnoses. Table 32.1 summarizes the location of pain associated with many of the causes of acute abdominal pain. Differentiating uterine from nonuterine pain can be difficult. One possible way to do so is to have the patient lie supine and then roll to the left or the right. If the pain shifts when she lies on her side, it is more likely to be of uterine origin. If it remains in the same location, consider an intraabdominal or retroperitoneal process.

Acute abdominal pain exacerbated by movement and coughing is generally consistent with peritoneal inflammation or irritation due to an infectious process or visceral rupture. Colicky pain refers to pain that is wavelike, with spasms that crescendo and decrescendo in a somewhat rhythmic pattern. This type of pain is characteristic of intestinal disorders, especially small bowel obstruction. It may also be consistent with adnexal torsion. Steady or constant pain is characteristic of a distended gallbladder or kidney.

The nature of the onset of the pain, the chronological sequence of events in the patient's history, and the duration of pain are important diagnostic elements. Associated symptoms may narrow the diagnosis. Fever and chills may suggest an infectious etiology. Pain followed by nausea and emesis is more characteristic of appendicitis while viral or bacterial enteritis may present with gastrointestinal complaints followed by pain.

Severity of pain does not necessarily correlate with the severity of disease and is not always useful in diagnosis. In most patients, it is appropriate to give analgesia while the evaluation of acute pain is ongoing. A history of radiation of pain may also be helpful. For instance, acute obstruction of the intravesicular portion of the ureter is characterized by severe suprapubic and flank pain that radiates to the labia or inner aspect of the upper thigh. Pain referred to the abdomen from the thorax can be a difficult diagnostic problem and an intrathoracic etiology should be considered in every patient with acute abdominal pain.

Physical examination of the abdomen, pelvis, and rectum are critical components of evaluation of the pregnant woman with abdominal pain. The examination should be gentle but thorough. Examination begins with observation of the patient's appearance and activity. The patient with peritoneal inflammation may minimize motion and lie with hips flexed to reduce pain. Patients with urinary colic from calculi usually move around. Vital signs are essential. Hypotension and tachycardia suggest hypovolemia, which may be due to dehydration or blood loss. Fever suggests an infectious process.

The fetal status should also be evaluated in a manner appropriate for gestational age. The uterus should be monitored for contractions with a tocodynamometer because preterm labor may occur in this clinical setting. If viable, the fetus should be assessed by means of a nonstress test (NST) followed by a biophysical profile if the NST is not reactive. Fetal tachycardia due to a maternal fever may resolve with fever reduction measures.

Gentle examination of the abdomen may reveal tenderness, involuntary guarding and rebound tenderness, which are characteristic of peritoneal inflammation of any etiology. Abdominal distention may occur with peritoneal inflammation or bowel obstruction. Palpation should be directed to the detection of possible abdominal masses as well as tenderness. Auscultation may reveal decreased or absent bowel sounds consistent with peritonitis or ileus. High-pitched bowel sounds and rushes may be heard if obstruction is present. Patients with findings consistent with generalized peritonitis, with guarding and rebound tenderness in all four quadrants of the abdomen, are commonly said to have a "surgical abdomen" and may require operative evaluation to arrive at the correct diagnosis.

Pelvic examination is often of limited value after the first trimester. Ultrasound is usually essential to rule out a pelvic mass in acute abdominal pain during pregnancy. The rectal examination may be helpful in further clarifying pelvic pathology and testing for occult blood at the time of the examination may help recognize gastrointestinal bleeding.

Laboratory and imaging evaluation

Table 32.2 lists many of the laboratory and imaging studies generally useful in evaluating the pregnant woman with acute abdominal pain. Laboratory examinations may be of great value, but rarely establish a definitive diagnosis. Not all are indicated in all women and their use should be predicated by the differential diagnosis determined from the history and physical

Table 32.2 Studies that may be useful in acute abdominal pain in the pregnant patient

---

Laboratory testing
Serum quantitative beta hCG
Urinalysis: assess for pyuria, hematuria, glucosuria, ketones
Urine culture and sensitivity: assess for urinary tract infection
Cervical cultures: assess for gonorrhea, chlamydia infection
Complete blood count and differential: assess for leukocytosis, anemia
Glucose
Serum ketones: assess in patients who may have diabetic keoacidosis
Liver function tests, total and direct bilirubin: assess for liver, gallbladder disease
Amylase, lipase: assess for pancreatic disease
Electrolytes, BUN, creatinine: assess metabolic state, renal function
Other specific tests when indicated (e.g., hemoglobin electrophoresis, ANA)
Imaging (scans with radiation exposure are generally second line)
Pelvic ultrasound: assess pregnancy, adnexa, uterus
Abdominal ultrasound: assess gallbladder, appendix, liver, free fluid
Renal ultrasound: assess kidneys for hydronephrosis, calculi
Chest radiograph: assess lungs, heart silhouette
Abdominal X-ray series: assess bowels if perforation, obstruction suspected
CT or MR scans as indicated

---

examination. Studies that are usually indicated include complete blood count, urinalysis, urine culture, and electrolytes.

Imaging may be helpful. Magnetic resonance imaging and ultrasound scans are considered safe in pregnancy and can be used without reservation. In general, examinations with ionizing radiation exposure are avoided, particularly in the first trimester. As a general rule, no single imaging study provides enough radiation exposure to the fetus to cause damage. Accumulative doses should not exceed 5 rad. A CT scan of the abdomen exposes the fetus to about 3.5 rad. Radioactive isotopes should also be avoided in pregnancy.

Treatment

Appropriate treatment of acute abdominal pain in the pregnant patient will be dictated by the differential diagnosis. In most cases, management will be unchanged from that employed in nonpregnant patients.

Acute appendicitis

Acute appendicitis is the most common cause for surgery for abdominal pain in pregnancy, occurring in about 1 in 3000 pregnancies. Appendicitis occurs more often in the middle trimester and perforation of the appendix is skewed toward later pregnancy. This probably reflects both the difficulty and delay of diagnosis in later pregnancy. The clinical presentation of appendicitis during pregnancy is not greatly different from that in the nonpregnant woman. Most patients will complain of abdominal pain, nausea and vomiting. Anorexia is not a consistent finding in pregnancy and diarrhea may be present. The presence of fever may be less common in pregnancy and white blood counts may be just mildly elevated although the majority of women will have a left shift. Imaging plays a crucial role in diagnosis. Ultrasound is usually performed first due to its low cost and safety, but technical issues due to pregnancy make ultrasound unreliable in some cases. Magnetic resonance imaging has taken on an important role and is usually diagnostic. Treatment is expedient appendectomy. Tolerance of a significant rate of normal appendixes is necessary to prevent the serious maternal and fetal morbidity associated with perforation. Antibiotics are generally administered prior to and after surgery. Tocolysis may be indicated.

Ovarian cysts and adnexal torsion

Ovarian cysts may cause acute abdominal pain due to rupture. Adnexal torsion may occur with normal adnexae, but more often occurs with adnexal cystic lesions, neoplastic lesions or hyperstimulated ovaries. The majority of torsions occur in the first half of the pregnancy. Ovarian torsion usually presents with unilateral pelvic pain, possibly with vomiting. Ultrasound may demonstrate a pelvic mass and absent flow on Doppler evaluation. Adnexal torsion represents a surgical emergency due to the potential danger of permanent destruction of the organs involved, peritonitis, or even death. The traditional approach has been surgical removal of the adnexa. However, untwisting and preservation of the ovary is usually successful even with an apparently necrotic ovary or tube.

Cholecystitis/cholelithiasis

Asymptomatic cholelithiasis occurs in 3–4% of pregnant women and is the cause of over 90% of cases of cholecystitis in pregnancy. Cholecystitis during pregnancy is uncommon, with 5–10 cases per 10,000 births. Steady and severe right upper quadrant pain is often the presenting symptom. Fever, leukocytosis, nausea, vomiting, and anorexia may also be present. Ultrasonography will show gallstones in almost all cases. Medical treatment is preferred in pregnancy. Initial treatment consists of no oral intake, intravenous hydration, bed rest, pain relief and antibiotics if febrile. Most women respond to this approach and avoid surgical treatment during pregnancy. Surgery, if needed for failed medical management, is best performed in the second trimester.

Urinary tract infection

Acute cystitis is very common in gravid women. It may occur alone or in conjunction with pyelonephritis. Acute uncomplicated cystitis is manifested primarily by dysuria, with associated frequency, urgency, suprapubic pain and/or hematuria. Fever, flank pain, costovertebral angle tenderness and nausea or vomiting suggest pyelonephritis and warrant more aggressive diagnostic and therapeutic measures. Pyelonephritis is identified in 1–2% of all pregnancies. Treatment includes parenteral antibiotics and intravenous hydration. Close monitoring for complications such as renal impairment, hematological abnormalities, septic shock and pulmonary dysfunction is critical in the pregnant patient. Prophylactic antibiotics may be indicated for the remainder of the pregnancy.

Urinary calculi

Stones or calculi of the urinary tract usually cause severe abdominal pain associated with nausea, but sometimes present with milder symptoms during pregnancy. With ureteral obstruction, flank pain is present which may radiate to the ipsilateral groin and percussion may elicit tenderness over the costovertebral angle. Hematuria is usually present. Ultrasound examination may demonstrate hydroureter, hydronephrosis or calculi. In most cases of renal or ureteral calculus, the stone eventually passes, thus supportive treatment with intravenous hydration and pain control is usually sufficient. Lithotripsy is contraindicated in pregnancy.

Pancreatitis

Acute pancreatitis complicates 1 in 1000 to 10,000 pregnancies. Gallbladder disease is the most common cause; medications, infection and hyperlipidemia are less frequent causes. Signs and symptoms are similar to those in the nonpregnant woman. Medical management includes bowel rest, pain relief and correction of fluid and electrolyte imbalances. Patients with pancreatic abscess, ruptured pseudocyst or hemorrhagic pancreatitis may require surgery while they are still pregnant.

Hepatitis

Viral hepatitis is the most common serious, nonobstetric liver disease in pregnant women. Although pregnancy has little influence on the presentation or course of hepatitis, hepatitis carries significant implications to the pregnancy, fetus and neonate depending on the type and gestational age. Management is generally unchanged during pregnancy. See Protocol 23.

Uterine leiomyomata

Acute pain from myomata during pregnancy is usually due to degeneration secondary to inadequacy of blood supply to the myoma. Pain and tenderness are generally localized and can be severe. Low-grade fever and leukocytosis can occur. Preterm labor may be initiated due to irritation of adjacent myometrium. Ultrasound is helpful in making the diagnosis. Management is nonsurgical with use of analgesics and observation for preterm labor.

Intraabdominal hemorrhage

Acute abdominal hemorrhage, other than from ectopic pregnancy, is uncommon during pregnancy, but may rarely occur. It has been reported with rupture of the aorta, splenic artery and endometriotic lesions. Evaluation with imaging studies usually demonstrates the presence of a hemoperitoneum. Management is almost always surgical.

Pelvic inflammatory disease

Acute endometritis, salpingitis, and/or oophoritis are not common in pregnancy, but do occasionally occur, even with the development of tubo-ovarian abscesses. Findings of cervical gonorrhea or Chlamydia or imaging studies consistent with tubo-ovarian complexes or pyosalpinges support the clinical diagnosis. Many clinicians think that PID is not possible during pregnancy, but this is incorrect and may lead to missed diagnoses and inappropriate treatment.

Conclusion

The ability to distinguish an acute process that requires surgical intervention or referral to a specialist is based on the clinical skills of the provider. This requires a complete history, careful physical examination, judicious use of laboratory and radiologic studies, and frequent reevaluation until a firm diagnosis is reached. The primary care clinician should have a low threshold for seeking advice from a surgeon, obstetrician or other specialist. The difficulties of diagnosing abdominal pain in pregnancy are well known. Prompt clinical diagnosis and surgical intervention when indicated are necessary to minimize maternal and fetal morbidity and mortality.

Suggested reading

Dewhurst C, Beddy P, Pedrosa I. MRI evaluation of acute appendicitis in pregnancy. *J Magn Reson Imaging* 2013;37:566–75.

Diegelmann L. Nonobstetric abdominal pain and surgical emergencies in pregnancy. *Emerg Med Clin N Am* 2012;30:885–901.

Hasiakos D, Papakonstantinou K, Kontoravdis A, Gogas L, Aravantinos L, Vitoratos N. Adnexal torsion during pregnancy: report of four cases and review of the literature. *J Obstet Gynaecol Res* 2008;34(4 Pt 2):683–7.

Khandelwal A, Fasih N, Kielar A. Imaging of acute abdomen in pregnancy. *Radiol Clin N Am* 2013;51:1005–22.

Kilpatrick CC, Orejuela FJ. Management of the acute abdomen in pregnancy: a review. *Curr Opin Obstet Gynecol* 2008;20(6):534–9.

Upadhyay A, Stanten S, Kazantsev G, Horoupian R, Stanten A. Laparoscopic management of a nonobstetric emergency in the third trimester of pregnancy. *Surg Endosc* 2007;21(8):1344–8.

PROTOCOL 33

Gallbladder, Fatty Liver, and Pancreatic Disease

Jeffrey R. Johnson
Women and Children's Hospital, Buffalo, NY, USA

Clinical significance

Disorders of the gallbladder are common during pregnancy. Cholestasis (also known as intrahepatic cholestasis of pregnancy or IHCP) affects about 1 in 500 pregnancies, can recur during subsequent pregnancies, and there appears to be a mother–daughter correlation in disease incidence. It is related to a history of oral contraceptive use as well, and may be related to elevated estrogen levels. Incidence varies across ethnic groups, from less than 1% patients of Western and Central European descent, to 15% in some ethnic groups of South America.

Gallstones are seen in up to 4% of pregnancies, the majority being asymptomatic. Pigmented stones comprise 15% and mixed pigmented and cholesterol also comprise about 15% of stones. Increased formation of gallstones is associated with being female (four times more likely than in males), increasing age, obesity, a diet high in fat, diabetes, high parity and exogenous hormone administration, particularly estrogen. About 90% of cases of cholecystitis are associated with stones while 10% are acalculous and are due to infection, trauma, malignancy, tuberculosis or parasitic infections.

Acute fatty liver of pregnancy (AFLP) is rare, affecting 1 in 15,000 pregnancies. It is a particularly aggressive form of liver dysfunction: maternal mortality is 18–25%, and perinatal morbidity and mortality are related to gestational age at delivery. It is seen more commonly with a male fetus or multiple gestations. Its typical presentation is the third trimester or within 48 hours postpartum. AFLP has been associated with preeclampsia, although AFLP is not considered part of the preeclampsia/gestational hypertension disease spectrum.

Protocols for High-Risk Pregnancies: An Evidence-Based Approach, Sixth Edition.
Edited by John T. Queenan, Catherine Y. Spong and Charles J. Lockwood.
© 2015 John Wiley & Sons, Ltd. Published 2015 by John Wiley & Sons, Ltd.

Acute pancreatitis is a rare complication in pregnancy, occurring in between 1 per 1000 and 1 per 3000 pregnancies. Most are due to gallstones, which is different than in nonpregnant cases, which are primarily alcohol-related. Hypertriglyceridemia is a rare but important cause of pancreatitis in pregnancy, and can be difficult to treat. It is more common in 20- to 30-year-old primigravidas in the third trimester. Pancreatitis due to hypertriglyceridemia carries a 10% mortality rate for both mother and fetus. There is also an association of AFLP and pancreatitis, and the prognosis is especially poor in these patients. A summary of these conditions is found in Table 33.1.

Pathophysiology

Cholestasis results from a decrease in excretion of bile acids, causing hepatic canalicular plugging without evidence of necrosis. There may be mutations in the bile acid transporter gene, which impairs the transport and excretion of bile acids. Estrogen is also known to have effects on the bile acid transport mechanism, and cholestasis is often seen in cases of high estrogen such as oral contraceptive use, multiple gestations, and third trimester of

Table 33.1 Summary of gallbladder, fatty liver, and pancreatic disease in pregnancy

	Cholestasis	Cholelithiasis	AFLP	Pancreatitis
Incidence	1:500	4%	1:15,000	1:3000
Pathophysiology	Decreased bile acid secretion	Supersaturation of cholesterol and lipids; increased progesterone	Unknown; may be assoc. with LCHAD mutations	Cholelithiasis; also alcohol, infectious, medications, trauma
Diagnosis	Unrelenting pruritis; occasional rash; elevated bile salts with normal LFTs; U/S not useful	RUQ pain, esp. after fatty meals; colicky RUQ pain if stone in ducts; U/S useful	Elevation in LFTs; abnormal clotting profile; low glucose, elevated ammonia; U/S useful	Elevated amylase, lipase; physical exam; U/S and MRI useful
Treatment	Ursodeoxycholic acid; adjuvant cholestyramine or prednisone in refractory cases	Pain control (avoid morphine), IV hydration, dietary change; cholecystectomy	Supportive in ICU; clotting factor replacement; delivery	Bowel rest and NGT decompression; antibiotics if indicated

AFLP, acute fatty liver disease of pregnancy; LCHAD, long chain 3-hydroxyacyl-coenzyme A dehydrogenase; LFTs, liver function tests; U/S, ultrasound; RUQ, right upper quadrant; MRI, magnetic resonance imaging; IV, intravenous; ICU, intensive care unit; NGT, nasogastric tube.

pregnancy. The bile acids are hydrophobic, resulting in deposition of bile salts in the dermal layer of the skin, leading to extreme pruritis. Due to the hydrophobic nature of bile acids, they also readily cross the placenta, and may result in fetal complications.

Seventy percent of gallstones are comprised of cholesterol, and gallstones form from supersaturation of cholesterol and lipids. Pregnancy is associated with stone formation, due to high levels of circulating sex hormones, as well as increasing progesterone. As progesterone levels rise through the first half of gestation there is an overall decrease in motility of smooth muscle, including the gallbladder. This results in decreased emptying and an increase in biliary sludge, which forms a nidus for stone formation.

The etiology of AFLP remains unclear, but is no longer thought to be a part of the preeclampsia spectrum of disease. In a mother who is heterozygous for an autosomal recessive mutation in the long chain 3-hydroxyacyl-coenzyme A dehydrogenase (LCHAD) in mitochondria, and has a fetus that is homozygous for the LCHAD mutation, fatty acid accumulates, resulting in a significant increase in risk for development of AFLP. These pregnancies may be at increased risk for fetal growth restriction and poor neonatal outcomes. Management in a tertiary center with availability of maternal and neonatal intensive care is recommended. Concomitant preeclampsia in up to 40% of cases further compromises maternal liver function, and increases free radical and hydrogen peroxide production, further damaging the liver. The risk of recurrence is less than 5%, but if it is recurrent, then testing for the LCHAD defect is warranted.

The majority (80%) of cases of pancreatitis in pregnancy are due to cholelithiasis. Increasing rates of obesity among females, as well as higher levels of steroid synthesis and breakdown during pregnancy, are both etiologic factors contributing to the development of cholelithiasis. Other causes of pancreatitis in decreasing order of frequency are: alcohol, infections (mumps, coxsackie B, tuberculosis), drugs (corticosteroids, acetaminophen, nitrofurantoin, and flagyl), trauma, post-surgical iatrogenic, and idiopathic.

Hypertriglyceridemia is recognized as a rare but important cause of pancreatitis. It is thought that the decreased activity of lipoprotein lipase, which initiates catabolism of triglyceride-rich proteins, plays the major role in development of pancreatitis in this group of patients. The decreased activity of lipoprotein lipase is related to the increased insulin resistance seen in the second and third trimesters. This decrease in lipoprotein lipase activity can make treatment in these patients particularly problematic.

Diagnosis

Cholestasis is most commonly diagnosed with extreme, unrelenting, miserable pruritis that does not respond to any of the usual antihistamine or topical steroid therapy. The onset of pruritus often precedes any laboratory abnormalities. The palms and soles are particularly affected. There is occasionally a nonspecific rash on the trunk, face, and legs. The liver enzymes are normal to minimally elevated, with a normal to minimally elevated total bilirubin. There is an elevation in bile acid levels when tested. Although not recommended during pregnancy, hepatic biopsy will show deposition of bile in the canaliculi, without surrounding hepatic necrosis. Ultrasonography of the right upper quadrant is not helpful.

Cholelithiasis is usually asymptomatic; however, there may be right upper quadrant pain, particularly after a fatty meal. Severe symptoms occur when a stone enters the cystic or common bile duct. There is a sudden onset of right upper quadrant pain, which may radiate to the mid-epigastrium or right scapula; there is nausea with rapid progression to vomiting and anorexia. The serum alkaline phosphatase is an excellent predictor of obstructive cholelithiasis in the nonpregnant patient, but is less useful during pregnancy due to placental production of alkaline phosphatase. However, an elevated hepatic alkaline phosphatase can be determined by exposing the sample to heat in the laboratory, as the placental fraction of alkaline phosphatase is heat-stable. Ultrasonography is sensitive and specific for cholelithiasis, detecting more than 95% of gallstones. It is also useful to find evidence of obstruction of the cystic or common bile duct by looking for ductal dilatation. Ultrasonography will detect gallbladder wall thickening or pericystic fluid collections, which are evidence for cholecystitis. The risk of preterm labor with cholecystitis is increased. The fetal loss rates are less than 5% in appropriately treated cases.

AFLP can initially present with vomiting, followed by a rapid progression in sequence of right upper quadrant pain, coma, hepatic failure with disseminated intravascular coagulation, and death. Hepatomegaly is not a feature of AFLP. A severe coagulopathy is nearly always present, with an abnormal INR due to absence of vitamin K-dependent clotting factors. An elevated INR will differentiate AFLP from HELLP syndrome, which may also have an associated coagulopathy, but does not result in an elevation in INR. Patients may develop hepatorenal syndrome or diabetes insipidus. Liver enzymes are elevated but less than 500 U/L. There is hypoglycemia and also increased serum ammonia levels. Ultrasonography of the liver will demonstrate fatty infiltration of the liver. Computed tomography scanning is neither sensitive nor specific for AFLP, and is not recommended. Magnetic resonance imaging which is T_2 weighted is very sensitive for fatty infiltration of the liver, but not specific to AFLP.

Pancreatitis may present with nausea and vomiting, low-grade fever and leukocytosis. Abdominal examination usually reveals tenderness in the epigastric area, occasionally radiating to the flank or shoulders. There is rarely guarding or rebound tenderness. Computed tomography scanning is best avoided during the second and third trimester due to the concerns of radiation exposure. Ultrasonography may be performed, but the gravid uterus may interfere with adequate visualization of the pancreas. Ultrasonography may demonstrate a large pancreatic cyst or pseudocyst. Magnetic resonance imaging may reveal cystic changes in the pancreas, as well as obstruction of the common bile duct by a stone. Ileus is a frequent clinical and radiological finding. Elevated amylase, especially three times the normal range, is the most common laboratory abnormality. Other abnormalities may include elevated lipase and liver enzymes, particularly if obstruction due to a gallstone is present. Serum alkaline phosphatase may be elevated in cases of cholelithiasis, and differentiation between placental and hepatic alkaline phosphatase can be made by determining the heat-stable versus total alkaline phosphatase.

Treatment

The majority of pregnancies affected with cholestasis are uncomplicated. There is a marginally increased rate of premature labor and postpartum hemorrhage, and stillbirth. No specific monitoring or interventions have been shown to be helpful in predicting adverse outcomes. Maternal therapy should be directed both at alleviating the pruritic symptoms and decreasing bile acids. An effective therapy in most cases is with ursodeoxycholic acid which allows binding of the bile acids into salts, making them hydrophilic, so that they may be excreted in the feces. Relief may take 48 to 72 hours after initiating therapy. Cholestyramine is marginally effective, and is best used as an adjuvant therapy if ursodeoxycholic acid is not completely effective. Corticosteroids have been shown to be an effective third agent in cases that are otherwise refractory. Antihistamines provide some symptomatic relief, as does hydroxyzine. The limitations for both these therapies are their side effects, particularly sedation.

Cholelithiasis is treated with intravenous hydration and withholding oral nutrition for several days. A low-fat diet, once feedings are reestablished, is essential. Pain medications are given parenterally initially, and meperidine is the drug of choice. Morphine should be avoided as it precipitates spasms of the sphincter of Oddi, and can exacerbate symptoms. Antibiotics are indicated if there is concomitant cholecystitis. The risk of preterm labor is significantly elevated, and antipyretics and tocolytics are indicated. Surgical intervention is indicated after 48 hours of antibiotics. Nonpregnant patients are often managed conservatively with antibiotics for first episode cholecystitis. However, sepsis and acute respiratory distress syndrome are increased during pregnancy from cholecystitis, and surgical intervention is recommended for first episode cholecystitis in pregnancy. Nonsurgical medical therapy (bile acid therapy, dissolution with methyl terbutyl ether, or lithotripsy) is not recommended in pregnancy. Laparoscopic cholecystectomy has been shown to be safe in multiple reports, and may often be the primary mode of treatment. Seventy percent of patients with significant stones will have a relapse of symptoms. Laparoscopic cholecystectomy is preferred for initial management if there is a high probability of recurrence, if the episodes are repeated, or for evidence of perforation. The laparoscopic approach is best used through about 24 weeks of gestation, but may be performed by experienced operators even in the third trimester. The open approach is best avoided if possible due to the increased risk of postoperative complications such as thromboembolic complications, and long healing periods associated with the open technique. Laparoscopic cholecystectomy is the second most common nonobstetric surgical procedure performed during pregnancy, after appendectomy. If there is obstruction of the common bile duct, endoscopic retrograde cholangiopancreatography (ERCP) may also be safely performed in pregnancy. There is no increased rate of prematurity seen with ERCP performed in the second or third trimesters, although the loss rate may be elevated with first trimester ERCP. The rate of post-ERCP pancreatitis is higher (15%) than in the nonpregnant population. Post-ERCP pancreatitis responds readily to conservative medical management including decompression with a nasogastric tube and limited oral intake.

Treatment for AFLP is directed toward immediate recognition and delivery. Vaginal delivery is preferred due to the risks of bleeding with abdominal delivery, although cesarean delivery may be preferred if the induction was to be prolonged. Regional anesthesia is preferable due to both the potential for hepatotoxicity with inhaled agents, and also the ability to monitor maternal levels of consciousness. These patients are best served in an intensive care setting in a tertiary medical center. Clotting factor replacement is essential to survival, as disseminated intravascular coagulation is the cause for mortality in the majority of patients. Hepatic failure is also a potential concern. Careful monitoring of serum glucose and electrolytes is essential. Liver transplantation has been used in some cases, although with intensive support these patients do recover without transplantation.

Most cases of acute pancreatitis resolve spontaneously. Approximately 10% of patients may be critically ill and require treatment in an intensive care unit. The general management is bowel rest, and nasogastric suction in cases associated with ileus. Adequate intravenous hydration and electrolyte monitoring is essential due to fluid and electrolyte loss associated with large pancreatic cysts or prolonged vomiting. A low-fat elemental enteral nutrition program is essential in the treatment of pancreatitis regardless of etiology with meperidine, as morphine may cause spasm of the sphincter of Oddi and exacerbate symptoms of biliary colic. Antibiotics are indicated only if infection is suspected. Cases associated with large or a high number of stones may not respond to conservative management. The rate of relapse can be as high as 70%. In 68 ERCPs performed between 2000 and 2006, indications were recurrent biliary colic, abnormal liver function testing and dilated bile duct. The median fluoroscopy time was 1.45 minutes, and there were no complications related to the procedure (perforation, post-spincterotomy bleeding, cholangitis, or maternal or fetal loss). However, 11 patients (16%) developed post-ERCP pancreatitis. All were managed successfully with conservative therapy. The term pregnancy rate was 90% overall, although patients who underwent ERCP in the first trimester had the highest loss rate of 20%. ERCP in pregnancy was associated with a higher rate of post-procedure pancreatitis than in the general population. Cases due to hypertriglyceridemia are best managed with enteral feeding of a low-lipid diet, and generally do not respond to routine nasogastric suctioning and intravenous fluids alone. Careful attention to glucose is mandated due to an increase in glycemic indices. Plasmapheresis has been reported, but is considered largely investigational, and should not be routinely performed. In general, pregnancy does not have an adverse effect on pancreatitis, and delivery does not improve the clinical course in most cases. Fetal monitoring is suggested, particularly in the third trimester.

Complications

The bile acids may have a direct depressive or toxic effect on the fetal myocardium, and twice-weekly nonstress testing after 32 weeks is advocated in many centers despite the lack of evidence of benefit. Cholestasis is one of the few obstetric indications for early delivery at 37 weeks without amniocentesis to determine fetal pulmonary maturity, to avoid the risk of stillbirth. Cesarean delivery is reserved for the usual obstetric indications.

The primary complications associated with pancreatitis in pregnancy are maternal, due to fluid and electrolyte imbalances. Complications due to obstruction are no higher than in the nonpregnant population, but may include perforation by the stone in rare cases. There is a slightly higher rate of preterm labor and delivery as with any peritoneal inflammatory response, which can cause increased uterine irritability.

Conclusion

Gallbladder disorders may occur more frequently during pregnancy. Cholestasis presents with maternal symptoms and is associated with increased stillbirth and pregnancy complications. Monitoring and therapy are guided both to decreasing maternal symptoms and preventing perinatal complications.

Cholelithiasis is more commonly seen due to increasing obesity as well as diets high in fats. It is best treated during pregnancy surgically, and evaluation for concomitant cholecystitis is required for optimal management. Surgical interventions during pregnancy have been shown to be safe, and should not be withheld if it is the appropriate management.

AFLP presents an unusual and rare constellation of findings, and can be life-threatening. Optimal and early treatment is essential for maternal survival, but fortunately is rare and tends not to recur.

Pancreatitis is an unusual obstetric complication, and is commonly due to stone obstruction of the cystic or common bile duct. Diagnosis is usually made by a combination of clinical findings, and radiological studies such as ultrasound or magnetic resonance imaging. Treatment is conservative in the majority of cases, although surgical intervention is warranted in some cases. ERCP has been shown to be safe in pregnancy, and may be used when appropriate. Pancreatitis due to hypertriglyceridemia is rare and should be treated with low-lipid enteral feeding. Morbidity and mortality due to hypertriglyceridemic pancreatitis is elevated for both mother and fetus if inappropriately diagnosed or treated.

Suggested reading

American College of Obstetricians and Gynecologists. Multifetal gestations: twin, triplet, and higher-order multifetal pregnancies. Practice Bulletin No. 144. American College of Obstetricians and Gynecologists. *Obstet Gynecol* 2014;123:1118–32.

Crisan LS, Steidl ET, Rivera-Alsina ME. Acute hyperlipidemic pancreatitis in pregnancy. *Am J Obstet Gynecol* 2008;198:e1–3.

Glantz A, Marschall HU, Lammert F, Mattsson LA. Intrahepatic cholestasis of pregnancy: a randomized controlled trial comparing dexamethasone and ursodeoxycholic acid. *Hepatology* 2005;42:1399–405.

Guntupalli SR, Steingrub J. Hepatic disease and pregnancy: an overview of diagnosis and management. *Crit Care Med* 2005;33(10 Supple):S332–9.

Kayatas SE, Eser M, Cam C, *et al.* Acute pancreatitis associated with hypertriglyceridemia: a life-threatening complication. *Arch Gynecol Obstet* 2009 Aug 6 [Epub ahead of print].

Ko H, Yoshida EM. Acute fatty liver of pregnancy. *Can J Gastroenterol* 2006;20(1):25–30.

Moldenhauer JS, O'Brien JM, Barton JR, *et al.* Acute fatty liver of pregnancy associated with pancreatitis: a life-threatening complication. *Am J Obstet Gynecol* 2004;190:502–5.

Natarajan SK, Thangaraj KR, Eapen CA, *et al.* Livery injury in acute fatty liver of pregnancy: possible link to placental mitochondrial dysfunction and oxidative stress. *Hepatology* 2010;51:191–200.

Petrov MS, Zagainov VE. Influence of enteral versus parenteral nutrition on blood glucose control in acute pancreatitis: a systematic review. *Clin Nutr* 2007;26:514–23.

Rakheja D, Bennett MJ, Foster BM, *et al.* Evidence for fatty acid oxidation in human placenta, and the relationship of fatty acid oxidation enzyme activities with gestational age. *Placenta* 2002;23:447–50.

Tang SJ, Mayo MJ, Rodriguez-Frias E, *et al.* Safety and utility of ERCP during pregnancy. *Gastrointest Endosc* 2009;69(3):453–61.

PART IV
Obstetric Problems

First Trimester Vaginal Bleeding

John T. Queenan Jr

Department of Obstetrics and Gynecology, University of Rochester Medical Center, Rochester, NY, USA

Clinical significance

Vaginal bleeding in the first trimester of pregnancy is a very common problem. One in four women will experience vaginal bleeding during pregnancy and this accounts for 1–2% of all Emergency Room visits. When vaginal bleeding occurs in the first trimester, it places the patient at a true crossroad. Many causes are benign and the patient will continue with a normal pregnancy. However, first trimester bleeding can also be the presenting sign of spontaneous abortion, ectopic pregnancy, or gestational trophoblastic disease. Clinicians need to have a high index of suspicion based on history, risk factors, and early symptoms to determine which patients merit prompt evaluation. Early recognition and appropriate therapy are essential to minimize the morbidity and mortality that arise from some causes of first trimester bleeding.

Pathophysiology

Implantation begins 5–7 days after fertilization and hCG can be detected in maternal serum 8–10 days after ovulation. The invasion of trophoblast into the endometrium and maternal vasculature can result in vaginal spotting. Placental development is an ongoing process involving continuing invasion by extravillous cytotrophoblasts as they remodel the maternal vasculature. Implantation bleeding typically resolves by the 13th week of gestation.

The high circulating levels of estrogen and progesterone in pregnancy bring about several changes that can cause bleeding or spotting. The vaginal pH becomes more acidic altering the vaginal flora that leads to physiologic discharge and occasionally vaginitis. The cervix becomes more friable and

Protocols for High-Risk Pregnancies: An Evidence-Based Approach, Sixth Edition.
Edited by John T. Queenan, Catherine Y. Spong and Charles J. Lockwood.
© 2015 John Wiley & Sons, Ltd. Published 2015 by John Wiley & Sons, Ltd.

receives increased blood flow in the first trimester. As a result, the patient is more likely to see spotting after intercourse.

Starting at the time of missed menses when hCG levels are approximately 100 IU/L, serum hCG concentration will double every 1.4–2.1 days. By 8–10 weeks of gestation, hCG will reach a plateau between 50,000 and 100,000 IU/L. One diagnostic tool to evaluate first trimester bleeding is based on the knowledge that serum hCG levels rise at a predictable rate in a normal pregnancy. Nonviable and ectopic pregnancies will frequently exhibit a slower rate of rise. In contrast, trophoblastic disease produces hCG levels that can be 3–100 times above the normal level.

Diagnosis and treatment

When a reproductive age female presents with vaginal bleeding in the first trimester of pregnancy, the following initial evaluation should be performed.

1 Obtain vital signs. Verify pregnancy and Rh status.
2 Document the menstrual, gynecologic, sexual and birth control history. Inquire about any history of infertility or use of fertility drugs.
3 Complete a physical examination with inspection for lacerations, cervical lesions or signs of infection, uterine size, open cervical os, adnexal masses, abdominal tenderness, and peritoneal signs.
4 Obtain serum quantitative hCG and transvaginal sonography.
5 Treat or follow as suggested by clinical presentation.

The etiology of first trimester bleeding may be readily apparent on ultrasound examination such as viable pregnancy, ectopic pregnancy, miscarriage, or trophoblastic disease. If the location of a gestation cannot be determined after transvaginal sonography, this is termed pregnancy of unknown location (PUL) and close follow up is warranted.

Any woman of reproductive age who presents with vaginal bleeding in the first trimester with or without pain is at risk for ectopic pregnancy. Prior to widespread use of transvaginal sonography, ectopic pregnancy was responsible for up to 6% of all maternal deaths in the United States.

Vaginal bleeding when there is a viable intrauterine pregnancy

There are many reasons for vaginal bleeding in the first trimester other than ectopic pregnancy or impending miscarriage. A friable cervix, recent intercourse, and implantation bleeding are examples. If sonography confirms a viable gestation, it is prudent to look for reasons that explain the presence of bleeding: cervicitis, vaginitis, subchorionic hematoma, vanishing twin, trauma, cervical polyps or, rarely, cancer.

The clinician should be familiar with the milestones of normal pregnancy. Transvaginal sonography with a transducer frequency of at least 5 MHz should be used. A gestational sac should be detectable by 5.5–6.0 weeks if the gestational age is known. Alternatively, a gestational sac should be visible by transvaginal ultrasound when hCG is above the discriminatory zone of 1500–2000 IU/L. Each institution should determine their own discriminatory zone: the hCG level above which all intrauterine pregnancies can be seen by transvaginal sonography for the specific hCG assay and ultrasound equipment used.

If a patient exhibits a normal fetal heart rate (FHR), gestational sac size greater than or equal to 12 mm or a yolk sac of 2–6 mm on post-conception day 33–36, then the odds of a viable ongoing pregnancy are over 90%. Prognosis improves with increasing gestational age but is worse with the presence of subchorionic hematoma, low FHR, and increasing severity of vaginal bleeding.

Bleeding before 20 weeks of gestation in a pregnancy with cardiac activity and a closed cervix is a threatened abortion by definition. Management should be conservative. Pelvic rest is the traditional advice but this recommendation is not evidence-based. Strict bed rest or vaginal progestin therapy has not been shown to improve outcomes.

The finding of an intrauterine pregnancy on ultrasound generally excludes the diagnosis of ectopic pregnancy. The chance of a heterotopic pregnancy is 1:4000, unless conception occurred in an assisted reproductive technology (ART) cycle, which has a risk of 1:1000.

Early pregnancy loss

Miscarriage will be the outcome in 15–20% of all clinically recognized pregnancies. It can occur at any time in the first half of pregnancy but most often occurs in the first 13 weeks. About one-half of those who experience bleeding in the first trimester will miscarry. Aneuploidy is responsible for at least 50–60% of early losses.

The presence of a gestational sac greater than 18 mm without a yolk sac or fetal pole confirms an anembryonic pregnancy (formerly termed blighted ovum). Cardiac activity should be present when the crown rump length (CRL) exceeds 5 mm. Absence of cardiac activity at this CRL size indicates embryonic demise (formerly termed missed abortion). Many have advocated this cutoff of 5 mm but a large multicenter study recently suggested there are still false positives at this point. Thus, to minimize the chance of inadvertent interruption of a viable pregnancy that has been misdiagnosed

Table 34.1 Early pregnancy milestones

Gestational age (weeks)	Ultrasound finding	Comment
4.0 to 5.0	Gestational sac	Visible when hCG is >1500–2000
5.0 to 6.0	Yolk sac	Visible when gestational sac is >10 mm
5.0 to 6.0	Fetal pole	Visible when gestational sac is >18 mm
5.0 to 6.2	Cardiac activity	Present when crown rump length is >7 mm

as an early pregnancy loss, they suggest a cutoff of 25 mm for the mean gestational sac size and of 7 mm for the CRL. A repeat scan is performed in 1 week to determine viability with certainty. Table 34.1 summarizes early pregnancy milestones.

A normal pregnancy should follow a predictable growth pattern. The CRL should increase by at least 1 mm per day. The hCG level should rise at least 53% over a 2-day interval. Slow FHR can be suggestive of impending early pregnancy failure but FHR is slower than one might expect in early pregnancy; FHR is normally 100 bpm or more prior to 6.2 weeks and 120 bpm or more from 6.3 weeks.

Once early pregnancy failure has been confirmed, treatment options include dilatation and curettage (D&C), manual vacuum aspiration, expectant management, or medical management using misoprostol.

Ectopic pregnancy

The goal is early detection and treatment so as to minimize morbidity and mortality as well as preserving future fertility. A high index of suspicion should be applied to patients at risk. Women are at higher risk if they have a history of prior ectopic, tubal surgery, tubal infections, smoking, ART or conceive with an intrauterine device (IUD) in place.

There is universal agreement that transvaginal sonography and serial hCG levels are essential in the diagnosis of ectopic pregnancy. If gestational age is known, the absence of a gestational sac with yolk sac and embryonic pole by 5.5–6.0 weeks of gestation is highly suggestive of an ectopic pregnancy. If dates are not known, the absence of an intrauterine pregnancy when hCG is above the discriminatory zone is also highly suggestive. Prompt treatment is indicated once a pregnancy is seen in an ectopic location.

When ultrasonography does not detect an intrauterine pregnancy, a thorough examination of other structures should be performed. Although 90% of ectopic pregnancies will occur in the fallopian tube, pathologic implantation can also occur in the cervix, within a cesarean scar, in the interstitial portion of the tube. Free fluid in the cul de sac or an adnexal mass in addition to the corpus luteum is also highly suggestive. Patients with heterotopic pregnancy are at greater risk for hypovolemic shock due to delay in recognition; this diagnosis should always be considered in patients who have conceived via ART.

If diagnosis cannot be made by ultrasonography, then a repeat hCG in 48 hours can be used if the patient is clinically stable. The hCG level should increase by at least 53%. If serum hCG is rising then the patient should be followed with serial hCG levels and ultrasound repeated once in the discriminatory zone. If an intrauterine pregnancy cannot be identified, then ectopic pregnancy is likely.

Many ectopics will resolve without intervention either by regression or tubal abortion. Expectant management is reserved for those compliant and reliable patients with a declining pattern of hCG starting at less than 1000 IU/L.

Treatment of an ectopic pregnancy can be done medically with Methotrexate or surgically by laparoscopy. Early and accurate diagnosis can enable medical management over surgical intervention, enable conservative surgery versus extirpative surgery, and can conserve future fertility.

Pregnancy of unknown location

When the hCG is below the discriminatory zone, the location of a pregnancy after transvaginal sonography can be uncertain. There is a clear consensus that a woman with a PUL should be followed closely until a final diagnosis can be made. A conservative approach is wise to safeguard against intervention that might interrupt an early but viable intrauterine pregnancy. Serial hCG levels are followed and ultrasound is repeated within 1 week. The management of PUL may vary due to a lack of consensus on standardized protocols; follow up should be individualized in relationship to the level of suspicion for ectopic pregnancy.

If the hCG does not rise at least 53% over a 2-day interval, then a viable pregnancy has been virtually excluded. This finding would not discriminate ectopic from early pregnancy failure and uterine evacuation is sometimes needed to reach a definitive diagnosis.

Declining hCG levels point to a pregnancy that is resolving spontaneously. Although reassuring, it is does not completely exclude ectopic pregnancy and these patients should be followed until their hCG levels are negative.

Molar pregnancy

Identifying a characteristic ultrasonographic pattern can make the diagnosis of a complete mole. The complete mole will not have a fetus present. There is a heterogenous echogenic mass in the uterus with many distinct anechoic spaces corresponding to hydropic chorionic villi. This appeared as a "snowstorm" image on older ultrasound machines. Grape-like clusters are seen grossly, and hCG levels may be helpful. The diagnosis of a partial mole can be a challenge since a gestational sac and embryo are present. The placenta is usually abnormal with multiple anechoic cystic spaces and the fetus is growth restricted. A karyotype analysis may reveal a triploid conception. Management involves prompt evacuation of the uterus. Delay in diagnosis and lack of appropriate follow up can increase the risk for metastatic disease.

Follow up after a pregnancy loss

Several important issues should be addressed after pregnancy loss. Women who are Rh-negative should receive 50 µg of anti D immune globulin. Contraception should be discussed and offered. The emotional impact of pregnancy loss at any gestational age can be devastating. Sympathy and reassurance are part of being compassionate to patients in this circumstance. Grief counseling should be offered.

Conclusion

Through the integration of history, physical examination, hCG levels and transvaginal ultrasound examination, a physician can usually arrive at the etiology of first trimester vaginal bleeding. The appropriate management plan can be initiated and the patient's care can be tailored to her needs. The complications associated with first trimester bleeding that impact maternal morbidity and mortality can be minimized.

Suggested reading

Abdallah Y, Daemen A, Kirk E, *et al*. Limitations of current definitions of miscarriage using mean gestational sac diameter and crown-rump length measurements: a multicenter observational study. *Ultrasound Obstet Gynecol* 2011;38:497–502.

American College of Obstetricians and Gynecologists. *Prevention of Rh D alloimmunization. Practice Bulletin 4*. ACOG: Washington, DC; 1999.

Banhart K, van Mello N, Bourne T, *et al*. Pregnancy of unknown location: a consensus statement of nomenclature, definitions, and outcome. *Fertil Steril* 2011;95:857–866.

Barnhart KT, Sammel MD, Rinauldo PF, Zhou L, Hummel AC, Guo W. Symptomatic patients with an early viable intrauterine pregnancy: hCG curves redefined. *Obstet Gynecol* 2004;104:50–55.

Berg CJ, Chang J, Callaghan WM, Whitehead SJ. Pregnancy-related mortality in the United States, 1991–1997. *Obstet Gynecol* 2003;101:289–96.

Seeber BE. What serial hCG can tell you, and cannot tell you, about an early pregnancy. *Fertil Steril* 2012;98:1074–77.

The Practice Committee of the American Society for Reproductive Medicine. Medical treatment of ectopic pregnancy: a committee opinion. *Fertil Steril* 2013;100:638–644.

PROTOCOL 35

Cervical Insufficiency

John Owen

Department of Obstetrics and Gynecology, Division of Maternal-Fetal Medicine,
University of Alabama at Birmingham, Birmingham, AL, USA

Introduction

Traditional teaching depicted the cervix as competent or incompetent; however, current evidence suggests that cervical "competence" is rather one anatomic component of a more complex *spontaneous preterm birth syndrome* that also involves the uterus (i.e., contractions) and the chorioamnion (e.g., premature membrane rupture, PROM) (Romero *et al.* 2006). Although some women whose poor obstetric history suggests a dominant cervical factor actually have physical examination evidence of poor cervical integrity, the vast majority of women who are diagnosed clinically with cervical insufficiency have normal cervical anatomy, both between pregnancies and in early gestation. The clinical presentation of cervical insufficiency more likely results from a process of *premature cervical ripening* (in the absence of clinical labor or chorioamnion rupture) due to one or more underlying factors, including local inflammation (e.g., from bleeding or subclinical infection), hormonal effects or even genetic predisposition. If and when the mechanical (and secondarily, the immunological) integrity of the cervix is compromised, other pathways to prematurity may be stimulated, appearing clinically as the preterm birth syndrome. Thus, the term "cervical insufficiency" may be evolving into a convenient label to describe a more complex, but poorly understood process of pathological premature cervical ripening. The more contemporary usage of the term may characterize a clinical situation where the spontaneous preterm birth syndrome appears to have a dominant cervical component.

Diagnosis of cervical insufficiency

The clinical diagnosis

Simply defined, cervical insufficiency is the inability of the uterine cervix to retain a pregnancy through the second trimester. The *clinical*

Protocols for High-Risk Pregnancies: An Evidence-Based Approach, Sixth Edition.
Edited by John T. Queenan, Catherine Y. Spong and Charles J. Lockwood.
© 2015 John Wiley & Sons, Ltd. Published 2015 by John Wiley & Sons, Ltd.

diagnosis of cervical insufficiency is confidently made in women with recurrent "painless" cervical dilation and spontaneous midtrimester birth, usually of a liveborn who succumbs to extreme prematurity. Generally diagnoses of exclusion, other obvious causes of spontaneous preterm birth (e.g., labor, abruption) are excluded. Since there are few, if any, proven or even practical objective criteria (other than the rare gross cervical malformation) for an interval diagnosis, a careful review of the history and past obstetric records is essential. In many instances the records are unavailable or incomplete, and many women are unable to provide an accurate history. Even with excellent records and a reliable history, clinicians might have divergent opinions about the clinical diagnosis, save for the most classic circumstances. Confounding factors in the history or physical examination might either support or refute the diagnosis, depending on their perceived importance. Clearly, the physician managing a patient who suffers a spontaneous midtrimester birth is in the optimal position to document the events and findings and to assess whether clinical criteria for cervical insufficiency were present (e.g., hour-glassing membranes). However, because the preterm birth syndrome may involve other anatomic components, it should not be surprising that some women with cervical insufficiency have antecedent chorioamnion rupture or eventually develop clinically apparent uterine activity; vaginal bleeding may occur with cervical dilation. Acute chorioamnionitis might also preclude the diagnosis of insufficiency; however, if premature cervical ripening and occult dilation caused loss of the mucus plug and compromised the normal immunological barrier between the vaginal flora and chorioamnion, intrauterine infection might simply be the culminating clinical event (Jones, 1998), and subclinical intrauterine infections are commonly seen in cases of silent cervical dilation, described below. Thus as a diagnosis of exclusion, the extent to which other causes should be excluded has never been completely defined; however, antiphospholipid syndrome and fetal aneuploidy, for example, are well-characterized causes of midtrimester fetal loss and likely do not involve a dominant cervical component.

Physical examination

Physical examination criteria include a gross cervical malformation (classically from birth trauma) or destructive cervical procedures (e.g., trachelectomy). In cases of insufficiency in evolution, criteria are based primarily on case series and comparative studies of women who present with "silent" cervical dilation of at least 2 cm with visible membranes at or beyond the internal os on speculum examination. Interestingly, in most cases cervical length has been maintained, and little effacement is recognized; effacement might be more characteristic of preterm labor. At times clinicians may choose to follow selected patients with serial pelvic examinations in order to detect earlier changes on palpation which may also suggest the diagnosis. Common accompanying symptoms may include a sensation of pelvic pressure, vaginal discharge, urinary frequency, and the absence of regular painful contractions. Termed *acute cervical insufficiency* by most investigators, it provides insight into the natural history of this condition.

Sonography

Numerous investigators have suggested that cervical insufficiency may be a sonographic diagnosis, and clearly there is a relationship between (shortened) cervical length and reproductive performance, chiefly characterized by a spontaneous preterm birth, but not typically the clinical presentation of cervical insufficiency (Honest *et al.* 2003). These observations support the concept of premature cervical ripening. Various sonographic findings, including shortened cervical length, funneling at the internal os and spontaneous or fundal pressure-induced dynamic changes, have been used to support the diagnosis of cervical insufficiency and to select patients for treatment, usually cerclage. Since the possible additive effects of funneling and dynamic changes have been shown to be equivocal (when controlling for cervical length), the most commonly cited criterion for "short cervix" is a midtrimester length less than 25 mm. However, since this finding represents the population 10th percentile and has very poor predictive value for preterm birth in low-risk women, it was an inappropriate sonographic diagnostic criterion for cervical insufficiency.

However, it is also well documented that women with progressively shorter cervical lengths have correspondingly higher rates of preterm birth, but uncommonly develop complete cervical dilation (i.e., acute cervical insufficiency) as described in the next section. Notably, the relationship between obstetric history and cervical length is compelling, because the predictive accuracy of shortened cervical length for spontaneous preterm birth is appreciably higher in women with a history of a prior spontaneous preterm birth, especially an early birth prior to 34 weeks of gestation (Owen *et al.* 2001). Thus, defining appropriate diagnostic criteria for the sonographic diagnosis of insufficiency and the prescription for an effective intervention has been extremely problematic; it is likely that many women were inappropriately given this diagnosis and received an ineffective therapy.

Patient selection for cerclage

History-indicated (a.k.a. prophylactic) cerclage

Women who meet criteria for the clinical diagnosis of cervical insufficiency should be counseled regarding the risks and benefits of cerclage.

Although no randomized trials have been performed in women with a typical history, numerous case series using historic control populations have been summarized (Cousins 1980; Branch 1986) and suggest that, prior to cerclage, perinatal survival ranged from 7% to 50% but that, with cerclage, survival increased to a range from 63% to 89%. Since older series used a metric of perinatal survival and not birth gestational age, the effect on pregnancy prolongation and neonatal morbidities was never properly assessed. Associated risks appear to be low, but include those associated with anesthesia; generally a regional technique is chosen. Contraindications include active cervicitis, certain fetal problems (e.g., anomaly, oligohydramnios), and hemorrhage. Appropriately selected candidates generally undergo surgery at around 14 weeks after sonographic confirmation of a normal fetus.

Physical-examination-indicated (a.k.a. emergent) cerclage

The use of cerclage in the clinical setting of acute cervical insufficiency has been investigated through the use of both case series (absent control populations) and retrospective cohort studies where pregnancy outcomes following the uncontrolled use of cerclage were compared to the outcomes of women with similar examination findings who did not undergo surgery and were usually managed expectantly with bed rest. Only one small randomized trial of cerclage for acute cervical insufficiency has been published comprising 23 patients (Althuisius *et al.* 2003), which showed a significant benefit to cerclage. Collectively, these reports demonstrate a clinically significant benefit from the use of physical examination-indicated cerclage, considering both pregnancy prolongation and neonatal morbidity outcomes.

Women who present with prolapsing membranes at or beyond the external os represent an extraordinarily high-risk and surgically challenging group. Various techniques have been suggested to reduce the membranes at surgery and include combinations of Trendelenberg positioning, therapeutic amnioreduction, uterine relaxants and bladder filling, as well as manual replacement and intraoperative support using a 30–60 mL Foley catheter balloon. These techniques are used empirically and have not been systematically compared to determine the best strategy or combinations. As expected, increasing amounts of dilation and effacement greatly increase the surgical complexity and may even cause the obstetrician to abandon the case; iatrogenic membrane rupture is the most common serious complication. Many clinicians also recommend a preoperative observation period of 12–24 hours to rule out active clinical infection and preterm labor, well-known contraindications to cerclage. Recently, the potential utility of analyzing amniotic fluid harvested in women with acute cervical insufficiency has been investigated. It is clear that a subgroup of these women will have biochemical evidence of inflammation and infection, but whether these results can be used to improve perinatal outcomes has not been demonstrated. Thus, amniotic fluid analysis for patient selection remains investigational (Airioldi et al. 2009).

Ultrasound-indicated (a.k.a. rescue or urgent) cerclage

As of this writing, five randomized trials of cerclage in women with shortened cervical length have been published. Of appreciable interest was a subsequent patient-level meta-analysis of the initial four trials that demonstrated that cerclage benefit was limited to women with singletons *and* a prior preterm birth (Berghella et al. 2005).

In the fifth trial, investigators sought to confirm the importance of obstetric history (Owen et al. 2009). This was the largest trial to date of (McDonald) cerclage for shortened cervical length in high-risk women and included 302 women with singletons and at least one prior spontaneous preterm birth prior to 34 weeks of gestation. Using a cervical length cut-off of less than 25 mm, preterm birth prior to 35 weeks was lower in the cerclage group, 32% vs 42% in the no-cerclage group. While this difference was not statistically significant, previable birth and perinatal mortality were significantly lower in the cerclage group. The importance of obstetric history in selecting women for ultrasound-indicated cerclage was then reaffirmed in a subsequent meta-analysis (Berghella et al. 2011). In summary, the clinical significance of obstetric history in selecting women for ultrasound-indicated cerclage seems irrefutable, and cervical ultrasound surveillance is now appropriate for women with a prior spontaneous preterm birth.

Can cervical ultrasonography be used to avoid cerclage?

In a systematic review of studies that included women with suspected cervical insufficiency, pregnancy outcomes of ultrasound-indicated versus history-indicated cerclage were compared (Blikman et al. 2008). Five of the six reports selected for the review showed similar pregnancy outcomes (spontaneous preterm birth prior to 24 weeks of gestation) between the ultrasound-indicated and the history-indicated cerclage groups. A recent meta-analysis of three randomized trials comparing history-indicated and ultrasound-indicated cerclage demonstrated similar rates of preterm birth and that surgery could be avoided in 58% when sonographic cervical surveillance was utilized (Berghella and Mackeen 2011). Based on this systematic review and meta-analysis, women with suspected, but nonclassic cervical insufficiency may undergo midtrimester cervical length assessment to optimize candidate selection.

Cerclage technique

McDonald cerclage is favored by many obstetricians because of its simplicity in placement (and removal in anticipation of vaginal birth). Under regional anesthesia and with adequate visualization of the cervix, a nonabsorbable suture is placed in a circumferential pattern as close as possible to the bladder reflection anterior and just below the reflection of rectum posterior. Though originally described with four needle insertions, the actual number of penetrations may vary depending on the size of the ectocervix and the penetration depth of the curved needle and its size. Choice of suture varies but includes Mersilene and Prolene. Some prefer Mersilene 0.5 mm tape, which is technically more difficult to place, but is believed by some surgeons to have a theoretic advantage over suture; regardless, no suture type has been shown to be superior.

The Shirodkar cerclage also has strong proponents, although comparative studies have not confirmed its superiority. This technique has the theoretic advantage of placing the Mersilene tape higher along the cervical canal. Special training and experience are required. The initial step is similar to one used in vaginal hysterectomy whereby the bladder and rectum are dissected off the cervix and displaced upward. An Allis clamp grasps and stabilizes the cervical tissue at 3 and 6 o'clock. Then the tape, threaded on an aneurysm needle, is placed medial to the clamp and buried with its securing knot with a separate line of suture under the mucosal edges left from the anterior and posterior dissection. Not surprisingly, removal of a Shirodkar stitch can be challenging and has been associated with an increased risk of cesarean.

Benson originally described an abdominal technique for women whose anatomy prohibited a vaginal approach. Women with cervical hypoplasia, prior cone or large LEEP biopsies or extensive cervical damage from failed cerclage or birth trauma may be selected for this procedure. An increasingly common indication is prior failed transvaginal cerclage (Debbs *et al.* 2007). Originally placed via laparotomy, these have been successfully placed and removed with laparoscopy. Most have been placed in the first trimester, after viability has been established, although interval placement has also been reported. Appropriate candidate selection and placement are generally relegated to specialty centers.

Cerclage removal

In the absence of urgent indications, transvaginal cerclage is removed in the early term period (e.g., 37 weeks). The McDonald stitch can generally be removed as an outpatient, but some bleeding may occur and can generally be managed with local pressure; some sedation is desirable to improve patient tolerance of the procedure. Removal of a Shirodkar stitch usually involves tissue dissection and appreciable risk for bleeding; thus removal as an inpatient with anesthesia available is preferred.

Urgent indications for preterm removal include labor, bleeding, and non-reassuring fetal status. Cervical change in the setting of painful contractions with cerclage in place may be more difficult to appreciate, but serial examination can confirm labor. If tocolytics are prescribed and deemed ineffective, the suture should be removed to avoid cervical laceration. Bleeding at the suture line should in itself prompt removal with suspected labor.

Since many women who undergo cerclage are also at risk for developing other components of the preterm birth syndrome, in addition to spontaneous labor, PROM may also occur. Importantly, no series has found a significant benefit from cerclage retention, and one investigator documented increased neonatal death (largely due to infection) with cerclage retention. A recently published 10-year, multicenter randomized clinical trial of immediate versus delayed removal was halted due to poor patient accrual after only 56 of the planned 142 were recruited (Galyean *et al.* 2014). Though underpowered, there was neither significant benefit nor risk to cerclage retention, although both latency period and peripartum infection rates favored immediate removal. Whether cerclage should be retained while corticosteroids are administered to enhance fetal maturation with concurrent broad-spectrum antibiotic administration has been considered, but if this plan is chosen, the weight of available evidence indicates that stitch should be removed after 48 hours.

Adjunctive therapies

Commonly used adjuncts to cerclage are perioperative prophylactic antibiotics and tocolytics, although active genital infection and preterm labor are widely considered absolute contraindications. Published series and trials suggest that investigators are increasingly likely to prescribe prophylaxis in women undergoing ultrasound-indicated and especially physical-examination-indicated procedures, as compared to history-indicated cases. Lack of randomized trials confirming that these pharmacological adjuncts improve perinatal outcomes suggests that these recommendations are empiric. The authors of a recent review of the evidence (Berghella *et al.* 2013) concluded that tocolytics may be considered in either ultrasound-indicated or physical examination-indicated cerclage but recommend against antibiotics. Although intraamniotic bacterial colonization is common in women with acute cervical insufficiency, this is considered a contraindication to physical examination-indicated cerclage and whether antibiotic therapy improves outcomes in these women has not been investigated. We do recommend screening for and treating known cervical pathogens prior to placing history-indicated and ultrasound-indicated stitches since this is part of standard prenatal care, although this practice has never been formally evaluated in the setting of cerclage. We will empirically prescribe a short course of indomethacin for women with postoperative symptomatic uterine activity.

The use of progesterone congeners, most commonly 17α-hydroxyprogesterone caproate, has been widely investigated for the prevention of recurrent preterm birth. Since most women who are candidates for either history-indicated or ultrasound-indicated cerclage have delivered a prior preterm infant, administration of progesterone beginning in the midtrimester is widely recommended. Less clear and in need of further investigation is whether there is an interaction between progesterone and cerclage in selected patients, rendering progesterone unnecessary or possibly heightening its efficacy. Investigations into whether progesterone congeners begun in the early midtrimester limit cervical shortening and thus the need for ultrasound-indicated cerclage in high-risk women are inconclusive.

Also in need of further investigation is the use of vaginal pessary for preterm birth prevention in women with suspected cervical insufficiency. The results of a recent randomized trial of 380 women (Goya *et al.* 2012) with short cervical length less than 25 mm confirmed a significant reduction in preterm birth with a "cerclage pessary" (not approved for use in the United States as of this writing) compared to no intervention; however, the trial did not focus on high-risk women with a history of spontaneous preterm birth. Thus, it remains to be demonstrated whether a particular pessary design will be shown to have similar efficacy to either history-indicated or ultrasound-indicated cerclage for cervical insufficiency; several clinical trials of pessary for preterm birth prevention are currently in progress.

Bed rest has not been demonstrated to improve pregnancy outcomes for numerous types of pregnancy conditions in controlled studies, and yet it continues to be widely prescribed in women with cervical insufficiency. A recent secondary analysis of a randomized trial of 17-α hydroxyprogesterone caproate for short cervix less than 30 mm found higher rates of preterm birth in women who were placed on activity restriction (Grobman *et al.* 2013). Some clinicians have even justified cerclage placement by suggesting that this mechanical support permits women to expand their physical activities; evidence for this is also absent. The recommendation for post-cerclage pelvic rest seems more practical, leaving activity recommendations individualized and based on maternal symptoms and pelvic findings.

Summary

Contemporary lines of evidence tell us that cervical insufficiency is a poorly defined entity, lacking objective and reproducible criteria. It may be more effectively conceptualized as simply one factor in the complex syndrome of spontaneous preterm birth. Deciding whether an individual patient has a significant (and treatable) component of insufficiency requires significant clinical judgment. Herein are presented evidence-based guidelines for the selection of patients who would reasonably benefit from cerclage.

Suggested reading

Airioldi J, Pereira L, Cotter A, Gomez R, Berghella V, Prasertcharoensuk W, *et al*. Amniocentesis prior to physical exam-indicated cerclage in women with midtrimester cervical dilation: results from the expectant management compared to physical-exam-indicated cerclage international cohort study. *Am J Perinatol* 2009;26:63–8.

Althuisius SM, Dekker GA, Hummel P, van Geijn HP. Cervical incompetence prevention randomized cerclage trial: Emergency cerclage with bed rest versus bed rest alone. *Am J Obstet Gynecol* 2003;189:907–10.

Berghella V, Mackeen AD. Cervical length screening with ultrasound-indicated cerclage compared with history-indicated cerclage for prevention of preterm birth. *Am J Obstet Gynecol* 2011;118:148–55.

Berghella V, Odibo AO, To MS, Rust OA, Althuisius SM. Cerclage for short cervix on ultrasonography, meta-analysis of trials using individual patient-level data. *Obstet Gynecol* 2005;106(1):181–9.

Berghella V, Rafael TJ, Syychowski JM, Rust OA, Owen J. Cerclage for short cervix on ultrasonography in women with singleton gestations and previous preterm birth: a meta-analysis. *Obstet Gynecol* 2011;117:663–71.

Berghella V, Ludmir J, Simonazzi G, Owen J. Transvaginal cervical cerclage: evidence for perioperative management strategies. *Am J Obstet Gynecol* 2013;201:181–92.

Blikman MJC, Le T, Bruinse HW, van der Heijden GJMG. Ultrasound-predicated versus history-predicated cerclage in women at risk of cervical insufficiency: a systematic review. *Obstet Gynecol Surv* 2008;63:803–12.

Branch DW. Operations for cervical incompetence. *Clin Obstet Gynecol* 1986;29:240–54.

Cousins LM. Cervical incompetence 1980: a time for reappraisal. *Clin Obstet Gynecol* 1980;23:467–79.

Debbs RH, Guilleremo ADV, Pearson S, Sehdev H, Marchiano D, Ludmir J. Transabdominal cerclage after comprehensive evaluation of women with previous unsuccessful transvaginal cerclage. *Am J Obstet Gynecol* 2007;197:317.e1–4.

Galyean A, Garite T, *et al*. Removal versus retention of cerclage in preterm premature rupture of membranes: A randomized controlled trial. *Am J Obstet Gynecol* 2014;210 S0002–9378(14)00347-0.

Goya M, Pratcorona L, Merced C, Rodó C, Valle L, Romero A, *et al*. Cervical pessary in pregnant women with a short cervix (PECEP): an open-label randomised controlled trial. *Lancet* 2012;379:1800–6.

Grobman WA, Gilbert SA, Iams JD, Spong CY, Saade G, Bercer BM, *et al*. Activity restriction among women with a short cervix. *Obstet Gynecol* 2013;121:1181–6.

Honest H, Bachmann LM, Coomarasamy A, Gupta JK, Kleijnen J, Khan KS. Accuracy of cervical transvaginal sonography in predicting preterm birth: a systematic review. *Ultrasound Obstet Gynecol* 2003;22:305–322.

Jones G. The weak cervix: failing to keep the baby in or infection out? *Br J Obstet Gynaecol* 1998;105:1214–15.

Owen J, Yost N, Berghella V, Thom E, Swain M, Dildy GA, Miodovnik M, Langer D, Sibai BM. McNellis D for the National Institute for Child Health and Human Development Maternal Fetal Medicine Unit Network. Mid-trimester endovaginal sonography in women at high risk for spontaneous preterm birth. *JAMA* 2001;286:1340–8.

Owen J, Hankins G, Iams JD, *et al.* Multicenter randomized trial of cerclage for preterm birth prevention in high-risk women with shortened midtrimester cervical length. *Am J Obstet Gynecol* 2009;201:375.e1–8.

Romero R, Espinoza J, Kusanovic JP, *et al.* The preterm parturition syndrome. *Br J Obstet Gynecol* 2006;113:17–42.

PROTOCOL 36
Nausea and Vomiting

Gayle Olson
Department of Obstetrics & Gynecology, University of Texas Medical Branch, Galveston, TX, USA

Clinical significance

Nausea and vomiting during pregnancy (NVP) continue to challenge women and their providers. Approximately 85% of women experience some degree of NVP while up to 2% will be afflicted with the more severe condition of hyperemesis gravidarum (HG). HG, typically described as vomiting, dehydration, acid–base disturbance, weight loss due to vomiting, ketonuria and electrolyte disturbances, is seen in no more than 2% of cases.

In addition, approximately 35% of gravidas with nausea and vomiting will consider their symptoms severe enough to limit activities of daily living. This disruption in quality of life further extends to loss of time at work, ineffectiveness at home or on the job and deterioration in relationships.

Unfortunately, because NVP can be so common, symptoms and, therefore, treatment risk being minimized by both patients and healthcare providers, resulting in progression to more severe levels before therapy is initiated.

Pathophysiology

The pathophysiology of NVP has not been clearly identified but is most likely multifactorial. Hypotheses include psychological factors, evolutionary adaptation, hormone alterations, genetic inheritance, infection, and gastrointestinal tract dysfunction. Psychological conditions have not been identified as a cause of NVP, but women in the throes of severe NVP may experience anxiety and other psychosocial morbidity. Increased estrogen and human chorionic gonadotropin (hCG) concentrations during pregnancy have been shown to be associated with nausea and vomiting in a dose-dependent fashion. Finally, gastrointestinal motility

Protocols for High-Risk Pregnancies: An Evidence-Based Approach, Sixth Edition.
Edited by John T. Queenan, Catherine Y. Spong and Charles J. Lockwood.
© 2015 John Wiley & Sons, Ltd. Published 2015 by John Wiley & Sons, Ltd.

is diminished by pregnancy, and gastric emptying time is prolonged which may exacerbate symptoms. Heartburn and acid reflux have been identified in several studies as contributors to the severity of NVP. Women treated for their heartburn and reflux demonstrated increased overall well-being as well as decreased symptoms on objective scoring scales. *Helicobacter pylori*, a gram-negative flagellated spiral bacterium, also plays a role in the severity of symptoms. The evidence of this association is strong enough for related reviews to recommend testing for *H. pylori* when NVP is excessive or extends beyond the expected gestational age (Clark *et al.* 2012).

Risk factors for NVP include an increased placental mass as seen with molar gestation or multiple gestations, a family history or personal history of HG, and a history of motion sickness or migraines. Body mass index (BMI) has also been investigated as a risk factor for NVP. In a retrospective study, Cedergren *et al.* noted underweight women (BMI < 20 kg/m^2) were more likely to be afflicted with severe NVP/HG than normal weight women (RR, 1.19; 95% CI, 1.14–1.24) and require hospitalization (RR, 1.43; 95% CI, 1.33–1.54).

Diagnosis

Nausea and vomiting most often will begin early in pregnancy at 4–5 weeks of gestation, peak around 9–10 weeks and subside by 16 weeks. A small proportion of women will continue to experience symptoms past 16 weeks until the end of the pregnancy. For many women the symptoms will manifest in the morning, hence the term morning sickness. However, a number of pregnant women experience their most severe symptoms at other times of the day, and the failure of nausea to be restricted to the morning in no way invalidates the complaint. When the start of symptoms falls outside the above gestational age range, is accompanied by other complaints or remains persistently severe in spite of adequate treatment, other underlying conditions should be considered and excluded (Table 36.1). In addition, symptoms and findings not associated with simple NVP include abdominal or epigastric pain, fever, headache, cough, goiter and an abnormal neurological examination.

Nausea and vomiting of pregnancy exists as a spectrum of symptoms ranging in severity from mild and self-limited to severe and debilitating. Mild NVP consists of nausea for less than 1 hour and a frequency of vomiting/retching up to twice a day. When the nausea symptoms persist for 6 hours or more with five or more episodes of vomiting/retching NVP may be considered severe. HG, at the severest end of this spectrum is characterized by nausea and vomiting plus weight loss (5% of body weight),

Table 36.1 Differential diagnosis of nausea and vomiting

System	Diagnosis
Gastrointestinal	Gastroenteritis
	Hepatitis
	Peptic ulcer disease
	Pancreatitis
	Appendicitis
	Helicobacter pylori infection
	Herniation or obstruction after bariatric surgery
	Biliary tract disease
Genitourinary tract	Pyelonephritis
	Ovarian torsion
	Kidney stones
Metabolic disease	Diabetic ketoacidosis
	Hyperthyroidism
Neurological disorders	Pseudotumor cerebri
	Vestibular lesions
	Migraines
	Tumors of the central nervous system
	Ventriculoperitoneal shunt malfunction
Psychological	Drug toxicity or intolerance
	Depression
Pregnancy-related	Preeclampsia
	Acute fatty liver

Source: Adapted from ACOG Practice Bulletin No. 52 and 105.

ketonuria, electrolyte disturbances, especially hypokalemia, muscle wasting and dehydration.

Scoring systems have been developed and validated by various investigators to assess the severity of nausea and vomiting (Rhodes score, pregnancy-unique quantification of emesis and nausea (PUQE) and modified-PUQE). The PUQE and modified-PUQE were designed for use during pregnancy and are simplified when compared to the older "gold standard" Rhodes system. The PUQE scoring system focuses and quantifies the three main symptoms of NVP: nausea, vomiting, and retching. A score of 3 suggests no symptoms while 15 is considered severe and provides a rationale to guide drug therapy (Koren *et al.* 2005).

Initial laboratory tests can be considered, as listed in Table 36.2. Additional testing can thereafter be tailored by suspicions for other underlying medical conditions. The structural homology of hCG with TSH contribute to the appearance of transient hyperthyroidism in early pregnancy. This transient hyperthyroidism usually subsides by 20 weeks of gestation. Propylthiouracil is not recommended and does not contribute to a decrease in

Table 36.2 Initial laboratory evaluation

Complete blood count
Urinalysis, ketones
TSH, Free T3, Free T4 (if history suggests thyroid disease)
LDH, AST, ALT, amylase, lipase
Serum blood urea nitrogen, creatinine
Serum sodium, potassium, chloride, magnesium

nausea. True primary hyperthyroidism will typically predate the pregnancy and rarely presents with vomiting.

Women may experience anxiety and demoralization due to NVP. Demoralization, a normal response to illness, is characterized by sadness, fear, irritability, passive aggressive behavior and an active struggle with illness which should be distinguished from depression. An in-depth discussion with the patient can usually determine this distinction.

Treatment

Treatment of NVP varies with the severity of the disease and can begin with nonpharmacological choices including dietary/lifestyle modification and vitamin/herbal supplementation, followed by pharmacological antiemetic therapy. Nonpharmacological therapy includes increased rest and avoidance of foods and odors that trigger symptoms (perfumes, smoke, petroleum products). Adjustment in eating habits may include small, frequent snacks with a focus on bland and dry foods or foods high in protein. Spicy, fatty, and acidic foods may need to be eliminated. High-protein meals have been shown to alleviate nausea and vomiting better than carbohydrate or fatty meals.

Acupressure has been used to alleviate symptoms of nausea and vomiting by applying pressure at the Neguian P6 acupoint. This point is located approximately 2 in. proximal to the wrist crease between the flexor carpi radialis and palmaris longus tendons (Niebyl 2010).

Ginger root, a common spice and flavorer, has also been used for treatment. Ozgoli *et al.* randomized women to ginger 250 mg four times a day for 4 days versus placebo with an improvement in nausea (85% versus 56%; $P = 0.01$) and a decrease in vomiting (50% versus 9%; $P = 0.05$). Ginger extracts at doses up to 1 g/day have been shown to be more efficacious at reducing nausea than vitamin B_6 (pyridoxine). ACOG recommends the use of vitamin B_6 (10–25 mg orally every 8 hours) alone or in combination with doxylamine succinate as first-line therapy (ACOG Practice Bulletin 52, 2004).

Table 36.3 Pharmacological agents for use in nausea and vomiting in pregnancy

Class	Drug name	Risk factor category
H$_1$ receptor antagonist	Doxylamine (Unisom)	A
	Dimenhydrinate (Dramamine)	B$_m$
	Cetirizine (Zyrtec)	B$_m$
	Meclizine (Antivert)	B$_m$
	Hydroxyzine (Vistaril, Atarax)	C
	Diphenhydramine (Benadryl)	B$_m$
H$_2$ receptor antagonist	Cimetidine	B$_m$
	Ranitidine	B$_m$
Anticholinergics	Scopolamine	C$_m$
Dopamine antagonists	Metoclopramide (Reglan)	B$_m$
Phenothiazines	Promethazine (Phenergan)	C
	Prochlorperazine (Compazine)	C
	Chlorpromazine (Thorazine)	C
Serotonin antagonist	Ondansetron (Zofran)	B$_m$
Steroids	Methylprednisolone	C

Source: Adapted from ACOG Practice Bulletin No. 52 and 105.

Diclectin (delayed release pyridoxine hydrochloride 10 mg + doxylamine succinate 10 mg) was studied in comparison to placebo in a double-blind randomized multicentre placebo-controlled trial. Diclectin significantly decreased symptoms of NVP and improved the quality of life compared to placebo.

When nonpharmacological approaches fail, breakthrough therapy using pharmacological agents is needed. The most common categories for use are antihistamines, dopamine antagonists, phenothiazines, and serotonin antagonists (see Table 36.3). Treatment decisions must be individually prescribed; however, treatment algorithms have been proposed to facilitate a rational use of first-line and breakthrough therapy (Fig. 36.1).

Complications

Though rare, persistent vomiting for 3 or more weeks may result in a deficiency of vitamin B$_1$ (thiamine). Thiamine deficiency can be further exacerbated by fluid resuscitation with a dextrose infusion resulting in acute encephalopathy. Also known as Wernicke encephalopathy, this syndrome is characterized by the classic triad of ophthalmoplegia, gait ataxia and mental confusion, or less commonly by memory loss, apathy, altered consciousness and vision changes (Niebyl 2010). The condition is easily treatable and reversible in a majority of cases; however, untreated

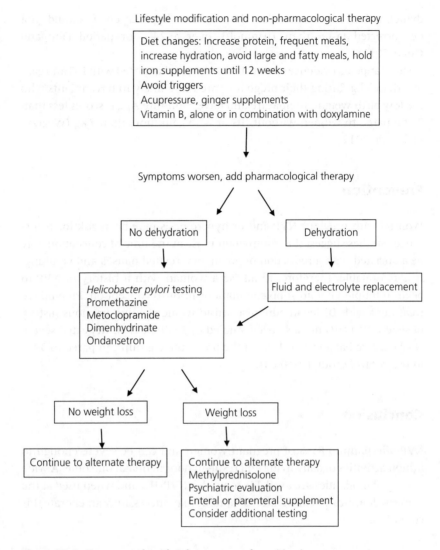

Lifestyle modification and non-pharmacological therapy

> Diet changes: Increase protein, frequent meals, increase hydration, avoid large and fatty meals, hold iron supplements until 12 weeks
> Avoid triggers
> Acupressure, ginger supplements
> Vitamin B, alone or in combination with doxylamine

Symptoms worsen, add pharmacological therapy

No dehydration

Dehydration

> *Helicobacter pylori* testing
> Promethazine
> Metoclopramide
> Dimenhydrinate
> Ondansetron

Fluid and electrolyte replacement

No weight loss

Weight loss

Continue to alternate therapy

> Continue to alternate therapy
> Methylprednisolone
> Psychiatric evaluation
> Enteral or parenteral supplement
> Consider additional testing

Figure 36.1 Treatment algorithm for nausea and vomiting in pregnancy.

encephalopathy has been associated with a fetal loss rate up to 37%. For this reason some would recommend empirically supplementing vitamin B_1 for women with prolonged NVP/HG of greater than 3 weeks in duration (Clark *et al.* 2012; Wegrzyniak *et al.* 2012). Supplementation of thiamine can be administered orally, 1.5 mg/day or intravenously as 100 mg diluted in 100 cc normal saline and infused over 30 minutes weekly (Wegrzyniak *et al.* 2012).

Rapid correction of hyponatremia resulting from HG can result in the severe complication of central pontine myelinolysis or osmotic dymelination syndrome. For this reason, hyponatremia should not be corrected faster than 10 mmol/L over a 24-hour period (Tan and Omar 2011).

There appears evidence that women who are diagnosed with HG and gain less than 7 kg during their pregnancy are more likely to have infants who are low birth weight, premature and have 5-minute Apgar scores less than 7 compared to women without HG or who gain more than 7 kg (Wegrzyniak *et al.* 2012).

Prevention

Women with previous NVP and/or hyperemesis may be at risk for recurrence. Studies suggest that multivitamin use at the time of conception may be associated with a reduction of pregnancy-related nausea and vomiting. It is reasonable, therefore, to advise a woman with a history of NVP to begin multiple vitamin supplementations prior to conception. Preemptive treatment with Diclectin administered to women with a previous history of severe NVP/HG has also been studied by Maltepe *et al*. Repeated severe NVP occurred at a rate of 15% in the preemptive group compared to 39% in the control group ($P < 0.04$).

Conclusion

NVP affects up to 85% of pregnant women and can be severe enough to inhibit activities of daily living and result in poor neonatal outcome. A wide variety of modalities are available to use for NVP/HG and when used at the earliest identification of signs or symptoms may successfully ameliorate this condition.

Suggested reading

American College of Obstetricians and Gynecologists. Nausea and vomiting of pregnancy. ACOG Practice Bulletin No. 52. American College of Obstetricians and Gynecologists. *Obstet Gynecol* 2004;103:803–15. (Reaffirmed 2013).

American College of Obstetricians and Gynecologists. Bariatric Surgery and Pregnancy. ACOG Practice Bulletin No. 105. American College of Obstetricians and Gynecologists. *Obstet Gynecol* 2009;113:1405–13. (Reaffirmed 2013).

Briggs GG, Freeman RK, Yaffe SJ, editors. *Drugs in Pregnancy and Lactation: A Reference guide to fetal and neonatal risk*. 9th ed. Philadelphia, PA: Lippincott Williams & Wilkins; 2011.

Cedergren M, Brynhildsen J, Josefsson A, Sydsjö G. Hyperemesis gravidarum that requires hospitalization and the use of antiemetic drugs in relation to maternal body composition. *Am J Obstet Gynecol* 2008;198:412.e1–412.e5.

Clark S, Costantine M, Hankins G. Review of NVP and HG and early pharmacotherapeutic intervention. *Obstet Gynecol Int* 2012;2012:252676.

Koren G, Piwko E, Ahn E, *et al.* Validation studies of the Pregnancy Unique-Quantification of Emesis (PUQE) scores. *Obstet Gynecol* 2005;25(3):241–44.

Maltepe C, Koren G. Preemptive treatment of nausea and vomiting of pregnancy results of a randomized controlled trial. *Obstet Gynecol Int* 2013;2013:809787.

Niebyl J. Nausea and vomiting in pregnancy. *N Engl J Med* 2010;363:1544–50.

Ozgoli G, Goli M, Simbar M. Effects of ginger capsules on pregnancy, nausea, and vomiting. *J Altern Complem Med* 2009;15:243–46.

Tan PC, Omar SZ. Contemporary approaches to hyperemesis during pregnancy. *Curr Opin Obstet Gynecol* 2011;23(2):87–93.

U.S. National Library of Medicine. National Institute of Health, Health and Human Services. Drug Information Portal Mobile Site. Druginfo.nlm.nih.gov, 2014.

Wegrzyniak L, Repke J, Ural S. Treatment of hyperemesis gravidarum. *Rev Obstet Gynecol* 2012;5(2):78–84.

PROTOCOL 37

Fetal Death and Stillbirth

Robert M. Silver

Department of Obstetrics & Gynecology, Division of Maternal-Fetal Medicine,
University of Utah Health Sciences Center, Salt Lake City, UT, USA

Overview

The death of an advanced pregnancy is an extremely difficult medical and emotional challenge for clinicians and families. The problem is common, as pregnancy loss occurs in about 12% of clinically recognized pregnancies. Most of these are spontaneous abortions that happen early in gestation. However, approximately 3% of pregnancies result in fetal death. Thus, obstetric providers will care for many women with the condition. Traditionally, the term "missed abortion" referred to the presence of a nonviable pregnancy *in utero* prior to 20 weeks of gestation. It is more useful to distinguish between pre-embryonic pregnancy loss (gestational sac without an embryo – previously referred to as "blighted ovum"), embryonic demise (embryo without cardiac activity at less than 10 weeks of gestation), and fetal demise (fetus without cardiac activity after 10 weeks of gestation). These terms refer to fetal loss that occurs prior to the onset of labor. Nonviable pregnancies after 20 weeks of gestation are traditionally referred to as stillbirths. Fetal death or stillbirth that occurs during the labor process is referred to as intrapartum fetal death or stillbirth.

Pathophysiology and etiology

There is no single pathophysiological mechanism that explains all cases of fetal death. There are a myriad of causes and in many cases an etiology is never determined. Causes and risk factors of fetal loss include genetic problems such as chromosomal abnormalities, syndromes and single gene mutations, birth defects, bacterial infections, viral infections, fetal–maternal hemorrhage, red cell alloimmunization, hypertension, diabetes, renal disease, thyroid disease, antiphospholipid

Protocols for High-Risk Pregnancies: An Evidence-Based Approach, Sixth Edition.
Edited by John T. Queenan, Catherine Y. Spong and Charles J. Lockwood.
© 2015 John Wiley & Sons, Ltd. Published 2015 by John Wiley & Sons, Ltd.

syndrome, substance abuse, disorders unique to multiple gestation, abruption, and uterine anomalies such as uterine septum. Umbilical cord accidents are often attributed as the cause of fetal death, but this is difficult to prove. Common features of some of these conditions include placental insufficiency, fetal anemia, cardiac insufficiency, and hypoxia. The frequency of these disorders varies among populations and also with gestational age. For example, chromosomal abnormalities are more common in pregnancy loss during the first trimester, while antiphospholipid syndrome is more strongly associated with second or third trimester losses. Many cases of intrapartum fetal death are due to preterm labor, often with cervical insufficiency, chorioamnionitis and preterm premature rupture of membranes, usually at a previable gestational age. A majority of women in the United States with fetal deaths have incomplete or inadequate evaluations for possible causes (see Section "Follow up").

Diagnosis

Women may note the cessation of signs and symptoms associated with pregnancy or absence of previously perceived fetal movements. On physical examination, the uterus may be smaller than expected, and fetal heart tones are inaudible. After 10 weeks of gestation, the hand-held Doppler to detect fetal heart tones may further assist in the diagnosis. Real-time ultrasonography confirms the absence of fetal movements and/or absence of fetal heart or aortic pulsations. In cases of pre-embryonic loss, there are specific sonographic criteria that can be used to confirm that the pregnancy is not viable. In cases of very early pre-embryonic loss, serial sonograms may be required to make a definitive diagnosis. Vaginal bleeding or uterine cramping will only occur in a subset of women with pregnancy loss. It is unclear why some, but not all, cases of pregnancy loss will present with bleeding or labor. Also, fetal death may precede bleeding or cramping by an extended and variable period of time.

Treatment

A significant part of the treatment of families with pregnancy loss is dealing with their (almost universal) feelings of failure and personal guilt. It is crucial to provide reassurance that there was nothing they did to cause the loss, nor anything they could have done to prevent it. They should be offered bereavement services, counseling, support groups, etc. Making every effort to determine an etiology (see Section "Follow up") is also very important for most couples. If a cause of pregnancy loss is determined it facilitates grieving and helps to bring "emotional closure" for the couple. It is also critical for counseling regarding subsequent pregnancies.

In all cases of pregnancy loss, the couple should be offered the options of uterine evacuation (either surgical or medical) or expectant management. Both of these options are medically safe for most women, and the decision may be made on an emotional basis. Many women have strong feelings about wanting to proceed immediately, while others desire as natural a process as possible. Most women will eventually pass the products of conception or labor after a period of expectant management. In general, the later in gestation, the less likely patients are to elect expectant management.

Expectant management

There are some theoretical risks of expectant management including intrauterine infection and maternal coagulopathy. These risks have prompted some authorities to advise delivery within 2 weeks of the demise and to institute surveillance for infection and coagulopathy. Examples of such surveillance include weekly visits for counseling and support and examination for evidence of rupture of membranes, infection, cervical dilation and/or bleeding. Determination of weekly complete blood count, platelet count, and fibrinogen level after 3 weeks of expectant therapy also has been advised. This latter recommendation is based on a reported 25% chance of consumptive coagulopathy if a dead fetus remains in utero for longer than 4 weeks. However, the risk appears to be less than originally reported and is limited to stillbirths. The vast majority of women with fetal deaths after 20 weeks of gestation do not choose prolonged expectant management. Although the aforementioned surveillance is not medically harmful, it is of unproven efficacy and is not required in the absence of symptoms, especially in cases less than 20 weeks of gestation. Patients should be advised to report symptoms associated with infection or bleeding.

Dilation and curettage (uterus 12 weeks of gestation in size or less)

1 Admit to the hospital, day operating room, office, or clinic.
2 Obtain baseline hematocrit if there is concern for baseline anemia. Obtain blood type if unavailable.
3 Administer misoprostol 4 hours prior to the procedure in order to facilitate cervical instrumentation. A typical dose is 200 mg placed in the posterior fornix (may be placed by patient) or taken orally as a lozenge.
4 Perform dilation and evacuation.
5 Discharge home after conscious sedation/anesthesia has worn off and the patient exhibits minimal vaginal bleeding.
6 Administer RhD immune globulin if the patient is RhD negative.

7 Schedule a follow-up visit in 2 weeks.

8 Prescribe NSAIDs or mild narcotics.

Dilation and evacuation (uterus between 13 and 22 weeks of gestation in size)

1 Admit to the hospital, day operating room, office, or clinic.

2 Obtain baseline hematocrit and blood type and screen.

3 Place laminaria at least 4–6 hours prior to the procedure.

4 Administer misoprostol 4 hours prior to the procedure in order to facilitate cervical instrumentation. A typical dose is 200 mg placed in the posterior fornix (may be placed by patient) or taken orally as a lozenge.

5 Perform dilation and evacuation.

6 Discharge to home after conscious sedation/anesthesia has won off and the patient exhibits minimal vaginal bleeding.

7 Administer RhD immune globulin if the patient is RhD negative.

8 Schedule a follow-up visit in 2 weeks.

9 Prescribe NSAIDs or mild narcotics.

Dilation and evacuation at gestations beyond 22 weeks may be safely performed by a small number of experienced practitioners. Modifications to this protocol may be required for gestations beyond 22 weeks.

Induction of labor

Many patients wish to proceed with induction of labor rather than dilation and evacuation. This may be due to a late gestational age or a desire to deliver an intact fetus. In turn, this may allow for a higher quality postmortem examination of the fetus and placenta and may facilitate bereavement. The availability of prostaglandins has greatly improved our ability to successfully induce labor at early gestational ages. The appropriate dosing of prostaglandins is determined by (1) whether the fetus is viable and (2) the size of the uterus. Even in the presence of a nonviable fetus, lower dosing is required when the uterus is greater than 28 weeks of gestation in size due to the potential for uterine rupture. Prostaglandin E_{2a} has been the most commonly used drug for the induction of labor during the past 30 years. However, misoprostol has become the prostaglandin of choice for induction of labor in cases of fetal demise due to similar efficacy (compared with prostaglandin E_{2a}) with fewer side effects. Misoprostol may be placed in the vaginal fornix or taken orally as a lozenge. The interval to delivery is shorter on average when the drug is administered vaginally. Adverse effects of prostaglandins include nausea, vomiting, diarrhea, or pyrexia. There may be only minimal changes in cervical dilation with strong uterine contractions. Delivery often occurs suddenly, after only minimal cervical dilation. Contraindications to the use of misoprostol include active cardiac, pulmonary or renal disease, and glaucoma. Also, the drug (or any prostaglandin product) should not be used for labor induction in cases of prior uterine scar if the uterus is greater than 26 weeks gestational size.

Fetal demise (uterus less than 28 weeks of gestation in size)

1 Admit the patient to the hospital.
2 Obtain baseline laboratory values of complete blood cell count (CBC) and type and screen. Consider assessment of platelet count and fibrinogen level if the fetus has been dead for over 4 weeks duration.
3 Misoprostol is administered at a dose of 200 mg placed in the posterior fornix. This is repeated every 4 hours until delivery of the fetus and placenta. Up to 400 mg given every 2 hours may be safely used at this gestation. However, it does not shorten the interval to delivery compared with 200 mg given every 4 hours. The misoprostol also may be given orally (taken as a lozenge) at a dose of 200 to 400 mg every 2–4 hours. This route of administration requires (on average) a few hours longer to cause delivery compared with vaginal administration. However, it is preferred by some patients or providers. There is substantial risk for retained placenta, especially prior to 20 weeks of gestation. This risk can be diminished by allowing the placenta to spontaneously deliver. Patience and the avoidance of pulling on the cord are essential. Additional doses of misoprostol can be administered (at appropriate intervals) to promote uterine contractility between delivery of the fetus and placenta.
4 Vital signs should be assessed per routine for labor and delivery.
5 Epidural anesthesia can be utilized.
6 Narcotics, antiemetics, and antipyretics should be used as needed.
7 If vital signs are stable and the patient is not bleeding excessively, she may be discharged from the hospital in 6 to 24 hours. Many women wish to leave the hospital as soon as it is medically safe so as to avoid further emotional distress. If possible, patients suffering fetal demise should receive postpartum care on a nonmaternity ward.
8 Parents should be encouraged to spend time with their infant and offered pictures, hand and foot prints, casts, etc.
9 Administer RhD immune globulin to RhD-negative mothers.
10 A follow-up visit (2 to 6 weeks) and bereavement services should be offered.

Fetal demise (uterus greater than 28 weeks of gestation in size)

1 Admit the patient to the hospital.

2 Obtain baseline laboratory values of CBC and type and screen. Consider assessment of platelet count and fibrinogen level if the fetus has been dead for over 4 weeks duration.

3 Misoprostol is administered at a dose of 25 mg placed in the posterior fornix. This is repeated (at a dose of 25–50 mg) every 4 hours until delivery of the fetus and placenta. The misoprostol also may be given orally (taken as a lozenge) at a dose of 25 mg every 4 hours. This route of administration requires (on average) a few hours longer to cause delivery compared with vaginal administration. There is substantial risk for retained placenta, especially prior to 20 weeks of gestation. This risk can be diminished by allowing the placenta to spontaneously deliver. Patience and the avoidance of pulling on the cord are essential. Additional doses of misoprostol can be administered (at appropriate intervals) to promote uterine contractility between delivery of the fetus and placenta.

4 In the presence of a favorable cervix (Bishop score of 6 or more), either before or after the administration of one or more doses of misoprostol, oxytocin may be infused per usual protocol for induction of labor.

5 Vital signs should be assessed per routine for labor and delivery.

6 Epidural anesthesia can be utilized.

7 Narcotics, antiemetics, and antipyretics should be used as needed.

8 If vital signs are stable and the patient is not bleeding excessively, she may be discharged from the hospital in 12 to 24 hours. Many women wish to leave the hospital as soon as it is medically safe so as to avoid further emotional distress. If possible, patients suffering fetal demise should receive postpartum care on a nonmaternity ward.

9 The parents should be encouraged to spend time with their infant and offered pictures, hand and foot prints, casts, etc.

10 Administer RhD immune globulin to RhD-negative mothers.

11 A follow-up visit (2 to 6 weeks) and bereavement services should be offered.

If the duration of fetal death is more than 4 weeks or is unknown, obtain blood fibrinogen levels and complete blood and platelet counts. Because fibrinogen levels are elevated up to 450 mg/dL in pregnancy, normal blood fibrinogen level (300 mg/dL) may be an early signs of consumptive coagulopathy. Significant coagulopathy does not occur until fibrinogen levels fall to less than 100 mg/dL. Subsequent tests showing elevated prothrombin time and thromboplastin time, decreased fibrinogen and platelet count, and the presence of fibrin degradation products confirm the diagnosis of a consumptive coagulopathy. Manifestations of the coagulopathy are variable and may include localized bleeding, petechiae, or minor generalized bleeding or no evidence of bleeding. Upon diagnosis of a clotting deficit, continue monitoring clotting mechanisms and deliver the patient by the most appropriate means. If the clotting defect is severe or there is evidence of bleeding, replenish blood volume and depleted clotting factors with blood component therapy before inducing labor and delivery. Again, this complication of fetal demise is extremely rare. Thus, it is unnecessary to order extensive and serial laboratory studies in the absence of clinical bleeding and if an initial coagulation screen is normal.

Diagnostic evaluation

The most important and useful tests in the work-up of fetal death are perinatal autopsy, placental histology, karyotype and chromosomal microarray. If possible, these tests should be performed in all cases. Also, a test for fetal–maternal hemorrhage should be done since it is only helpful for a few weeks after the demise. The remaining tests can be accurately performed at a later date, and need only be done if prompted by clues in the clinical story, autopsy, etc.

1 Autopsy should be offered and encouraged. If the family does not consent to autopsy, consider magnetic resonance imaging, X-ray and/or gross evaluation by a trained dysmorphologist (typically a pediatric geneticist). This can provide valuable information in lieu of autopsy.

2 The placenta should undergo gross and microscopic evaluation.

3 Although cost may be an issue, fetal karyotype should be considered. This may be of greater emotional value in patients with recurrent pregnancy loss, or with second or third trimester losses. Although abnormal karyotypes are common in first trimester losses (relative to losses later in gestation), they are usually due to *de novo* nondisjunctional events that do not tend to recur. Tissues that remain alive despite in utero death (either placental tissue or tissues that remain alive at low oxygen tension) are most likely to provide cells for chromosome analysis. Examples include chorionic plate (near the insertion of the umbilical cord), fascia lata, and the nape of the neck. Techniques such as chromosomal microarray allow for the assessment of chromosomal abnormalities, even in cases wherein cells will not grow in culture. Therefore, it is appropriate to perform in cases of cell culture failure. In addition, microarray can identify abnormalities not revealed by standard karyotype. Thus, it is an attractive approach to genetic testing in cases of pregnancy loss. At present, it costs more than karyotype and may not be feasible in all cases. However, it will probably eventually replace karyotype as a first-line genetic test for fetal death due to a much lower failure rate.

4 Obtain a Kleihauer-Betke (or flow cytometry) to assess for fetal–
maternal hemorrhage. Ideally this should be accomplished soon after
the diagnosis of fetal demise, although it is probably valuable for a few
weeks after delivery. In addition to determining a potential cause for the
demise, excessive fetal–maternal hemorrhage may require additional
dosing of RhD immune globulin in RhD-negative individuals.

5 Clinical data should be assessed for evidence of hypertension, renal
disease, infection, occult rupture of membranes, cervical insufficiency,
abruption, etc.

6 Clinically overt diabetes and thyroid disease are associated with fetal
death. However, the utility of screening for asymptomatic disease with
glycosylated hemoglobin and/or TSH is uncertain and is not routinely
advised.

7 Antibody screen should be obtained (if unavailable from the prenatal
record).

8 Several investigators report an association between heritable thrombophilias such as the factor V Leiden mutation, the 2010A prothrombin
gene mutation, hyperhomocysteinemia, protein C deficiency, protein S
deficiency and antithrombin III deficiency and fetal death. However,
the association is controversial and routine screening is not currently
advised for isolated cases of fetal demise. Consider testing in cases of
recurrent fetal death or thromboembolism.

9 Consider testing for antiphospholipid syndrome with lupus anticoagulant screen and testing for anticardiolipin antibodies if there is evidence
of placental insufficiency, and/or the patient has recurrent pregnancy
loss, thromboembolism, or autoimmune disease.

10 TORCH titers are recommended by some authorities. However, clinical
utility is low and the test is not advised in routine cases. Careful autopsy
and placental evaluation may be more valuable in the diagnosis of fetal
infection.

11 Serological screen for syphilis should be assessed.

12 Toxicology screen should be considered if the clinical data (such as
abruption or hypertensive crisis) raise suspicion for illicit drugs.

13 Consideration should be given to assessment of the uterine cavity after
the patient fully recovers (3 months postpartum). Clinical evidence of
cervical insufficiency, second trimester losses and evidence of placental
insufficiency increase the likelihood of finding a uterine abnormality.

Follow up

The patient should be offered a postpartum visit at 1–2 weeks to assess
emotional well-being and to offer support and psychological counseling.

Another visit should be scheduled at 6–8 weeks postpartum. At this time, data should be available from diagnostic testing so that obstetric counseling may be accomplished. In some cases, further evaluation may be appropriate.

The risk of recurrent fetal death is estimated to be 2–10 times increased over baseline. Also, there is an increased rate of obstetric complications such as preeclampsia, fetal growth impairment, and preterm birth in subsequent pregnancies. No interventions are proven to improve obstetric outcome. However, antenatal surveillance and/or elective delivery at term may provide emotional benefit and have the potential to reduce subsequent complications.

Suggested reading

American College of Obstetricians and Gynecologists. Management of Stillbirth. ACOG Practice Bulletin No. 102. American College of Obstetricians and Gynecologists. *Obstet Gynecol* 2009;113:748–61.

Korteweg FJ, Erwich JJ, Timmer A, *et al.* Evaluation of 1025 fetal deaths: a proposed diagnostic workup. *Am J Obstet Gynecol* 2012;206:53e1–56.

Reddy UM. Prediction and prevention of recurrent stillbirth. *Obstet Gynecol* 2007;110:1151–64.

Reddy UM, Page GP, Saade GR, Silver RM, Thorsten VR, Parker CB, Pinar H, Willinger M, Stoll BJ, Heim-Hall J, Varner MW, Goldenberg R, Bukowski R, Wapner RJ, Drews-Botsch CD, O'Brien B, Dudley DJ, Levy B for the Eunice Kennedy Shriver National Institute of Child Health and Human Development (NICHD) Stillbirth Collaborative Research Network (SCRN). Genetic abnormalities in stillbirth: comparison of karyotype and microarray testing. *N Engl J Med* 2012;367:2185–93.

Silver RM, Varner MV, Reddy UM, *et al.* Work-up of stillbirth: a review of the evidence. *Am J Obstet Gynecol* 2007;196:433–44.

Silver RM. Fetal death. *Obstet Gynecol* 2007;109:153–67.

Silver RM, Branch DW, Goldenberg R, Iams JD, Klebanoff MA. Nomenclature for pregnancy outcomes: time for a change. *Obstet Gynecol* 2011;118:1402–8.

The Stillbirth Collaborative Research Network Writing group – corresponding author Silver RM, Bukowski R, Carpenter M, Conway D, Coustan D, Dudley DJ, Koch MA, Goldenberg R, Rowland Hogue CJ, Parker CB, Pinar H, Reddy UM, Saade GR, Silver RM, Stoll B, Varner MW, Willinger M. Causes of death among stillbirths. *JAMA* 2011;306:2459–68.

The Stillbirth Collaborative Research Network Writing group Silver RM, Bukowski R, Carpenter M, Conway D, Coustan D, Dudley DJ, Koch MA, Goldenberg R, Rowland Hogue CJ, Parker CB, Pinar H, Reddy UM, Saade GR, Silver RM, Stoll B, Varner MW, Willinger M. Association between stillbirth and risk factors known at pregnancy confirmation. *JAMA* 2011;306:2469–79.

PROTOCOL 38

Abnormal Amniotic Fluid Volume

Thomas R. Moore

Department of Reproductive Medicine, Division of Perinatal Medicine, University of California at San Diego, San Diego, CA, USA

Overview

Adequate amniotic fluid volume is necessary for proper fetal growth and development. Severe and longstanding oligohydramnios, especially prior to 20 weeks of gestation, inhibits lung growth and promotes limb positional defects such as club foot and arm contractures. Thick meconium, deep variable fetal heart rate decelerations, and low birth weight centile are common findings in the term or post-term gestation complicated by low amniotic fluid. Perinatal mortality has been reported to be increased 13-fold to 47-fold in the presence of marginal to severe oligohydramnios, respectively. Presence of oligohydramnios in the second trimester carries a 43% perinatal mortality rate. Table 38.1 contains some figures for oligohydramnios and perinatal morbidity. When amniotic fluid is essentially absent (anhydramnios), lethal outcomes are as high as 88%. Similarly, excessive amniotic fluid, polyhydramnios, has a twofold to fivefold increase in perinatal mortality (Chauhan *et al.* 1999).

Table 38.1 Correlation of oligohydramnios and perinatal morbidity

Antepartum AFI less than 5.0 cm	Relative risk*	95% confidence interval
Risk of cesarean delivery for fetal distress	2.22	1.47–3.37
Risk of Apgar score less than 7 at 5 minutes	5.16	2.36–11.29

AFI, amniotic fluid index.
*Pooled relative risks from meta-analysis.
Source: Chauhan *et al.*, 1999. Adapted with permission of Elsevier.

Protocols for High-Risk Pregnancies: An Evidence-Based Approach, Sixth Edition.
Edited by John T. Queenan, Catherine Y. Spong and Charles J. Lockwood.
© 2015 John Wiley & Sons, Ltd. Published 2015 by John Wiley & Sons, Ltd.

Physiology of normal amniotic fluid volume

Amniotic fluid volume is normally regulated within a surprisingly narrow range. Studies of normal human pregnancies have shown that the amniotic fluid volume rises linearly from early gestation up to 32 weeks, whereupon it remains constant in the range of 700–800 mL until term. After 40 weeks of gestation, the volume declines at a rate of 8% per week. By 42 weeks, this volume decreases to about 400 mL (Fig. 38.1) (Brace and Wolf 1989).

Factors influencing amniotic fluid volume
Amniotic fluid production

Fetal urination is the predominant source of amniotic fluid after fetal kidney function begins at 10–12 weeks. This notion is confirmed by the almost complete absence of amniotic fluid with fetal renal obstruction or agenesis. Estimates of human fetal urine output from sonographic bladder measurements indicate urine production rate of 1000–1200 mL/day near term. Thus changes in fetal urine production have a major impact on amniotic fluid volume. Fetal lung fluid is an additional contributor to

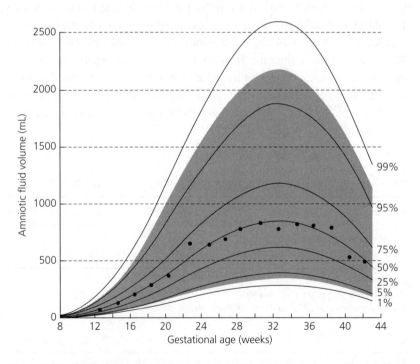

Figure 38.1 Normal amniotic fluid volume in pregnancy. Source: Brace and Wolf, 1989. Adapted with permission of Elsevier.

amniotic fluid volume, but comprises less than half of urine flow. Fetal urinary flow rates are reduced in conditions of placental insufficiency and hypoxia, and increased in the setting of fetal hydrops (e.g., twin–twin transfusion syndrome, fetal anemias). Thus sonographic assessment of placental and fetal cardiac function is an important adjunct to the workup of abnormal amniotic fluid volume.

Amniotic fluid removal

Fetal swallowing is the major mechanism by which fluid leaves the amniotic cavity and has been estimated at 500 mL/day from radio-labeled erythrocytes injected into the amniotic cavity, a rate considerably less than the volume flowing into the amniotic space from urinary output. Thus other paths must exist to balance amniotic fluid volume and these are *transmembranous fluid movement* across the amniotic membranes into the maternal circulation and *intramembranous movement* into the fetal circulation via the vessels on the fetal surface of the placenta. Unfortunately these pathways, well demonstrated in nonhuman species, cannot be measured or manipulated clinically. When evaluating cases of apparently high amniotic fluid volume, therefore, sonographic evaluation of fetal swallowing function is important. Problems with fetal swallowing can be inferred by failing to visualize a normal-sized stomach, noting anatomic anomalies of the fetal face and neck, potential esophageal obstruction due to a thoracic mass, or intestinal obstruction due to gastroschisis or segmental atresia.

Amniotic fluid volume changes with gestational age

Figure 38.1 demonstrates the changes in amniotic fluid volumes during gestation. Important features of this curve include: (1) amniotic fluid volume rises progressively during gestation until approximately 32 weeks; (2) from 32 to 39 weeks, the mean amniotic fluid volume is relatively constant in the range of 700–800 mL; (3) from 40 to 44 weeks there is a progressive decline in amniotic fluid volume at a rate of 8% per week, averaging only 400 mL at 42 weeks; (4) the variation in "normal" fluid volume below the mean value is modest. "Oligohydramnios" (the 5th percentile) is approximately 300 mL. However, variation in the upper range is almost threefold greater, with "polyhydramnios" (95th percentile) varying from 1700 to 1900 mL. Thus "abnormal" amniotic fluid volume should be determined after reference to a curve or table that includes gestational age as a variable (see Fig. 38.2).

Oligohydramnios
Diagnosis

Effective management of oligohydramnios begins with accurate diagnosis. Unfortunately, sonographic methods for determining amniotic fluid

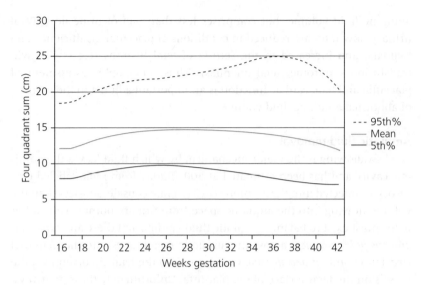

Figure 38.2 Amniotic fluid index percentiles during pregnancy. Source: Moore and Cayle, 1990. Adapted with permission of Elsevier.

volume such as amniotic fluid index (AFI) and maximal vertical pocket (MVP) perform best for identifying normal amniotic fluid volumes, while sonographic methods for identifying oligohydramnios are much less than optimal.

The AFI is calculated by summing the vertical amniotic fluid pocket depth in each of four quadrants of the uterus. Mild oligohydramnios should be suspected with an AFI of less than 7 cm. AFI values less than 5 cm are distinctly abnormal (less than 2% of normal pregnancies at term; Fig. 38.2). However, it should be noted that the lower 5th centile boundary for AFI varies significantly with gestational age. At term, an AFI of 5 cm has been used as a common cut-off value to define oligohydramnios. Particular care should be taken in measuring the AFI when amniotic fluid volume appears to be low. Intraobserver and interobserver errors have been shown to average between 5 and 10 mm, respectively, or approximately 3–7% overall but the error can be as high as ±30% for an AFI below 7 cm. To minimize this error in patients with decreased amniotic fluid, the AFI measurements should be done in triplicate and averaged. It is also important to avoid measuring into narrow, slit-like amniotic fluid pockets. All amniotic fluid pockets should have a width of at least 1 cm and no intervening structures should be visible (e.g., umbilical cord, fetal limbs or digits). Similar conventions apply to measuring the MVP: care must be taken to survey the entire uterus and visualize the deepest pocket at least 1 cm in width. For the diagnosis of oligohydramnios, the absence of an MVP of 2 cm in depth is commonly used.

Table 38.2 Comparison of use of amniotic fluid index or mean vertical pocket in antepartum testing

AFI vs MVP	Relative risk	95% CI
NICU admission	1.04	0.85–1.26
Umbilical artery pH less than 7.1	1.1	0.74–1.65
Diagnosis of oligohydramnios	2.39	1.73–3.28
Induction of labor	1.92	1.5–2.46
Cesarean delivery	1.09	0.92–1.29
Cesarean delivery for fetal distress	1.46	1.08–1.96

AFI, amniotic fluid index; MVP, maximum vertical pocket; CI, confidence interval; NICU, neonatal intensive care unit.
Source: Data from Nabhan et al., 2008.

For documentation of relative amniotic fluid volume at the time of diagnostic sonography, the AFI is most commonly employed and referenced to the values in Fig. 38.2. However, for determining the presence or absence of oligohydramnios as part of antepartum testing, a significant body of evidence suggests that the MVP can be used with equivalent or even superior effectiveness. A systematic review of five randomized controlled trials comparing AFI and MVP by Nabhan and Abdelmoula (2008) determined that MVP measurement during fetal biophysical surveillance seems a better choice since the use of the AFI increases the rate of diagnosis of oligohydramnios and the rate of induction of labor with equivalent results in peripartum outcomes (Table 38.2).

Table 38.3 is a tabulation of the average and upper/lower 5% boundary values for both the AFI and MVP during gestation reported by Magann et al. (2000).

Evaluation
Rule out ruptured membranes

The workup of oligohydramnios is generally initiated by careful sonography and physical examination. Near term, ruptured membranes as the cause of oligohydramnios can reliably be confirmed by examination of the fluid in the vaginal fornix. However, chronic leakage of amniotic fluid may be difficult to detect especially in the second trimester. If a normal-sized fetal bladder is observed in the presence of oligohydramnios, the most likely cause is premature rupture of membranes (PROM). Prior to 20 weeks of gestation, sterile speculum or biochemical tests may be negative or equivocal, and the patient may not be sure whether vaginal moisture represents amniotic fluid or cervical mucus. Although instillation of a dye such as indigo carmine may provide unequivocal proof of PROM, such invasive

Table 38.3 Diagnostic categories of ultrasonographic amniotic fluid volume assessment

Week of gestation	20	21	22	23	24	25	26	27	28	29	30	31	32	33	34	35	36	37	38	39	40	41
Maximum vertical pocket (cm)																						
5th Percentile	3	3	3	3	3	3	3	3	3	3	3	3	3	3	3	3	3	3	2	2	2	2
50th Percentile	4	5	5	5	5	5	5	5	5	5	5	5	5	5	5	5	5	5	4	4	4	4
95th Percentile	7	7	7	7	7	7	7	7	7	7	7	7	7	7	7	7	7	7	7	7	6	6
Amniotic fluid index (cm)																						
5th Percentile	5	5	6	6	6	7	7	7	8	8	8	8	8	7	7	7	6	6	6	5	5	4
50th Percentile	8	9	9	10	11	11	12	13	13	13	14	14	14	13	13	12	12	11	10	9	9	8
95th Percentile	11	12	13	14	15	16	17	18	19	19	20	20	21	21	20	20	19	19	18	17	16	15

Source: Magann et al., 2000. Adapted with permission of Elsevier.

procedures rarely affect management except in cases of previable PROM (prior to 23 weeks).

Assess fetal urinary tract anatomy and function

If there is no evidence of PROM, detailed assessment of fetal urinary tract anatomy is in order since renal and ureteral anomalies are the most common causes of severe oligohydramnios. Sonographic evaluation should include the renal dimensions and morphology of the parenchyma, dimensions of the renal pelvis and morphology of the urinary bladder. Bilateral renal agenesis is typically associated with severe oligohydramnios and is usually detectable after 16 weeks of gestation. However, unilateral or bilateral ureteropelvic junction obstruction or polycystic kidney disease may not be detectable until late in the second trimester and is usually associated with less severe oligohydramnios. Unilateral urinary obstruction rarely causes measurable decrement in amniotic fluid volume. Since urinary tract defects are commonly found in aneuploid fetuses, amniocentesis should be offered if these findings are present.

Assess fetal growth and placental function

In the absence of PROM and urinary tract anomalies, uteroplacental insufficiency should be considered. Oligohydramnios may result from poor placental function associated with maternal hypertension, chronic placental abruption, and autoimmune states such as systemic lupus and antiphospholipid syndrome. In such cases, fetal abdominal circumference growth typically lags that of the head. Increased placental vascular resistance evident on umbilical artery Doppler studies may help corroborate the diagnosis of oligohydramnios due to placental insufficiency. The risk of fetal asphyxia and death is high when severe oligohydramnios accompanies intrauterine growth restriction (IUGR). Intensive fetal testing and hospitalization should be considered in cases diagnosed after the point of fetal viability. After 32 weeks, severe oligohydramnios and fetal growth restriction should generally lead to evaluation for delivery.

Assess likelihood of pulmonary hypoplasia

Longstanding oligohydramnios predisposes to fetal pulmonary hypoplasia. Although the mechanism of this potentially lethal complication is not clear, inhibition of fetal breathing, loss of lung liquid because of reduction in amniotic pressure, and simple mechanical compression of the chest have been proposed. The end result is restricted lung growth leading to alveolar volume inadequate to support postnatal respiration. It appears that the risk of pulmonary hypoplasia is greatest when severe oligohydramnios is present from 16 to 20 weeks of gestation, the period of alveolar proliferation.

Although several methods have been proposed to predict pulmonary hypoplasia, no single criterion has adequate sensitivity and specificity for clinical decision making. Measurement of chest circumference, use of thoracic–head circumference ratio, calculating the lung area ratio [(chest area–cardiac area)/chest area] and thin-slice three-dimensional fetal lung volume/fetal body weight ratios have been proposed to assess the presence of pulmonary hypoplasia. However, in a review of 13 studies reporting on the prediction of lethal pulmonary hypoplasia, the estimated sROC curves for the chest circumference/abdominal circumference ratio and other parameters showed limited accuracy in the prediction of pulmonary hypoplasia (Laudy and Wladimiroff 2000). Thus in cases of mid-trimester PPROM, available evidence suggests caution in predicting lethality.

Treatment options
Delivery
Although the outcome of severe, longstanding oligohydramnios is at best guarded, lesser degrees of fluid restriction may be amenable to intervention. Data suggest that most of the perinatal morbidity associated with term and postdate pregnancy is confined to cases with an AFI of less than 5 cm and, particularly, those that lack a MVP of at least 2 cm. In such cases, continued expectant management and antepartum testing is likely to result in higher rates of meconium staining, fetal distress, low Apgar scores and cesarean delivery. However, in the preterm pregnancy, especially those less than 34 weeks of gestation, conservative measures and expectant management can be considered.

Amnioinfusion
At term, induction of labor in patients with severe oligohydramnios is associated with decreased perinatal morbidity but carries risk of prolonged labor and failed induction. One meta-analysis suggested that, in women with PROM and oligohydramnios, prophylactic transcervical saline infusion could improve neonatal outcome and lessen the rate of cesarean delivery, without increasing the rate of postpartum endometritis. However, a Cochrane Review (Novikova *et al.* 2012) found no differences in cesarean rate, cord arterial pH, oxytocin augmentation, neonatal pneumonia or postpartum endometritis. Prophylactic amnioinfusion was associated with increased intrapartum fever (risk ratio 3.48, 95% confidence interval 1.21 to 10.05). Other potential complications associated with amnioinfusion include inadvertent overdistention of the uterus, increased uterine contractions during the infusion, and the theoretical possibility of amniotic fluid embolus.

In the preterm pregnancy with intact membranes and oligohydramnios, the adverse consequences of prolonged fluid inadequacy could theoretically be reduced or eliminated by transabdominal amnioinfusion. However, a systematic review of trials reporting an impact of amnioinfusion on stillbirths (9 trials, $n = 1681$ women) and perinatal mortality (10 trials, $n = 3656$ women) revealed a nonsignificant reduction in risk associated with amnioinfusion (Chabra *et al.* 2007).

Maternal hydration

The interrelationship between amniotic fluid and maternal intravascular volumes has been demonstrated experimentally and clinically. Several studies have demonstrated increased fetal urine output following intravenous hydration of pregnant women. In a systematic review of randomized trials of maternal hydration by Hofmeyr and Gülmezoglu (2002), the AFI was significantly increased in women with oligohydramnios undergoing hydration vs controls (mean difference 2.01, 95% CI 1.43–2.60). When intravenous isotonic and hypotonic fluid infusions were compared with oral hydration, hypotonic but not isotonic IV infusion increased amniotic fluid volumes to a level similar to that of oral hydration. Thus in cases of isolated oligohydramnios (lacking evidence of coexisting fetal hypoxia or urinary tract anomalies), a trial of maternal oral hydration with 2 L of water, allowing at least 2 hours before reassessing amniotic fluid volume, is often effective.

Summary

Mild oligohydramnios (AFI 5–8 cm, MVP 2–3 cm) near term should be managed conservatively with frequent fetal surveillance and emphasis on maternal hydration as long as a 2×1 cm pocket of amniotic fluid is confidently demonstrable. Labor induction for significant oligohydramnios (absence of 2×1 cm pocket) at term is appropriate. Remote from term with oligohydramnios, fetal structural and chromosomal anomalies should be ruled out. If IUGR is present with oligohydramnios, the risk of fetal asphyxia and death is high. Such pregnancies should be managed aggressively with antenatal corticosteroids and early delivery unless lethal anomalies are present.

Polyhydramnios
Overview

Polyhydramnios is the pathological accumulation of excessive quantities of amniotic fluid. When polyhydramnios is diagnosed, a thorough examination for underlying abnormalities is indicated and the risk of adverse

Table 38.4   Clinical associations with polyhydramnios

Cause	Hill *et al.*, 1987 (*n* = 107) (%)	Many, 1995 (*n* = 275) (%)
Idiopathic	66	69
Diabetes mellitus	15	18
Congenital malformations	13	15
Rh incompatibility	1	
Multiple gestation	5	

Source: Data from Hill *et al.*, 1995.

pregnancy outcomes is increased. Clearly, as noted above in the discussion regarding amniotic fluid production and removal, polyhydramnios arises from either overproduction or under-removal or a combination of both. Since clinical ultrasound measurements of both fetal urinary flow and swallowing are not adequately precise for clinical measurement, the typical clinical associations with excess amniotic fluid have been catalogued (see Table 38.4).

Regarding the pathophysiological connection between polyhydramnios and its clinical associations, little is known with certainty. The link between the increased incidence of polyhydramnios with maternal hyperglycemia in diabetes has been proposed to arise from diuresis in the fetus in response to hyperglycemia. With associated anatomic abnormalities such as esophageal atresia, congenital diaphragmatic hernia and chest masses, fetal swallowing is impaired, contributing to polyhydramnios. Fetuses with central nervous system (CNS) anomalies such as anencephaly and holoprosencephaly may develop polyhydramnios from altered CNS function and altered swallowing function.

Fetal conditions associated with fetal anemia, cardiac overload or congestive heart failure often lead to polyhydramnios. Examples include the recipient twin in twin–twin transfusion syndrome, Rhesus isoimmunization, parvovirus infection and fetal–maternal hemorrhage. Regardless of etiology, polyhydramnios should be taken as a concerning finding, with perinatal mortality increased twofold to fivefold compared to pregnancies with normal amniotic fluid.

Diagnosis

Several criteria have been proposed as defining polyhydramnios which, by definition, is approximately 2–5% of the upper levels of sonographically measured AFI or MVP. As in oligohydramnios, the boundaries of normal and abnormal amniotic fluid vary with gestational age. In the third trimester, this coincides with MVP values above 7 cm, or AFI exceeding 21 cm (95th percentile, see Table 38.3). Others have advocated a more restrictive definition, such that only 1–2% of cases are defined. A commonly accepted cut-off for polyhydramnios is 24 cm (AFI) or 8 cm (MVP).

Evaluation
Sonography
Evaluate the fetus sonographically for cardiac failure, anemia or anomalies potentially altering fetal swallowing:
- Pericardial effusion, poor ventricular function, structural cardiac defect.
- Middle cerebral artery peak systolic velocity above 1.5 multiples of the median for gestational age.
- CNS defect, e.g., Arnold-Chiari malformation, holoprosencephaly.
- Thoracic mass, e.g., diaphragmatic hernia, pulmonary sequestration, cystic adenomatoid malformation.
- Gastrointestinal tract obstruction, e.g., duodenal atresia, esophageal atresia.
- Sonographic markers of aneuploidy.

Laboratory screening
Perform laboratory screening for:
- Gestational and preexisting diabetes.
- Rh isoimmunization
- Fetal infection (rubella, toxoplasmosis, parvovirus, CMV, syphilis).
- Thalassemia especially alpha-thalassemia.
- Kleihauer-Betke.
- Toxicology for substance abuse.

Amniocentesis
Consider amniocentesis for fetal karyotype.

Complications
Uterine distention can lead to a number of obstetrical complications including:
- Premature labor
- Preterm PROM.
- Malpresentation due to increased fetal mobility.
- Umbilical cord prolapse.
- Cesarean delivery.
- Placental abruption following PROM.
- Postpartum hemorrhage due to uterine overdistention.
- Maternal respiratory compromise due to mechanical pressure on the maternal diaphragm.
- Fetal mortality

Treatment options

It is not clear that any medical intervention improves the outcome of most cases of polyhydramnios. When a clear-cut etiology is evident, e.g., diabetes or isoimmunization, the underlying problem should be addressed. When polyhydramnios is caused by a congenital anomaly or is idiopathic, treatment is expectant and focused on closely monitoring fetal biophysical status and intervening for maternal or fetal complications. Importantly, a significant number of cases of mild polyhydramnios will resolve spontaneously.

Monitor cervical length for preterm labor

Since polyhydramnios is associated with increased risk of premature PROM and preterm birth, sonographic monitoring of cervical length may provide advanced warning of impending labor. Cervical length should be assessed as dictated by clinical circumstances and gestational age, but typically a cervical length measurement every 2 weeks from 24 to 33 weeks may provide guidance regarding when to admit the patient for antenatal corticosteroids. Finding a cervix less than 1.5 to 2.0 cm, especially with a positive cervical fetal fibronectin with gestational age less than 34 weeks should prompt evaluation for hospitalization and steroid treatment.

Labor management

Lacking significant maternal or fetal compromise, delivery should occur at term or when fetal lung maturity is documented. While a vaginal delivery is usually optimal, care must be taken during labor to ensure that the presenting part remains vertex and the obstetrical team is ready to manage complications of sudden uterine decompression including abruption, change to a nonvertex fetal position, umbilical cord prolapse and postpartum hemorrhage.

Amnioreduction

Amnioreduction, reducing amniotic fluid volume through large volume amniocentesis (100 mL to more than 1000 mL) may temporize difficult cases. Typical indications include maternal respiratory compromise or severe abdominal pain/contractions. While there are no trials conclusively demonstrating efficacy, amnioreduction is commonly performed in stage 1 or stage 2 twin–twin transfusion syndrome. Typically, amnioreduction volumes are aimed to reduce AFI or MVP to the upper-normal range. An 18-gauge needle is inserted sterilely into the uterine cavity under ultrasound guidance into a free pocket of amniotic fluid. Tubing is either connected to wall suction or a three-way stopcock to permit removal with a large syringe. Fluid should be removed no faster than 1000 mL over 20 minutes and the procedure is terminated when the AFI returns to the upper normal range. Complications of amnioreduction occur in 1–5% of cases and include chorioamnionitis, fetal bradycardia, placental abruption and preterm rupture of membranes. The procedure is repeated if symptoms recur and gestational age is less than 33 weeks.

Indomethacin

Indomethacin, a prostaglandin synthetase inhibitor, decreases fetal urine output through constriction of the fetal renal arteries. An important additional side effect of indomethacin is constriction of the fetal ductus arteriosus. Prior to 30 weeks, this effect is usually not significant but treatment after 30 weeks should be approached with caution and accompanied by daily sonographic assessment of fetal cardiac function. Use of indomethacin for polyhydramnios should generally be avoided in a fetus with IUGR or in discordant twins with one twin at or below the tenth percentile for estimated weight. The starting dose is 25 mg orally three times daily, but may be increased to as much as 150 mg daily. The AFI should be monitored daily and treatment stopped when the AFI returns to the upper normal range.

Biophysical monitoring of the fetus and amniotic fluid volume

Most cases of polyhydramnios resolve with advancing gestation. The frequency of monitoring of amniotic fluid volume should be determined by clinical circumstances and patient complaint. Usually every 2–3 weeks is adequate. However, because of the increased risk of fetal death with polyhydramnios, fetal biophysical status should be monitored carefully after the gestational age of viability. Typically, fetal movement counting is used nightly from 28 weeks and twice-weekly modified biophysical profiles utilized from 32 to 34 weeks onward.

Summary

Polyhydramnios occurs in 1–5% of pregnancies and is associated with significantly increased perinatal morbidity and mortality. A thorough laboratory and sonographic evaluation will aid in accurate recognition of the etiology and guide any subsequent therapy.

Suggested reading

Brace RA. Physiology of amniotic fluid volume regulation. *Clin Obstet Gynecol* 1997;40(2):280–9.

Brace RA, Wolf EJ. Normal amniotic fluid volume changes throughout pregnancy. *Am J Obstet Gynecol* 1989;161(2):382–8.

Cabrol D, Jannet D, Pannier E. Treatment of symptomatic polyhydramnios with indomethacin. *Eur J Obstet Gynecol Reprod Biol* 1996;66(1):11–15.

Chabra S, Dargan R, Nasare M. Antepartum transabdominal amnioinfusion. *Int J Gynecol Obstet* 2007;97:95–9.

Chauhan SP, Sanderson M, Hendrix NW, Magann EF, Devoe LD. Perinatal outcome and amnionitc fluid index in the antepartum and intrapartum periods: a meta-analysis. *Am J Obstet Gynecol* 1999;181:1473–8.

Darmstadt GL, Yakoob MY, Haws RA, *et al.* Reducing stillbirths: interventions during labour. *BMC Pregn Childbirth* 2009;9(Suppl 1):S6.

Dashe JS, McIntire DD, Ramus RM, Santos-Ramos R, Twickler DM. Hydramnios: anomaly prevalence and sonographic detection. *Obstet Gynecol* 2002;100(1):134–9.

Hill L, Breckle R, Thomas ML, Fires JK. Polyhydramnios:; ultrasonically detected prevalence and neonatal outcome. *Obstet Gynecol* 1987;69:21–25.

Hofmeyr GJ, Gülmezoglu AM. Maternal hydration for increasing amniotic fluid volume in oligohydramnios and normal amniotic fluid volume. *Cochrane Database Syst Rev* 2002;1:CD000134.

Laudy JA, Wladimiroff JW. The fetal lung. *II. Pulmonary hypoplasia. Ultrasound Obstet Gynecol* 2000;16:482–494.

Leung WC, Jouannic JM, Hyett J, Rodeck C, Jauniaux E. Procedure-related complications of rapid amniodrainage in the treatment of polyhydramnios. *Ultrasound Obstet Gynecol* 2004;23(2):154–8.

Magann EF, Chauhan SP, Doherty DA, Lutgendorf MA, Magann MI, Morrison JC. Review of idiopathic hydramnios and pregnancy outcomes. *Obstet Gynecol Surv* 2007;62(12):795–802.

Magann EF, Sanderson M, Martin JN, Chauhan S. The amniotic fluid index, single deepest pocket, and two-diameter pocket in normal human pregnancy. *Am J Obstet Gynecol* 2000;182:1581–8.

Many A, Hill LM, Lazebnik N, Martin JG. The association between polyhydramnios and preterm delivery. *Obstet Gynecol* 1995;86(3):389–91.

Moore TR, Cayle JE. The amniotic fluid index in normal human pregnancy. *Am J Obstet Gynecol* 1990;162:1168–73.

Moore TR, Piacquadio K. A prospective evaluation of fetal movement screening to reduce the incidence of antepartum fetal death. *Am J Obstet Gynecol* 1989;160:1075–80.

Nabhan AF, Abdelmoula YA. Amniotic fluid index versus single deepest vertical pocket as a screening test for preventing adverse pregnancy outcome. *Cochrane Database Syst Rev* 2008;(3):CD006593.

Novikova N, Hofmeyr GJ, Essilfie-Appiah G. Prophylactic versus therapeutic amnioinfusion for oligohydramnios in labour. *Cochrane Database Syst Rev.* 2012 Sep 12;9:CD000176.

Rossi AC, Prefumo F. Perinatal outcomes of isolated oligohydramnios at term and post-term pregnancy: a systematic review of literature with meta-analysis. *Eur J Obstet Gynecol Reprod Biol* 2013 Jul;169(2):149–54.

van Teeffelen AS, Van Der Heijden J, Oei SG, Porath MM, Willekes C, Opmeer B, Mol BW. Accuracy of imaging parameters in the prediction of lethal pulmonary hypoplasia secondary to mid-trimester prelabor rupture of fetal membranes: a systematic review and meta-analysis. *Ultrasound Obstet Gynecol* 2012 May;39(5):495–9.

PROTOCOL 39

Preeclampsia

Baha M. Sibai

Department of Obstetrics & Gynaecology and Reproductive Sciences, The University of Texas Medical School at Houston, Houston, TX, USA

Overview

Hypertension complicates 7–10% of pregnancies, of which 70% are due to gestational hypertension/preeclampsia and 30% are due to chronic essential hypertension. The rate of hypertensive disorders in nulliparous women approaches 29%.

Risk factors include:

- nulliparity
- obesity (BMI greater than 30 kg/m^2)
- multiple gestation
- family history of preeclampsia or eclampsia
- preexisting hypertension or renal disease
- previous preeclampsia or eclampsia
- diabetes mellitus or gestational diabetes
- Artificial conception
- Advanced maternal age (greater than 40 years)
- nonimmune hydrops
- antiphospholipid antibody syndrome or auto immune disease
- molar or partial molar pregnancy.

Preeclampsia rarely develops before 20 weeks of gestation. In this early stage, rule out underlying renal disease, molar pregnancy, and other medical disorders.

Pathophysiology

Preeclampsia is a disorder of unknown etiology that is peculiar to human pregnancy. The pathophysiological abnormalities in preeclampsia include

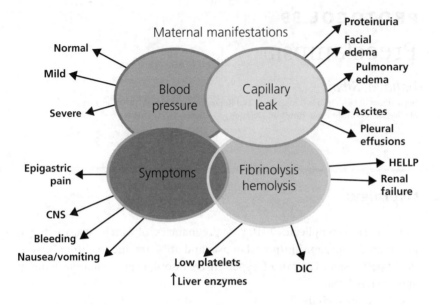

Figure 39.1   Signs and symptoms of preeclampsia and organ dysfunction.

inadequate maternal vascular response to placentation, endothelial dysfunction, abnormal angiogenesis, and exaggerated inflammatory response with resultant generalized vasospasm, activation of platelets and abnormal hemostasis. These abnormalities result in pathophysiological vascular lesions in peripheral vessels and utero-placental vascular beds, as well as in various organ systems, such as the kidneys, liver, lungs and brain. Consequently, these pregnancies, particularly those with preeclampsia and severe features, are associated with increased maternal and perinatal mortality and morbidity due to reduced utero-placental blood flow, abruptio placentae and preterm delivery. Recent evidence indicates that preeclampsia is an endothelial disorder. Thus, in some patients the disease may manifest itself in the form of either a capillary leak, fetal growth restriction, reduced amniotic fluid, or a spectrum of abnormal laboratory tests with multiple organ dysfunction (Fig. 39.1).

Diagnosis

Recently, the diagnosis of preeclampsia and its subtypes have been expanded and revised by the ACOG Task Force on Hypertension in Pregnancy:

Gestational hypertension

- Systolic blood pressure (BP) at least 140 mmHg, but less than 160 mmHg or
- Diastolic BP at least 90 mmHg, but less than 110 mmHg
- The above pressures should be observed on at least two occasions 4 hours apart, no more than 7 days apart
- BP readings can vary with the type of equipment used, cuff size, position of the arm, position of the patient, duration of rest period, obesity, smoking, anxiety, and the Korotkoff sound used to assess diastolic BP. Only Korotkoff sound V should be used to establish diastolic BP.

Severe hypertension

- Sustained elevations in systolic BP to at least 160 mmHg and/or in diastolic BP to at least 110 mmHg for at least 4 hours or once if patient is receiving antihypertensive medications.

Proteinuria

- 0.3 g or more in a 24-hour urine collection or protein: creatinine ratio 0.3 mg/mg or more.
- Protein excretion in the urine increases in normal pregnancy from approximately 5 mg/dL in the first and second trimesters to 15 mg/dL in the third trimester. These low levels are not detected by dipstick. The concentration of urinary protein is influenced by contamination with vaginal secretions, blood, bacteria, or amniotic fluid. It also varies with urine-specific gravity and pH, exercise and posture.
- Proteinuria usually appears after hypertension in the course of the disease process, but in some women it could appear before hypertension.

Edema

- Excessive weight gain greater than 4 lb/week (greater than 1.8 kg/week) in the second or third trimester may be the first sign of the potential development of preeclampsia.
- 39% of eclamptic patients do not have edema.

Preeclampsia

The Task Force classifies preeclampsia as preeclampsia with or without severe features. The term mild preeclampsia has been removed and should not be used. Preeclampsia is defined as gestational hypertension plus any of the following:

- Proteinuria as defined above or
- Any of the findings listed below for preeclampsia with severe features.

Preeclampsia with severe features

- Systolic BP at least 160 mmHg or diastolic BP at least 110 mmHg on two occasions at least 4 hours apart while the patient is on bed rest, or once if the patient receives antihypertensive therapy before that. It is recommended that severe BP values that are sustained for more than 30 minutes require immediate treatment.
- New onset persistent cerebral symptoms (headaches) or visual disturbances.
- Impaired liver function as indicated by abnormally elevated liver enzymes (twice normal levels), severe persistent right upper quadrant or epigastric pain unresponsive to medications and not accounted by alternative diagnosis, or both.
- Pulmonary edema.
- Thrombocytopenia (platelet count less than 100,000/µL).
- Progressive renal insufficiency (serum creatinine greater than 1.1 mg/dL).
- The amount of proteinuria, presence of oliguria, and fetal growth restriction have been removed from the diagnosis of severe disease.

Management

Delivery is the only available cure for preeclampsia. The ultimate goals of any management plan must be the safety of the mother first and then delivery of a live mature newborn that will not require intensive and prolonged neonatal care. The decision between immediate delivery and expectant management will depend on one or more of the following: maternal and fetal conditions at the time of evaluation, fetal gestational age, presence of labor or rupture of membranes, severity of the disease process, and maternal desire.

Mild hypertension or preeclampsia

Figure 39.2 provides a management algorithm for mild hypertension or preeclampsia.

37 weeks or more

- At 37 weeks or more of gestation, induction of labor is indicated. Induce also earlier for any signs of maternal-fetal distress (suspected abruption, confirmed fetal growth restriction, labor or rupture of membranes).
- Prostaglandins can be used for cervical ripening in those with Bishop score less than 6.

Management of mild HTN or preeclampsia

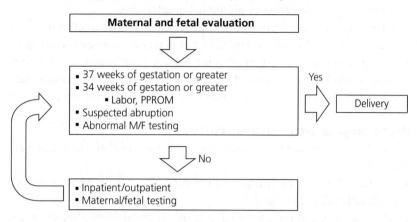

Figure 39.2 Recommended management of mild gestational hypertension or preeclampsia.

Less than 37 weeks

- In all patients, the maternal and fetal conditions should be evaluated.
- Outpatient management is possible if the patient's systolic BP is less than 155 mmHg and/or diastolic BP is less than 105 mmHg, with a platelet count more than 100,000/mL, normal liver enzymes and reassuring fetal testing. The patient should also have no subjective symptoms, and should be compliant and reliable.
- Whether the patient is in the hospital or being managed at home, the following should be observed:
  - Salt restriction, diuretics, antihypertensive drugs, and sedatives are not used.
  - Patient should have relative rest, twice weekly evaluation of protein (mild gestational hypertension only), twice weekly BP monitoring, 1–2 times per week fetal testing, and laboratory evaluation of hematocrit and platelets, and liver function tests, serum creatinine once a week. Patient should be educated about preeclampsia warning signs, such as headache, visual disturbances, epigastric pain, nausea and vomiting, and shortness of breath. Patient should be instructed about daily kick counts and labor signs or vaginal bleeding.
- Fetal testing should consist of at least weekly nonstress testing (NST) for gestational hypertension only, and twice weekly NST and measurement of amniotic fluid volume in those with preeclampsia. In addition, assessment of fetal growth by ultrasonography every 3 weeks. Testing is considered nonreassuring if:
  - NST is nonreactive with abnormal fetal biophysical profile

- NST shows repetitive late deceleration, repetitive variable decelerations, fetal tachycardia or prolonged deceleration.
- Oligohydramnios is present (AFI persistently less than 5.0 cm).
- Estimated fetal weight is less than 5th percentile for gestational age.
- Prompt hospitalization is needed for disease progression: acute severe hypertension, development of new symptoms, outpatient management unsatisfactory for the specific patient, or abnormal fetal testing.

Preeclampsia with severe features

Figure 39.3 provides a management algorithm for preeclampsia with severe features.

- Beyond 34 weeks: induction and delivery. There is no need for assessment of fetal lung maturity.
- 33 to 34 weeks: steroids for fetal lung maturity. Delivery after 48 hours.
- Hemolysis, elevated liver enzymes, low platelets (HELLP) syndrome: steroids for fetal lung maturity, then deliver after second dose.
- 23 weeks 0 days to 32 weeks 6 days: expectant management and steroids.
- Less than 23 weeks: offer termination with prostaglandin E_2 (PGE_2) vaginal suppository, laminaria and oxytocin (Pitocin), or dilatation and

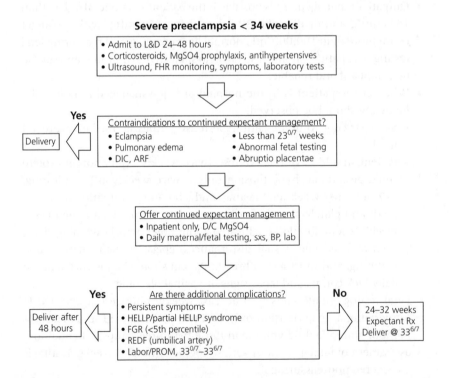

Figure 39.3 Recommended management of preeclampsia with severe features.

evacuation. Overall perinatal survival without termination is 6.7%. If patient does not elect to terminate, manage expectantly, but counsel about maternal risks and poor perinatal outcome.

Conservative management of preeclampsia with severe features

In a tertiary care center:

- Initial intravenous magnesium sulfate for 24 hours.
- Antihypertensives: intravenous boluses, then shift to oral administration, nifedipine, labetalol

   Hydralazine: 5 to 10 mg boluses every 20 to 30 minutes (maximum dose 25 mg)

   Labetalol: 20, 40, 80 mg boluses (maximum dose 220 mg), then 200 mg orally every 8 hours (maximum 800 mg every 8 hours)

   Nifedipine: 10 to 20 mg rapid acting orally every 20–30 minutes (maximum 50 mg), then 10–20 mg every 4–6 hours (maximum 120 mg/day). Oral long-acting nifedepine can also be used.
- Aim: Diastolic BP 90 to 100 mmHg and systolic BP 140 to 150 mmHg. Avoid normal BP because of the risk of decreased utero-placental perfusion. Adequate therapeutic response is expected in 12 hours.
- Give steroids for immature lungs and attempt to delay delivery at least for steroid benefit (48 hours).
- Daily fetal–maternal testing.

The majority of patients with severe preeclampsia managed conservatively will require delivery within 2 weeks of admission. Indications for delivery of these patients include the following:

- Maternal indications: thrombocytopenia or HELLP, disseminated intravascular coagulation (DIC), pulmonary edema, renal failure, eclampsia, uncontrolled severe hypertension, suspected abruptio placentae, labor or rupture of membranes, severe ascites; warning signs: persistent and severe headache, blurring of vision, epigastric pain.
- Fetal indications: Nonreassuring fetal heart rate tracing irrespective of gestational age or lung maturity, persistent severe oligohydramnios (largest vertical pocket 2 cm), severe fetal growth restriction (less than 5th percentile) with abnormal umbilical artery Doppler study, or gestational age greater than 34 weeks achieved.

HELLP

- Hemolysis: abnormal peripheral blood smear; increased bilirubin 1.2 mg/dL or higher; low haptoglobin levels.
- Elevated liver enzymes: increased lactic dehydrogenase or SGOT greater than twice the upper limit of normal.
- Low platelets: less than 100,000/μL.

- Occurs in 10% to 20% of preeclamptic patients with severe features.
- More frequent in whites and multiparas.
- Complaints of nausea and vomiting (50%), malaise of a few days' duration (90%), epigastric or right upper quadrant pain (65%), or swelling. Others will have vague abdominal pain, flank or shoulder pain, jaundice, hematuria, gastrointestinal bleeding, or gum bleeding.
- Onset antepartum in 70% of the cases and postpartum in 30% of the cases.
- In the postpartum period, the time of onset of the clinical manifestations may range from a few hours to one week, with the majority developing within 48 hours.
- Hypertension may be absent in 20% and mild in 30% of the cases.
- Proteinuria may be absent in 5% of cases.
- Temporary management of HELLP for 48 hours is only possible in the absence of DIC, particularly for benefit of corticosteroid administration.

Intrapartum management of preeclampsia with severe features and HELLP

- The first priority is to assess and stabilize maternal condition and then to evaluate fetal well-being. Finally, a decision must be made as to whether immediate delivery is indicated (Table 39.1).
- Intravenous magnesium sulfate: 4–6 g loading dose over 20 minutes (6 g in 100 mL 5% dextrose in water) followed by the maintenance dose of 2 g/h during labor and for 12 to 24 hours postpartum (40 g in 1 L lactated Ringer's solution at 50 mL/h or 20 g in 1 L lactated Ringer's solution at 100 mL/h). Remember that the risk of eclamptic convulsion in those with severe disease is less than 2%. For preeclampsia without severe features, the risk is less than 0.5%. For these women, it is appropriate not to give magnesium sulfate, but they should still receive close monitoring of BP and maternal symptoms to identify those that may progress to severe disease.
- For HELLP patients, type and cross-match with 2 units of blood. Have platelets available if the platelet count is below 50,000.
- Accurate measurement of fluid input and output: Foley catheter, restrict total intake to 100 mL/h to avoid pulmonary edema. If pulmonary edema is suspected, give 40 mg IV Lasix and obtain chest X-ray, and maternal echocardiography if needed.
- Frequent monitoring of pulse, BP, urine output, and respiration.
- Monitor for signs of magnesium toxicity and have a magnesium level drawn if needed; be ready to counteract magnesium toxicity with 10 mL of 10% calcium gluconate intravenously, and intubation if the patient develops respiratory arrest. Be ready to deal with convulsions.
- Continuous fetal monitoring.

Table 39.1 Management outline of antepartum HELLP syndrome

1 Assess and stabilize maternal condition
  a. Antiseizure prophylaxis with magnesium sulfate
  b. Treatment of severe hypertension
  c. Transfer to tertiary care center if appropriate
  d. Computed tomography or ultrasound of the abdomen if subcapsular hematoma of the liver is suspected

2 Evaluate fetal well-being
  a. 34 weeks of gestation or more→ delivery
  b. 24–34 weeks of gestation → steroids → delivery in 24–48 hours

Deliver if abnormal fetal assessment
Deliver if progressive deterioration in maternal condition

- Oxytocin induction and allow normal vaginal delivery for favorable cervix or gestational age of 30 weeks or beyond. If the cervix is unripe and gestational age is less than 30 weeks, consider elective cesarean delivery or cervical ripening with PGE_2.
- Anesthesia: intermittent small doses of Stadol IVP, 1 to 2 mg. Epidural anesthesia is preferred to general anesthesia in case of abdominal delivery if personnel skilled in obstetric anesthesia are available. Pudendal block and epidural are not advisable in HELLP patients as it might result in hematoma formation.
- If thrombocytopenia is present, it should be corrected before surgery: Transfuse with 6–10 units of platelets in all patients with a platelet count less than 40,000/μL.
- In HELLP patients to minimize the risk of hematoma formation: the bladder flap should be left open, a subfascial drain is used, and the wound is left open. The wounds can be successfully closed within 72 hours after drain removal.

Postpartum management

- Adequate observation of the mother in the recovery room for 12 to 24 hours under magnesium sulfate coverage. Remember that 25–30% of the eclampsia cases and 30% of the HELLP cases occur in the postpartum period. In addition, some women will develop new onset hypertension or preeclampsia for the first time postpartum. The majority will occur at 3–7 days postpartum. Therefore, patients with hypertensive disorders should have a BP recording at 3 days postpartum and again at 5–7 days after discharge.
- Most patients will show evidence of resolution of the disease process within 24 hours after delivery. Some, especially those with severe disease

in the midtrimester, HELLP, or eclampsia, require close monitoring for 2–3 days.

• By the time of discharge, most patients will be normotensive. If hypertension persists, antihypertensive medications are prescribed for 1 week, after which the patient is reevaluated. In addition, all patients should be given written instruction about signs and symptoms to report as well as a phone number to call in case of development of new symptoms or severe hypertension. Follow-up BP recordings can be done at home or in an office. Patients with preeclampsia with severe features and those with superimposed preeclampsia should not be prescribed nonsteroidal anti-inflammatory agents for pain or ergot derivatives.

Complications of preeclampsia and HELLP

Complications include abruptio placentae, pulmonary edema, acute renal failure, liver hematoma with possible rupture, pospartum hemorrhage, wound or intraabdominal hematomas, DIC and multiorgan failure, including liver, kidneys and lungs (adult respiratory distress syndrome). Neurologic-like eclampsia, hypertensive encephalopathy, ischemia, infarcts, edema and hemorrhage can also occur, as can cardiorespiratory arrest.

Follow up and maternal counseling

Women who develop preeclampsia in their first pregnancy are at increased risk (20%) for development of preeclampsia in subsequent pregnancies. The risk of preeclampsia in the sister of a patient with preeclampsia is 14%. With severe disease in a first pregnancy, the risk of recurrence is about 30%. With severe disease in the second trimester, the risk of recurrent preeclampsia is 50%. In 21% of cases, the disease also occurs in the second trimester. HELLP recurs in about 5% of cases.

There is increased risk of chronic hypertension and undiagnosed renal disease. This is especially true in patients with two episodes of preeclampsia in the second trimester. These patients should have adequate medical evaluation postpartum. There is also increased risk of fetal growth restriction in a subsequent pregnancy. Finally, women who develop hypertensive disorders in pregnancy are at increased risk for cardiovascular disease and metabolic syndrome later in life. Therefore, they should receive close monitoring for these complications.

Acknowledgement

The author would like to acknowledge the contributions of Hind N. Moussa, MD to this protocol.

Suggested reading

American College of Obstetricians and Gynecologists. *American College of Obstetricians and Gynecologists Task Force on Hypertension in Pregnancy. Hypertension in pregnancy*. Washington, DC: American College of Obstetricians and Gynecologists; 2013.

Koopmans CM, Biglenga D, Groen H, *et al.*, for the HYPITAT study group. Induction of labour versus expectant monitoring for gestational hypertension or mild pre-eclampsia after 36 weeks' gestation (HYPITAT): a multicentre, open-label randomised controlled trial. *Lancet* 2009;374:979–88.

Sibai BM. Diagnosis and management of gestational hypertension and preeclampsia. *Obstet Gynecol* 2003;102:181–92.

Sibai BM. Hypertension. In: Gabbe SG, Niebyl JR, Simpson JL, editors. *Obstetrics: Normal and Problem Pregnancies*. 5th ed. New York: Churchill Livingstone; 2009; p 945–1004.

Sibai BM. Diagnosis, controversies and management of the syndrome of hemolysis, elevated liver enzymes, and low platelet count. *Obstet Gynecol* 2004;103:981–91.

Sibai BM. Magnesium sulphate prophylaxis in preeclampsia: lessons learned from recent trials. *Am J Obstet Gynecol* 2004;190:1520–6.

Sibai BM, Barton JR. Expectant management of severe preeclampsia remote from term: patient selection, treatment, and delivery indications. *Am J Obstet Gynecol* 2007;196:514.e1–514.e9.

PROTOCOL 40

Fetal Growth Restriction

Henry L. Galan

Department of Obstetrics and Gynecology, University of Colorado School of Medicine, Aurora, CO, USA

Definition and clinical significance

Intrauterine growth restriction (IUGR), fetal growth restriction (FGR), and small for gestational age (SGA) are terms used interchangeably to identify a fetus that has not reached its growth potential. FGR was the preferred term in the recent practice bulletin of the American College of Obstetricians and Gynecologists and this term will be used in this chapter. IUGR is mostly commonly defined as an ultrasound estimated fetal weight (EFW) less than the 10th percentile for gestational age. SGA, originally defined by neonatologists, refers to actual birth weight less than 10th percentile for gestation. IUGR is a common complication of pregnancy affecting up to 8% of pregnancies in developed countries and up to 30% in underdeveloped countries. Approximately 30% of IUGR fetuses are at risk for increased perinatal morbidity and mortality, while 70% of IUGR fetuses are normal and not at risk (e.g., constitutionally small). Perinatal mortality is highest when birth weights are below the 3rd percentile. Furthermore, these IUGR babies are at increased risk for diseases in adulthood, including diabetes, stroke and death from coronary artery disease.

Pathophysiology

The etiology of IUGR is extensive and diverse in nature. About 40% of IUGR is due to maternal and fetal genetic contributions and 60% from the fetal environment. Table 40.1 shows the various causes of IUGR and relative contribution of each factor to IUGR that have been reported. The relative rates of contribution by each factor to IUGR are dependent on the definition of IUGR used and the gestational age at the time of IUGR diagnosis. For example, chromosomal and infectious causes will be more common in fetuses below the 3rd percentile and when the diagnosis of IUGR is made

Protocols for High-Risk Pregnancies: An Evidence-Based Approach, Sixth Edition.
Edited by John T. Queenan, Catherine Y. Spong and Charles J. Lockwood.
© 2015 John Wiley & Sons, Ltd. Published 2015 by John Wiley & Sons, Ltd.

Table 40.1   Etiologic factors for intrauterine growth restriction

Etiologic factors	Incidence (5)
Chromosomal and genetic disorders	5–20
Congenital/structural anomalies	5–10
Congenital infectious disease	5–10
Multiple gestation	<5
Inadequate maternal nutrition	<1–2
Environmental toxins (substance abuse and medication exposure)	5–10
Placental causes	10–20
Maternal vascular disorder	25–40

earlier in gestation. From a clinical standpoint, the overall contribution rates of the causes of IUGR listed in Table 40.1 are much lower when using the more broad IUGR definition of an EFW below the 10th percentile as recommended by the American College of Obstetricians and Gynecologists (ACOG). Seventy percent of fetuses below the 10th percentile are small for constitutional (normal) reasons, such as small parental size.

Several of the factors listed in the table (maternal vascular disorders, substance abuse, placental disorders) negatively impact fetal growth by way of uteroplacental dysfunction and, as a group, represent the major cause of IUGR. In normal circumstances, the spiral arteries respond to invading columns of the invasive cytotrophoblast cells by vascular muscle remodeling early in gestation, which changes these normally high resistance vessels to low resistance vessels. This accommodation by the spiral arteries together with placental branching angiogenesis (first and second trimester) and non-branching angiogenesis (second and third trimester) is responsible for the 600 cc/minute of uterine blood flow seen at term and for the establishment of normal placental blood flow needed for nutrient and waste exchange from the fetus and placenta. Failure of these processes can lead to suboptimal delivery of nutrient (oxygen, amino acids, carbohydrates, lipids) to the fetus and lead to a catabolic and hypoxic state in the fetus that can lead to accumulation of metabolic acids (lactic acid, uric acid, and ketoacids), and thus, fetal acidemia.

Diagnosis

The diagnosis of IUGR is dependent on accurate gestational dating, which begins with ascertainment of last normal menstrual period (LMP), cycle length, and use of hormonal contraception. Pregnancy wheels and ultrasound/computerized gestational age calculators of gestational age are based on a 280-day gestational period. Thus, patients with longer or shorter cycle length may have ultrasound dating that is several days off and may need their estimated date of confinement (EDC) adjusted accordingly. Fundal height assessments, part of the prenatal care visits, can be a useful screening of the overgrown or undergrown fetus; however, its sensitivity for the detection of IUGR varies broadly for a number of reasons including individual provider variation in measurement technique, increasing incidence of maternal obesity, amniotic fluid (AF) disorders, and fibroid uterus. Ultrasound remains the gold standard for confirming LMP gestational dating or establishing a firm EDC and for making the diagnosis of IUGR.

While a mean gestational sac diameter (MSD) can provide very early and accurate ultrasound dating (gestation age in days = MSD +30), it should not be used once the embryo pole is noted on the yolk sac and the crown-rump length (CRL) can be measured. The CRL is seen consistently transvaginally when 5 mm or more. Through studies of in vitro fertilization, the CRL is accurate to ±3 days. In general, a difference between LMP dating and ultrasound dating of ±5–7 days within the confines of the first trimester should be used to refute or confirm LMP dating of the pregnancy. In addition to the CRL, other standard biometric measurements used to determine the gestational age include the biparietal diameter (BPD), head circumference (HC), abdominal circumference (AC), and femur length (FL). A good time to transition away from the CRL and toward the other biometric measurements is approximately 14–15 weeks of gestation. Several formulas using a combination of BPD, HC, AC, and FL biometry can provide reasonable dating accuracy. In one study by Chervenak *et al.*, the individual parameters demonstrated 95% confidence intervals for gestational age that nearly approximated those of the CRL (+7.5 days for HC and +8.7 days for the FL) between 14 and 22 days. As gestational age progresses, the accuracy of these measurements decreases due to an increase in the variability of fetal growth. At 24–30 weeks, the variability in composite (combined biometry) gestational age is as high as 1.5 weeks and after 30 weeks it is about 2–3 weeks. Early dating of a pregnancy is best and generally should not be supplanted by an ultrasound done later in pregnancy as a growth disorder can otherwise be missed.

Over 50 formulas for EFW using combinations of the previously mentioned fetal biometry are available. Generally, the accuracy of the formula is higher based on an increased number of variables used. However, it has been shown that adding more biometry variables beyond the usual four variables mentioned (BPD, HC, AC, FL) does not increase accuracy significantly. The AC is generally incorporated into any of the published formulas as it reflects soft tissue growth and is the measurement most affected by growth disorders (e.g., IUGR, macrosomia). Several studies have shown that in experienced hands, the mean absolute error in EFW is 8–10%.

However, 20–30% of the time the absolute error can be in the range of 10–20%.

There are several other additional ultrasound clues that can be used to support growth disorders.

1 *Amniotic fluid (AF)*. The AF volume is an indirect measure of the fetal renal perfusion and vascular status; however, alone it is a poor screening method for IUGR since oligohydramnios is generally a late finding in IUGR. What has been described in both human IUGR and animal models of IUGR is a progressive and gradual reduction in AF volume that is due to redistribution of blood flow toward the fetal heart, brain and adrenal glands, and away from lungs, digestive tract, kidneys, and torso. In contrast, a normal or excess AF volume in the face of early-onset or severe IUGR could reflect an abnormal chromosomal arrangement in the fetus. AF volume can be measured by gestalt, the amniotic fluid index (AFI) or mean vertical pocket (MVP). In comparison to the AFI, the MVP measurement has been shown to result in fewer iatrogenic deliveries for low AF volume with no difference in perinatal morbidity.

2 *Placenta*. The placenta can be thickened sonographically in cases of aneuploidy or fetal hydrops. A placenta previa is considered a risk factor for IUGR. In cases where the fetus is small due to uteroplacental dysfunction, almost universally, the placenta is undersized as well. Other placental abnormalities can be suspected by ultrasound including circumvallate placentas, which are associated with IUGR. The placenta should be sent for pathologic examination following delivery of an IUGR fetus.

3 *Features of Aneuploidy or Fetal Infection*. Fetal karyotyping can be reserved for early-onset and severe IUGR or if there is a structural anomaly on ultrasound. If the patient declines amniocentesis, cell-free fetal DNA (cf fDNA) testing is a reasonable option, although its limitations need to be disclosed. TORCH infection testing can similarly be reserved for early-onset, severe IUGR with ultrasound findings suggestive of infection (hepatic and periventricular calcifications, ventriculomegaly). In general, testing IUGR fetuses for either karyotype or for fetal infection is of low yield and has been shown to not be cost-effective.

4 *Transcerebellar Diameter (TCD)*. The TCD has been shown in several studies to be spared of the growth reduction seen in other biometric measurements of the IUGR fetus.

Treatment

There is no current human evidence that any treatment halts or reverses the IUGR condition. Although smoking cessation has a beneficial effect on fetal growth when started prior to 20 weeks, anecdotal evidence suggests that eliminating the vasoactive substances by smoking cessation improves uteroplacental blood flow. Bedrest has not been show to halt the IUGR process or improve fetal growth, and is not recommended. In addition, bedrest is a risk factor for thromboembolic disease and maternal bone demineralization. Discontinuation of vigorous exercise is a reasonable recommendation. Several therapies have not been shown to be effective in IUGR including maternal oxygen administration, nitric oxide donors, baby aspirin, dietary changes, calcium channel blockers, antioxidant therapy, and omega-3 formulations. A baby aspirin has been shown to be effective in reducing the recurrence risk in a subsequent pregnancy. When delivery is anticipated due to fetal status, current recommendations are that the fetus destined to be delivered between 24 and 34 weeks of gestation receives glucocorticoid treatment.

Complications

The complications of IUGR are extensive and span the lifetime of the IUGR fetus. IUGR rates are disproportionately high among stillbirths. Approximately 50% of preterm stillbirths were growth restricted in a Norwegian study. Others have shown that birth weight below the 3rd percentile carries the highest risk of perinatal death regardless of whether the fetus is born prior to or after 37 weeks of gestation. Several large retrospective studies show that IUGR increases perinatal morbidity with an increase in virtually every major neonatal complication including respiratory distress syndrome, grade 3 or 4 intraventricular hemorrhage, sepsis, seizure activity, necrotizing enterocolitis, and retinopathy of prematurity. Children who are born with growth restriction have a higher risk of cerebral palsy, short stature, and cognitive delay. Fetal programming work has shown that as adults these IUGR fetuses have a higher incidence of hypertension, coronary artery disease, stroke, type 2 diabetes mellitus, and obesity. Other nonmedical complications that result from association with IUGR include an increased risk of low socioeconomic status, suicide, and financial distress in later life.

Surveillance

Upon making the diagnosis of IUGR, it is essential to initiate serial monitoring of fetal status. There are different monitoring techniques that are available for fetal surveillance that include serial fetal growth, Doppler velocimetry, biophysical testing (BPP), modified biophysical profile, AF volume, and fetal activity counts as perceived by the mother. Each of these tests serves a different role and they should be used collectively to ensure that continued intrauterine existence is safe for the fetus and better than being ex-utero. Surveillance modalities that test chronic status of the fetus include interval ultrasound assessment of growth and AF volume. Serial ultrasound evaluation of fetal growth should be performed at 2–3-week intervals. Intervals of less than 2 weeks are not useful as there is sufficient error in each parameter measured for calculating the EFW that the information is less interpretable and fetuses have also been noted to have growth spurts, which may be missed with shorter intervals. Lack of fetal growth beyond 32–34 weeks is an indication for delivery. AF volume is reflective of fetal renal perfusion and vascular volume status. A relationship between oligohydramnios and progressive worsening of both arterial and venous Doppler velocimetry findings has been previously reported, as well as an association with low Apgar scores. While oligohydramnios itself is not an indication for delivery of early IUGR fetuses, its presence is generally considered an indication for hospitalization for increased fetal surveillance. Beyond 34 weeks, oligohydramnios is an indication for delivery. However, there is currently no evidence from randomized trials assessing outcomes based on AF volume determinations.

The most commonly used antepartum surveillance tools for monitoring IUGR fetuses are the nonstress test (NST) and the BPP. The NST is a method of fetal heart rate (FHR) analysis that uses Doppler technology to record and trace the FHR concomitantly with contraction monitoring. NST reactivity is defined as two accelerations (15 bpm above baseline for 15 seconds duration) within a 20-minute window and this must occur within 40 minutes of monitoring. The presence of accelerations and/or good variability provides evidence of good fetal oxygenation and absence of acidemia at the time the test is performed and identifies a fetus at low-risk for stillbirth. Unfortunately, lack of accelerations and variability do not indicate with certainty that the fetus is hypoxemic or acidemic as the test carries a high false-positive rate. The frequency of surveillance testing in high-risk pregnancies is different for the BPP and NST. The BPP testing is performed weekly. The NST is performed twice per week with one assessment of AF per week (modified BPP). The BPP can be either an 8-point or 10-point BPP depending on whether a NST is added to the test. The potential advantage to the 10-point BPP is that one can view the FHR tracing and assess if there are any variable or late decelerations, which can still exist in a fetus that has normal oxygenation and acid–base status as well as a normal BPP and reactive tracing. One normally expects 80% of fetuses beyond 32 weeks to have a reactive NST, but in IUGR fetuses the rate of reactivity is lower. Several studies have shown that there is delay of CNS maturation including a delay in the normal decline of FHR with advancing gestation, a decrease in short-term and long-term variability and a delay in reactivity, especially in early IUGR. Thus, while the NST is generally preferred to the BPP for monitoring an IUGR fetus, a provider will often need to use the BPP as a secondary test for the evaluation of the IUGR fetus who has a nonreactive NST, especially in early gestation.

Pulsed-wave Doppler velocimetry can be used to assess changes in resistance in blow flow through various vascular beds (see Protocol 6). Use of umbilical artery Doppler velocimetry is the most important tool for surveillance of the IUGR fetus. When an IUGR pregnancy demonstrates an increase in the umbilical artery resistance indices, histologic examination shows that 30% of the placental villous vessels are abnormal. As placental disease deteriorates and the flow velocity waveforms show absent end-diastolic flow (AEDF) or reversed end-diastolic flow (REDF), placental examination shows that 60–70% of the villous vessels will be abnormal. Furthermore, the rate of hypoxemia has been reported to be as high as 50–80% by the time AEDF is apparent. There is Level 1 evidence to support the use of umbilical artery Doppler in IUGR and it is supported by ACOG. This is in contrast to the Level 2–3 evidence for NST due to the false-positive rates and lack of uniform evidence of clinical benefit of NST in IUGR surveillance. However, the umbilical artery Doppler and NSTs should be used together. Meta-analyses of randomized clinical trials (RCTs) have shown that the use of umbilical artery Doppler in conjunction with standard antenatal testing (BPP or modified BPP) reduces the risk of fetal demise by as much as 38%. No other individual surveillance tool or Doppler parameter has achieved this level of confirmation.

Doppler velocimetry has also been performed in a number of other vessels to evaluate the IUGR fetus, especially the middle cerebral artery (MCA) and the precardiac venous vessels. Doppler interrogation of the MCA vessel is able to detect changes in blood flow resistance in the cerebral circulation of the IUGR fetus. As described above, a common phenomenon in IUGR is the redistribution of blood flow away from nonvital structures toward the heart, brain and adrenal gland. In the cerebral circulation, this is reflected as an increase in diastolic velocity with a decrease in the various resistance indices (S/D ratio, PI and RI – see Protocol 6) and is referred to as the "brain-sparing" effect in IUGR. Several authors have reported that the brain-sparing effect identifies a group of IUGR fetuses prior to 34 weeks who have a higher risk of perinatal morbidity and mortality compared to those having an abnormal umbilical artery Doppler alone. The precardiac venous vessels have also been studied extensively in IUGR. In general, these "venous structures" principally refer to the ductus venosus (DV), hepatic veins (HV), and the inferior vena cava (IVC). The precardiac venous vessels have characteristic triphasic Doppler waveforms that reflect the central venous pressures due to cardiac function, while the peripheral venous vessels (umbilical vein and portal sinus) have steady flow velocity waveforms. As cardiac contractility and compliance are compromised in the late states of IUGR, abnormalities can be seen in the venous structures. More specifically, there is an increase in pulsatility indices and an impact on the a-wave (of the triphasic waveform) which reflects flow at the atrial kick where the foramen ovale and the christa dividens meet. The appearance of flow at the atrial kick is different depending on the vessel interrogated. Normally, flow at the atrial kick is forward for the DV, reversed for the IVC, and either absent or reversed in the HV. As cardiac function decreases, one can see either a reduced, absent or reversed flow at the atrial kick for the DV and increased reversal of flow in the IVC and HV. Hecher *et al.* and Rizzo *et al.* performed fetal blood sampling in fetuses that had reversal of flow in the DV or greatly reversed flow in the IVC and showed that this is consistent with an acidemic state in the fetus. While an abnormal MCA Doppler has been shown to identify an IUGR fetus at greater risk of morbidity than an abnormal umbilical artery alone and while venous Doppler abnormalities can identify the IUGR fetus at risk of acidemia, Doppler velocimetry of these vessels have not been vigorously tested in RCTs to show clinical benefit (Level 2 and 3 evidence). As such, their use is primarily relegated to specialized centers at the current time.

The frequency of surveillance of the IUGR and indications for hospitalization remains controversial. There is no consensus on how frequently to perform growth scans or umbilical artery Doppler velocimetry, or whether to perform modified NSTs or BPPs. However, in general, most experts would agree that surveillance should include ultrasound assessment of growth every 2–3 weeks, twice weekly testing with modified BPP, and umbilical artery Doppler every 1–2 weeks. Pregnant patients should be instructed on daily fetal activity counts with a low threshold to be seen if any fetal movement seems abnormal to them. Anecdotally, it is reasonable to have patients perform the kick counts twice daily and most patients are quite happy to do so. In otherwise isolated IUGR (e.g., normal AF, Doppler studies, anatomy survey, and antepartum testing), umbilical artery Dopplers can be performed at 2-week intervals. If umbilical artery Dopplers are abnormal or if the EFW or AC are below 5th percentile, weekly umbilical artery Dopplers should be performed. As additional complications occur, such as preeclampsia, AEDF, nonreactive NST, BPP of 4 or less, or oligohydramnios, hospitalization may be indicated so that monitoring frequency can be increased.

Management

Timing of delivery of the IUGR fetus is a challenge, as one must weigh the risk of continued intrauterine life and risk of end-organ injury compared to the risks associated with preterm delivery. Gestational age, EFW and fetal status are factors that contribute to delivery considerations in IUGR. If delivery is anticipated between 24 and 34 weeks, all efforts should be made to administer antenatal steroids, especially since complications of prematurity are magnified in the IUGR condition. The historic viability thresholds of 24 weeks gestation and 500 g for normally grown fetuses, does not apply in IUGR. In several retrospective studies, delivery of IUGR fetuses prior to 26–27 weeks with EFWs below 600 g carries a high probability of perinatal death. Other studies show that fetal survival and intact survival do not exceed 50% until after achieving 27 completed weeks, and that each additional week gained in utero substantially contributes to survival (reduction in perinatal mortality by 48% for each week gained below 30 weeks of gestation). Thus, gaining time in utero is a most critical goal and also appears to be more important than just the EFW.

One challenge that is encountered clinically is when fetal monitoring with the NST shows absent variability or occasional/repetitive decelerations or if the BPP drops to 4–6 in a fetus who is less than 26–27 weeks. While most patients would opt for intervention with delivery, the option of no intervention should be provided. In these instances where intervention is desired by patients, steroid administration should precede delivery. Although no randomized trials exist that show definitive clinical benefit, venous Dopplers may be helpful in determining whether the fetus is acidemic and perhaps influence delivery decisions. Results from the recently completed TRUFFLE study assessing the use of venous Dopplers in IUGR should be available soon.

Figure 40.1 shows an algorithm for the management of the IUGR fetus from the time of diagnosis. In general, delivery of FGR fetuses should be considered delivered upon entering the early term period at 37–39 weeks. If umbilical artery Dopplers are normal and testing continues to be normal and interval ultrasounds continue to show growth, this likely represents a constitutionally small fetus and delivery can be delayed until 38–40 weeks. If umbilical artery Dopplers show elevated indices of blood flow resistance with persistently forward diastolic flow (e.g., no evidence of AEDF or REDF), delivery at 36–37 weeks is recommended. The DIGITAT trial is the only RCT of IUGR fetuses near term where fetuses were either induced at 36 weeks or managed expectantly. While both groups showed higher NICU rates the earlier they delivered, there was no difference in perinatal morbidity between groups. Preeclampsia rates were doubled (7% versus 14%) in the expectant management group. There were no differences between the groups for neurodevelopmental outcome at 2 years of age. In late onset FGR (>34 weeks), umbilical artery Doppler waveforms may not show the abnormalities seen in early FGR, which suggests a difference in the pathophysiology of early versus late onset FGR. Recent data

Algorithm Guideline for Management of IUGR

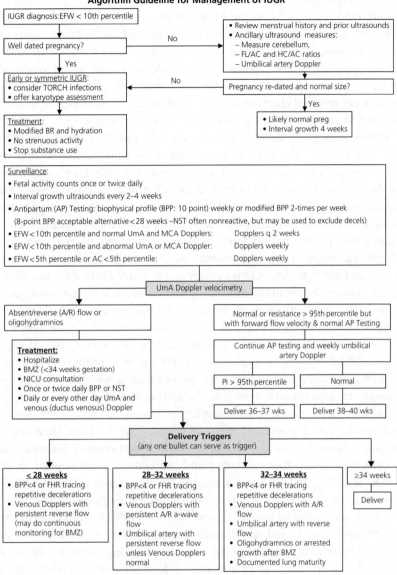

A/R, absent or reverse; BMZ, betamethasone

Figure 40.1 Algorithm for the management of the IUGR fetus from the time of diagnosis.

have emerged showing that in late FGR fetuses, the only Doppler abnormality detected may be in the MCA. In this group of fetuses, there are reported higher rates of fetal heart rate abnormalities in labor, cesarean rates, and adverse newborn neurologic outcomes. IUGR fetuses with AEDF in the umbilical artery can have delivery delayed until 32–34 weeks of gestation assuming other testing has continued to be reassuring and the patient has received glucocorticoid for fetal benefit. Continuing pregnancy beyond 34 weeks with AEDF present is not recommended.

Timing delivery for IUGR fetuses between 26 and 32 weeks of gestation presents a greater challenge as gestational age at delivery dictates perinatal morbidity. There are limited data to provide guidance for management of these IUGR fetuses. The only RCT for IUGR fetuses in this gestational period is the GRIT study where IUGR fetuses were randomized at a point in time when their providers were unsure of management to either immediate delivery (after steroid administration) or to expectant management. The mean number of days to delivery was 0.9 in the immediate delivery group and 4.9 in the expectant management group. There were no differences between either of the groups for immediate or long-term morbidity or mortality. While there were significant limitations of the GRIT study, it suggests that delaying delivery at least for a short period of time does not make a difference and that neurologic injury in IUGR may have already been established earlier in gestation. Several research groups have demonstrated that 50–70% of fetuses may demonstrate a sequence of Doppler changes in different fetal vessels as the fetal cardiovascular and placental circulation deteriorates. Use of Dopplers in vessels other than the umbilical artery, have not received rigorous testing in RCTs. Thus, their use is primarily based on retrospective review and expert opinion (Level 2 and 3 evidence). Given that morbidity and mortality is greatest prior to 29 weeks for IUGR fetuses (94% mortality in one study), tolerating AEDF and in some cases REDF in the umbilical artery may be warranted and has been accomplished for weeks in some reports. For IUGR fetuses in the 26–29-week time period with umbilical artery AEDF or REDF, persistent reversal of flow in the DV can be considered an indication for delivery as this has been shown to be a marker of fetal acidemia. Alternatively, if the DV in these fetuses shows forward flow, it can be reassuring for continuing the pregnancy. The threshold for delivery drops beyond 29 weeks with progressive improvement in survival and intact survival. Some experts have advocated for use of the DV in this time period to help with timing of delivery.

The route of delivery is not necessarily altered with IUGR. Taken as a group, the majority of IUGR fetuses can deliver vaginally. However, for the early and severely growth-restricted fetuses, especially with AEDF or REDF in the umbilical artery, cesarean delivery for FHR tracing abnormalities is much more common. In the GRIT RCT, the cesarean rate was 90%. In the presence of AEDF or REDF in the umbilical artery, oligohydramnios, severe IUGR (below 3rd percentile) or preeclampsia, an oxytocin contraction test prior to induction is a reasonable consideration.

Counseling

It is natural for patients to become anxious when first told that their pregnancy is complicated by IUGR. Emphasizing that 70% of fetuses below the 10th percentile are small for normal reasons helps to alleviate some of that anxiety. When discussing other possible etiologies of IUGR (Table 40.1), it is helpful to discuss that the majority of the 30% of causes reduce fetal growth by decreasing blood flow through the uterus and placenta. Other causes of reduced growth such as infectious and chromosomal abnormalities, while more severe, are less common. The risk of an IUGR in a future pregnancy depends on the cause of IUGR in a prior pregnancy and thus, it remains important to determine the cause. In general, the recurrence rate has been generally shown to be about 10% and taking a baby aspirin (81 mg) beginning early in the next pregnancy reduces the recurrence of IUGR. These points can be emphasized at the 6-week postpartum visit, at any future preconception visit, and early in the subsequent pregnancy.

Conclusion

Fetal growth restriction is a common complication of pregnancy that increases the risk of fetal demise and the newborn risk of perinatal morbidity and mortality compared to the normally grown newborn. Changes that occur to organ systems of the IUGR fetus and newborn predispose the fetus/newborn to chronic diseases later in life. Ultrasound modalities continue to be the mainstay for accurate pregnancy dating, diagnosis of IUGR and for management of the IUGR fetus. The only surveillance tool that has Level 1 evidence of improved outcomes is the Doppler of the umbilical artery; however, all other tools described are useful in providing an assessment of the global health of the fetus. Timing the delivery of the IUGR fetus remains the biggest challenge from a management standpoint with the threshold for delivery decreasing with advancing gestational age. Additional information on the use of multi-vessel arterial and venous Doppler interrogation should be forthcoming with completion of the TRUFFLE study in Europe.

Suggested reading

American College of Obstetricians and Gynecologists. Fetal Growth Restriction. Practice Bulletin. No 134. American College of Obstetricians and Gynecologists. *Obstet Gynecol* 2013;121:1122–33.

Barker DJP. Adult consequences of fetal growth restriction. *Clin Obstet Gynecol* 2006;49:270–83.

Baschat AA, Cosmi E, Bilardo CM, *et al*. Predictors of neonatal outcome in early-onset placental dysfunction. *Obstet Gynecol* 2007;109:253–61.

Berghella V. Prevention of recurrent fetal growth restriction. *Obstet Gynecol* 2007;110:904–12.

Boers KE, van Wyk L, van der Post JAM. Neonatal morbidity after induction vs expectant monitoring in intrauterine growth restriction at term: a subanalysis of the DIGITAT RCT. *Am J Obstet Gynecol* 2012;206:344e1–7.

Cruz-Martinez R, Figueras F, Hernandez-Andrade E, *et al*. Fetal brain Doppler to predict cesarean delivery for nonreassuring fetal status in term small-for-gestational age fetuses. *Obstet Gynecol* 2011;117:618–26.

Eixarch E, Meler E, Iraola A, *et al*. Neurodevelopmental outcome in 2-year-old infants who were small-for-gestational age term fetuses with cerebral blood flow redistribution. *Ultrasound Obstet Gynecol* 2008;32:894–9.

Fetal Growth Restriction. Practice Bulletin. No 134. American College of Obstetricians and Gynecologists. Obstet Gynecol 2013;121:1122-33.

Garite TJ, Clark R, Thorp JA. Intrauterine growth restriction increases morbidity and mortality among premature neonates. *Am J Obstet Gynecol* 2004;191:481–7.

Hecher K, Snijders R, Campbell S, Nicolaides K. Fetal venous, intracardiac, and arterial blood flow measurements in intrauterine growth retardation: Relationship with fetal blood gases. *Am J Obstet Gyneco* 1995;173:10–15.

McIntire DD, Bloom SL, Casey BM, *et al*. Birth weight in relation to morbidity and mortality among newborn infants. *N Eng J Med* 1999;340:1234–8.

Neilson JP, Alfirevic Z. Doppler ultrasound for fetal assessment in high-risk pregnancies. *Cochrane Database Syst Rev* 2005;(1):CD000073. Cochrane Library.

Oros D, Figueras F, Cruz-Martinez R, *et al*. Middle versus anterior cerebral artery Doppler for the prediction of perinatal outcome and neonatal neurobehavior in term small-for-gestational age fetuses with normal umbilical artery Doppler. *Ultrasound Obstet Gynecol.* 2010;35:456–61.

Resnik R, Creasy RK. Intrauterine growth restriction. In: Creasy RK, Resnik R, Lams JD, editors. *Maternal-fetal medicine: principles and practice*. 6th ed. Philadelphia (PA): Saunders; 2009.

Rizzo G, Capponi A, Arduini D. Romanini C. *The value of fetal arterial, cardiac and venous flows in predicting pH and blood gases measured in umbilical blood at cordocentesis in growth retarded fetuses*. 1995;102:963–9.

Rh and Other Blood Group Alloimmunizations

Kenneth J. Moise Jr
Department of Obstetrics, Gynecology and Reproductive Sciences, UT Health School of Medicine, Houston, TX, USA

Overview

Once a significant cause of perinatal loss, alloimmunization to red cell antigens is infrequently encountered today in obstetrical practice. Sensitization to the RhD antigen remains the leading cause of hemolytic disease of the fetus/newborn (HDFN) with an incidence of approximately 1 in 1200 pregnancies. Other significant red cell antibodies (see Table 41.1) are reported to complicate 1 in 300 pregnancies. After anti-D, anti-E is the next most frequent encountered antibody followed by anti-K and anti-c. Severe HDFN has been reported in 12% of pregnancies with anti-K, 4% with anti-c, and 1% with anti-E. Significant advances in diagnostic tools have occurred with the addition of genetic testing of the fetus and Doppler ultrasonography for the detection of fetal anemia.

Pathophysiology

The fetal–maternal interface was once thought to be an impervious barrier. However, more recent evidence suggests there is considerable trafficking of many types of cells between the fetus and its mother throughout gestation. In most cases, the antigenic load of incompatible antigen on the fetal erythrocytes and erythrocytic precursors is insufficient to stimulate the maternal immune system. However, in the case of a large antenatal feto-maternal hemorrhage, or a feto-maternal hemorrhage at delivery, B-lymphocyte clones that recognize the foreign red cell antigen are established. The initial maternal IgM antibody response is short-lived with a rapid change to IgG antibody.

Protocols for High-Risk Pregnancies: An Evidence-Based Approach, Sixth Edition.
Edited by John T. Queenan, Catherine Y. Spong and Charles J. Lockwood.
© 2015 John Wiley & Sons, Ltd. Published 2015 by John Wiley & Sons, Ltd.

Table 41.1 Non-RhD antibodies and associated hemolytic disease of the fetus or newborn

Antigen system	Specific antigen	Antigen system	Specific antigen	Antigen system	Specific antigen
Frequently associated with severe disease					
Kell	-K (K1)				
Rhesus	-c				
Infrequently associated with severe disease					
Colton	-Coa	MNS	-Mur	Scianna	-Sc2
	-Co3		-MV		-Rd
Diego	-ELO		-s	Other Ag's	-Bi
	-Dia		-sD		-Good
	-Dib		-S		-Heibel
	-Wra		-U		-HJK
	-Wrb		-Vw		-Hta
Duffy	-Fya	Rhesus	-Bea		-Jones
Kell	- Jsb		-C		-Joslin
	-k (K2)		-Ce		-Kg
	-Kpa		-Cw		-Kuhn
	- Kpb		-ce		-Lia
	-K11		-E		-MAM
	-K22		-Ew		-Niemetz
	-Ku		-Evans		-REIT
	- Ula		-G		-Reiter
Kidd	-Jka		-Goa		-Rd
MNS	-Ena		-Hr		-Sharp
	-Far		-Hro		-Vel
	-Hil		-JAL		-Zd
	-Hut		-Rh32		
	-M		-Rh42		
	-Mia		-Rh46		
	-Mta		-STEM		
	-MUT		-Tar		
Associated with mild disease					
Duffy	-Fyb	Kidd	-Jkb	Rhesus	-Riv
	-Fy3		-Jk3		-RH29
Gerbich	-Ge2	MNS	-Mit	Other	-Ata
	-Ge3	Rhesus	-CX		-JFV
	-Ge4		-Dw		-Jra
	-Lsa		-e		-Lan
Kell	- Jsa		-HOFM		
			-LOCR		

Source: Creasy *et al.*, 2004. Reproduced with permission of Elsevier.

Although the fetus of the sensitizing pregnancy often escapes the effects of the maternal antibody, subsequent fetuses are at risk for HDFN. Maternal IgG crosses the placenta and attaches to fetal erythrocytes that have expressed the paternal red cell antigen. These cells are then sequestered by macrophages in the fetal spleen where they undergo extravascular hemolysis producing fetal anemia. In cases of HDFN related to the Kell (anti-K1) antibody, in vitro and in vivo evidence suggest an additional mechanism for the fetal anemia – suppression of erythropoiesis. Hydrops fetalis is the most significant manifestation of the fetal anemia although its exact pathophysiology remains unknown. An elevated central venous pressure has been reported in these fetuses and may cause a functional blockage of the lymphatic system at the level of the thoracic duct as it empties into the left brachiocephalic vein. Reports of poor absorption of red cells transfused into the peritoneal cavity in cases of hydrops support this theory.

Management of the first alloimmunized pregnancy (Fig 41.1)

Obtain an antibody screen on all pregnant women at their first prenatal visit. If the antibody screen returns positive, the antibody should be identified to see if it has been associated with HDFN. If this is the case, an antiglobulin titer should be undertaken.

- Obtain an early ultrasound examination for pregnancy dating.
- Determine the paternal antigen status.
  - If negative and paternity is assured, no further evaluation is necessary.
  - If positive, serologic testing can be used in consultation with a blood bank pathologist to determine the paternal zygosity (homozygous or heterozygous) for most red cell antigens. The one exception is the RhD antigen where the lack of a "d" antigen is secondary to the nonexpression of the RHD gene. In this situation, testing for paternal zygosity should be undertaken through DNA methods at a reference laboratory.
- Repeat titers every month until 24 weeks of gestation; then every 2 weeks for the remainder of the pregnancy. Perform titers with the older tube technology (gel methods have not been correlated with clinical outcome and will usually result in values 1–2 dilutions higher than tube titers). Use an experienced blood bank; most commercial laboratories use enhancement techniques that will elevate titers.
- If the titer is 32 or greater (use a titer of 8 for the Kell antibody), there is a risk for fetal hydrops. Consult a maternal–fetal medicine specialist for further management.

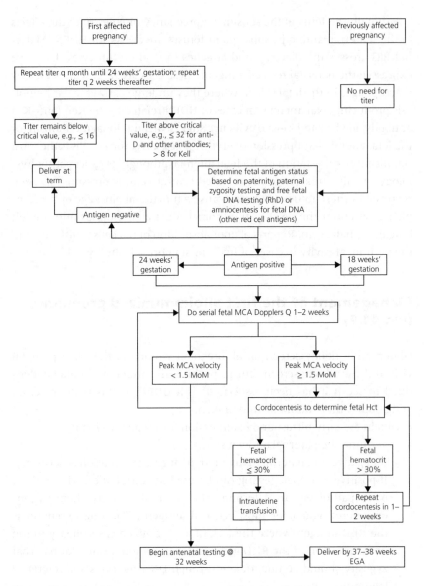

Figure 41.1 Algorithm for the management of the red cell alloimmunized pregnancy. Source: Moise & Argotti, 2012. Reproduced with permission of Lippincott Williams & Wilkins.

• In cases of a heterozygous partner for RhD, circulating cell-free fetal DNA (ccfDNA) in the maternal serum can now be used to test the antigen status of the fetus in a noninvasive fashion. For other red cell antigens, perform amniocentesis by 24 weeks of gestation to assess the fetal blood type through DNA analysis. Send maternal and paternal blood samples

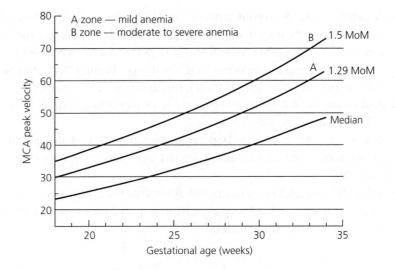

Figure 41.2   Middle cerebral artery peak systolic Doppler velocity. Source: Moise, 2002. Reproduced with permission of Lippincott Williams & Wilkins.

to the reference laboratory with the amniotic aliquot to minimize errors due to gene rearrangements in the parents. The antigen-positive fetus can be monitored for the development of anemia by ultrasonography using the peak middle cerebral artery (MCA) systolic velocity serially every 1–2 weeks.

- A value of greater than 1.5 multiples of the median (MOM) for gestational age is highly suggestive for fetal anemia (see Fig. 41.2).
- MCAs can be obtained as early as 18 weeks.
- If the MCA Doppler is greater than 1.5 MOM, perform cordocentesis with blood readied for intrauterine transfusion (IUT) for a fetal hematocrit of less than 30%.
- Initiate antenatal testing with nonstress testing or biophysical profiles at 32 weeks of gestation.
- Consider delivery by 37–38 weeks of gestation.

Management of a subsequent alloimmunized pregnancy

(Previously affected fetus that has undergone IUTs or an infant that has undergone neonatal transfusions)

- Maternal titers are *not* helpful in predicting the onset of fetal anemia after the first affected gestation.

- In cases of a heterozygous partner for RhD, ccfDNA in the maternal serum can now be used to test the antigen status of the fetus in a noninvasive fashion. For other red cell antigens, perform amniocentesis by 24 weeks of gestation to assess the fetal blood type through DNA analysis. If an antigen-negative fetus is found, no further testing is warranted.
- Begin serial MCA Doppler assessments at 18 weeks of gestation. Repeat at 1- to 2-week intervals.
- If a rising value for MCA Doppler greater than 1.5 MOM, perform cordocentesis with blood readied for IUT for a fetal hematocrit of less than 30%.
- If the MCA Doppler remains normal, follow the same protocol for antenatal monitoring and delivery as previously noted for the management of the first sensitized pregnancy.

Treatment

Since it was first introduced in 1963, the IUT of donor red blood cells has clearly contributed to the survival of countless fetuses with severe HDFN worldwide. Today, the direct intravascular transfusion (IVT) using the umbilical cord for access is the technique most widely used in the United States. Typically, a unit of donor red cells that has been recently donated and lacking the putative red cell antigen is used. The donor should be negative for antibody to cytomegalovirus. The unit is cross-matched to the pregnant patient and then packed to a final hematocrit of 75–85% to allow a minimal blood volume to be administered to the fetus during the IUT. The blood is then leukoreduced with a special filter and irradiated with 25 Gy to prevent graft-versus-host reaction.

The patient is usually admitted to the labor and delivery suite for an outpatient procedure. Conscious sedation is used in conjunction with local anesthetic. Prophylactic antibiotics are given but tocolytics are rarely required. Continuous ultrasonographic guidance is used to find the umbilical cord insertion. After the initial puncture of the umbilical vein, a sample of fetal blood is sent for hematocrit and other values. A small dose of a paralytic agent is administered to cause cessation of fetal movement. Donor red cells are then transfused based on the initial fetal hematocrit and formulas to calculate the fetoplacental blood volume using ultrasound-estimated fetal weight. A final sample is obtained to measure the fetal hematocrit at the conclusion of the procedure. After the procedure, the patient undergoes continuous fetal monitoring until there is resumption of fetal movement. Ultrasonography is performed the following day to assess fetal viability.

IUTs are rarely successful prior to 18 weeks of gestation; excellent rates of neonatal survival in today's nurseries have led most centers to limit IUTs to gestational ages of less than 35 weeks. If the fetus is severely anemic and the gestational age is less than 24 weeks, the fetal hematocrit is only partially corrected with the first IVT. A subsequent procedure is planned 48 hours later to correct the fetal hematocrit into the normal range. In other cases, the second procedure is usually planned 7–10 days after the first with an expected decrease in the fetal hematocrit of approximately 1%/day. Subsequent procedures are repeated at 2- to 3-week intervals based on fetal response.

After the last procedure, the patient is scheduled for induction of labor at 38–39 weeks of gestation to allow for fetal hepatic and pulmonary maturity. It is rare for these infants to require prolonged phototherapy or exchange transfusions. Breastfeeding is not contraindicated.

Outcome and follow up

In experienced centers, the overall perinatal survival with IUTs is 85–90%. Fetuses with hydrops have a markedly lower rate of survival, particularly if the hydrops does not resolve after two or three procedures. Suppression of fetal erythropoiesis results in prolonged bone marrow suppression after birth. These infants should be followed weekly with hematocrits and reticulocyte counts until there is evidence of reticulocytosis. Simple neonatal transfusions of red cells may be required in as many as 50% of cases, particularly if the neonate becomes symptomatic from its anemia.

Neurodevelopmental follow-up of neonates transfused by IVT indicates an increased rate of cerebral palsy (2.1%), severe developmental delay (3.1%) and bilateral deafness (1%). Severe hydrops was associated with an 11-fold increased risk for neurodevelopmental compromise.

Prevention

Only RhD alloimmunization can be prevented through the use of a specific immune globulin (RhIG). Although this product is manufactured from human serum, clinical trials are under way with synthesized polyclonal antibodies. Prevention of alloimmunization to other red cell antigens is currently not possible as specific prophylactic immune globulins are not available. In some countries, such as Australia, Kell-negative female children and women of reproductive age are cross-matched to receive Kell-negative blood when they require a transfusion. This policy has not been adopted in the United States due to the low frequency of the Kell antigen in the general population.

A blood type determination and antibody screening should be obtained at the first prenatal visit in all pregnant patients. Testing for "weak D," formerly "Du" antigen is being recommended in a new approach due to new genotyping capabilities and information. There are approximately 17,000 pregnant women per year with serological weak D phenotypes in the United States. They can be genotyped and if their RHD genotype is type 1, 2, or 3, they may be managed as RhD-positive because they will not develop antibodies if exposed to RhD-positive blood. Their clinical advantage is that RhIG is not indicated at 28 weeks of gestation or postpartum. Additionally, if a transfusion is necessary they may receive RhD-positive blood. This has particular import for travel in the Far East and Africa where if the need for a transfusion arises, RhD-negative blood is rare. The numerous other types of "weak Ds" may be susceptible to alloimmunization by exposure to Rh-positive blood and therefore they are managed as Rh-negative patients, receiving RhIG at 28 weeks of gestation and Rh-negative blood if a transfusion is necessary.

In RhD-negative patients with an initial negative antibody screen, a 300 microgram dose of RhIG should be administered at 28 weeks of gestation. If the patient's partner is determined to be RhD-negative and paternity is assured, this can be omitted. The rate of seroconversion prior to 28 weeks has been reported to be approximately 1 in 1000 pregnancies. A repeat antibody screen at 28 weeks is recommended by the American Association of Blood Banks (AABB), although the American College of Obstetricians and Gynecologists has left this to the discretion of the clinician. If an antibody screen is not done at 28 weeks, the rare Rh-alloimmunization will go undetected, as routine antibody screening is not done after RhIG administration. However, a recent analysis has not found the practice of repeat antibody testing to be cost-effective.

Although perhaps on the near horizon for the United States, ccfDNA determination for RHD has been incorporated into the antenatal prophylaxis algorithm in countries such as Denmark and the Netherlands and in regions of England, Sweden and France. In 40% of RhD-negative women who are pregnant, their fetus will be RhD-negative as well and therefore antenatal RhIG is unnecessary. ccfDNA evaluation as early as 10 weeks of gestation can be used to target only those women where antenatal RhIG is needed.

At the time of the delivery of an RhD-negative patient, cord blood should be tested for RhD typing. If the neonate is determined to be RhD-positive, a second dose of 300 microgram should be administered within 72 hours

Table 41.2   Other indications for Rhesus immune globulin administration

---

Spontaneous abortion
Threatened abortion
Elective abortion
Ectopic pregnancy
Hydatidiform mole
Amniocentesis
Chorionic villus biopsy
Placenta previa with bleeding
Suspected abruption
Fetal death
Blunt trauma to the abdomen (including motor vehicle accidents)
External cephalic version

---

of delivery. Routine screening of all women for excessive feto-maternal bleeding at the time of delivery should then be undertaken. Typically this involves a rosette test that is read qualitatively as positive or negative. If negative, one vial of RhIG (300 microgram) is given, as this will be sufficient to protect the patient from a 30 mL fetal bleed. If positive, the volume of the bleed is quantitated with a Kleihauer-Betke stain or fetal cell stain using flow cytometry. Blood bank consultation should then be undertaken to determine the number of doses of RhIG to administer. If RhIG is inadvertently omitted after delivery, some protection from sensitization has been shown with administration within 13 days. RhIG should not be withheld as late as 28 days after delivery if the need arises.

Additional indications for RhIG are listed in Table 41.2. The use of RhIG for threatened abortion has not been well studied. If minimal vaginal bleeding is noted, it can probably be omitted; however if significant clinical bleeding is present, a dose should be administered. Although a 50 microgram RhIG dose can be used up to 13 weeks of gestation, in practical terms most hospitals no longer stock this preparation and the cost is comparable to the standard 300 microgram dose. Repeat doses should be given at 12-week intervals if bleeding persists. A second indication for RhIg that is often overlooked is blunt trauma to the maternal abdomen, particularly at the time of a motor vehicle accident. Finally, if 300 microgram of RhIG are given late in gestation for external cephalic version or third trimester amniocentesis for fetal lung maturity, a repeat dose is unnecessary if delivery occurs within 3 weeks as long as a feto-maternal hemorrhage in excess of 30 mL is not documented. The use of a repeat dose of RhIG after 40 weeks of gestation or its use after postpartum tubal ligation remains controversial.

Conclusion

The prevention and treatment of HDFN secondary to rhesus alloimmunization represents a true victory of modern perinatal care. Advances in DNA
technology now allow for routine noninvasive RhD red cell typing of the
fetus from maternal serum. Maternal immunomodulation will probably
negate the need for IUT in the coming years.

Suggested reading

Abbey R, Dunsmoor-Su R. Cost-benefit analysis of indirect antiglobulin screening in
rh(d)-negative women at 28 weeks of gestation. *Obstet Gynecol* 2014;123:938–45.

Clausen FB, Christiansen M, Steffensen R, *et al.* Report of the first nationally implemented
clinical routine screening for fetal RHD in D- pregnant women to ascertain the requirement for antenatal RhD prophylaxis. *Transfusion* 2012;52:752–8.

Koelewijn JM, Vrijkotte TG, van der Schoot CE, Bonsel GJ, de Haas M. Effect of screening
for red cell antibodies, other than anti-D, to detect hemolytic disease of the fetus and
newborn: a population study in the Netherlands. *Transfusion* 2008;48:941–52.

Liley AW. Intrauterine transfusion of foetus in haemolytic disease. *BMJ* 1963;2:1107–9.

Lindenburg IT, Smits-Wintjens VE, van Klink JM, *et al.* Long-term neurodevelopmental
outcome after intrauterine transfusion for hemolytic disease of the fetus/newborn: the
LOTUS study. *Am J Obstet Gynecol* 2012;206:141 e1–8.

Mari G for the Collaborative Group for Doppler Assessment of the Blood Velocity in Anemic Fetuses. Noninvasive diagnosis by Doppler ultrasonography of fetal anemia due to
maternal red-cell alloimmunization. *N Engl J Med* 2000;342:9–14.

Moise KJ. Modern management of Rhesus alloimmunization in pregnancy. *Obstet Gynecol*
2002;100:600–11.

Moise KJ. Hemolytic disease of the fetus and newborn. In: Creasy R, Resnik R, Iams J,
editors. *Maternal-Fetal Medicine*. Philadelphia, PA: Saunders; 2004.

Moise KJ Jr.,, Argoti PS. Management and prevention of red cell alloimmunization in
pregnancy: a systematic review. *Obstet Gynecol* 2012;120:1132–9.

Moise KJ Jr.,, Boring NH, O'Shaughnessy R, *et al.* Circulating cell-free fetal DNA
for the detection of RHD status and sex using reflex fetal identifiers. *Prenat Diagn*
2013;33:95–101.

Radunovic N, Lockwood CJ, Alvarez M, Plecas D, Chitkara U, Berkowitz RL. The severely
anemic and hydropic isoimmune fetus: changes in fetal hematocrit associated with
intrauterine death. *Obstet Gynecol* 1992;79:390–3.

van Kamp IL, Klumper FJ, Oepkes D, *et al.* Complications of intrauterine intravascular
transfusion for fetal anemia due to maternal red-cell alloimmunization. *Am J Obstet
Gynecol* 2005;192:171–7.

Preterm Labor

Vincenzo Berghella

Department of Obstetrics and Gynecology, Division of Maternal-Fetal Medicine, Thomas Jefferson University, Philadelphia, PA, USA

Clinical significance

Preterm labor precedes approximately 50% of preterm births. Preterm birth is the foremost problem in obstetrics and accounts for most perinatal death. Preterm birth occurs in 11.5% (2012 data) of the approximately 4 million births in the United States. As such, there are over 500,000 preterm births in the United States each year. Over 75% of perinatal deaths related to preterm birth occur in babies born between 22 and 31 weeks of gestation. The rate of perinatal morbidity is also indirectly proportional to gestational age at birth (Table 42.1).

Pathophysiology

The pathophysiology of preterm labor is not well understood. At least four main mechanisms have been described: inflammation/infection, abruption (decidual bleeding), maternal and/or fetal stress, and excessive mechanical stretching of the uterus. Although arising from different pathways, and often more than just one, all spontaneous preterm births utilize a final common biochemical conduit that usually includes increased genital tract prostaglandin and protease production coupled with functional progesterone withdrawal related to progesterone receptor function. Disparities in preterm birth rates between racial groups may reflect both environmental stressors and differing genetic predispositions.

Diagnosis

Unfortunately, there are many differing definitions of preterm labor. The classic definition involves "uterine contractions (greater than 6/60 minute)

Table 42.1 Survival and major morbidities by gestational age at birth in 2008

GA (weeks)	Survival (%)	Chronic lung disease (%)	Severe IVH (%)	Necrotizing enterocolitis (%)	Severe ROP (%)
Less than 22	3.3	33.3	33.3	33.3	66.7
22	6.0	77.8	52.0	11.1	57.9
23	34.3	79.2	33.8	15.9	46.9
24	59.2	74.7	29.5	12.4	34.7
25	75.3	65.9	20.1	11.6	26.2
26	80.0	51.7	17.2	10.2	14.2
27	89.4	35.9	9.7	6.8	7.0
28	91.2	25.8	6.3	7.2	3.0
29	94.3	16.2	4.3	4.9	1.0
30	96.8	11.0	1.9	3.4	0.7
31	96.7	7.3	1.9	2.4	0.6
32	97.5	4.1	1.3	1.7	0.2
33	98.1	3.1	1.4	1.0	0.9
34	98.4	4.4	1.5	0.9	0.0

GA, gestational age.
Chronic lung disease is defined as need for oxygen therapy at 36 weeks of postmenstrual age.
Severe IVH: grades III and IV.
Necrotizing enterocolitis includes medical and surgical.
Severe ROP (retinopathy of prematurity) is defined as greater than grade 2.
Source: Data from Vermont Oxford Network 2007. Courtesy of Kevin Dysart, MD.

and documented cervical change by manual examination with intact membranes at 20–36 6/7 weeks of gestation." Most women with this diagnosis of preterm labor deliver at term (37 weeks or beyond) even without intervention. Transvaginal ultrasound (TVU) cervical length (CL) and fetal fibronectin (FFN) are currently the two tests with the best data for good prediction of preterm birth in women with preterm labor. Therefore, we like to add other criteria to the definition above: "in the presence of TVU CL less than 20 mm, or TVU 20–30 mm and positive FFN." The vast majority of women with these characteristics will deliver preterm. In contrast, women with preterm uterine contractions and manual cervical change but a TVU CL 30 mm or greater have a less than 2% chance of delivering within 1 week and less than 10% chance of delivering prior to 35 weeks of gestation.

Treatment

Preterm labor is better prevented than treated. The most important issues regarding management of a woman with true preterm labor are:

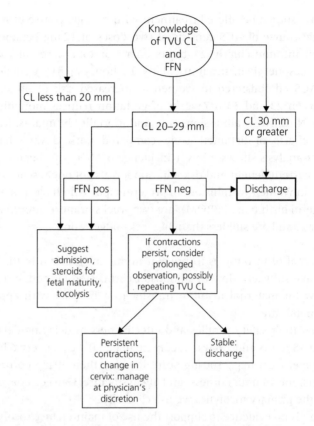

Figure 42.1 A proposed algorithm for combined cervical length (TVU CL) and fetal fibronectin (FFN) screening for women with symptoms of threatened preterm labor. TVU, transvaginal ultrasound; CL, cervical length; FFN, fetal fibronectin. Source: Ness *et al.*, 2007. Reproduced with permission of Elsevier.

- Treat only the women with true preterm labor and a real risk of preterm birth. A randomized trial by Ness *et al.* has shown benefit (reduction in preterm birth and quicker triage time) when women with threatened preterm labor are managed according to the algorithm shown in Fig. 42.1.
- Optimize fetal status:
  - *Transfer*: Assess for transfer to appropriate level hospital, usually with level III nursery.
  - *Corticosteroids for fetal maturity*: A course of antenatal corticosteroids (ACS) should be given to all women with true preterm labor, or at high risk for preterm birth within the next 7 days when between 23 and 34 weeks 6 days of gestation. All pregnant women between 23 0/7 and 33 6/7 weeks of gestation at high risk of preterm birth within

7 days should be offered treatment with a single course of ACS. This single course of ACS consists of two doses of 12 mg betamethasone given intramuscularly 24 hours apart; or four doses of 6 mg dexamethasone given intramuscularly 12 hours apart. A single course of ACS administered to women at increased risk of preterm birth between 23 and 33 6/7 weeks of gestation reduces morbidity (RDS, IVH, NEC, NICU admission, etc.) and mortality in infants. Regarding the effects of betamethasone compared with dexamethasone, a meta-analysis shows a lower incidence of IVH with betamethasone. The current benefit and risk data support use of one rescue courses of ACS in women with history of preterm labor who have a new risk for preterm birth (e.g., PPROM), are two weeks or more after first steroid course, and are still less than 34 weeks of gestation.

- Tocolysis:
  - The goal of tocolysis is to prevent imminent preterm birth, in order to have sufficient time to administer corticosteroids and, if necessary, allow for maternal in utero transfer to a hospital with appropriate neonatal care.
  - Given their safety profiles and effectiveness at delaying delivery for both 48 hours and 7 days, nifedipine (e.g., 20 mg po every 6 hours) or indomethacin (e.g., 100 mg po/pr loading, then 50 mg po/pr every 6 hours; for 48 hours or less, and always before 32 weeks of gestation) are the primary tocolytics we use clinically.
  - There is no evidence to support the use of maintenance tocolysis after successful arrest of preterm labor. There is not sufficient evidence to administer tocolysis once ACS have been administered.
- Magnesium for neuroprotection
  - Magnesium sulfate has been shown in five trials enrolling over 6000 women to significantly decrease cerebral palsy from 5.3% in placebo controls to 4.1%. The American College of Obstetricians and Gynecologists and the Society for Maternal Fetal Medicine have stated that "physicians electing to use magnesium sulfate for fetal neuroprotection should develop specific guidelines regarding inclusion criteria, treatment regimens (e.g., 4 mg loading dose, then 1gram/hour), concurrent tocolysis, and monitoring in accordance with one of the larger trials."
- Other interventions
  - There are insufficient data to recommend hydration, bed rest or decreased activity, progesterone or antibiotic therapy for prevention of preterm birth in women with preterm labor. Therefore, these interventions should be avoided, or reserved for clinical trials.

Complications

Preterm birth is associated with severe complications for the neonate. These include both short-term and long-term complications for the baby born too soon. Short-term, at times devastating, complications are listed in Table 42.1. Long-term complications include, among others, cerebral palsy, cognitive defects (e.g., low IQ), school difficulties, behavioral problems, and diminished long-term survival and reproduction.

Follow up

An episode of preterm labor usually does not give rise to a preterm birth. After administering ACS in the hospital, the woman can usually be discharged home. There are no interventions that are proven to prevent preterm birth between discharge and eventual delivery. Bed rest, frequent visits, and education on contractions have either been insufficiently studied or not proven beneficial so far. If the woman does have a preterm birth, postpartum counseling regarding how to prevent a recurrent preterm birth is extremely important.

Prevention

Prevention is of most importance. Several preventive interventions have been shown to be successful in reducing the risk of preterm birth (Table 42.2). These should be widely implemented, both at the local level (doctor–patient), and at the national level (government incentives and policies to assure implementation).

Conclusions

The incidence of preterm birth in the United States had increased more than 30% in the 20 years up to 2006. This was mostly due to increases in use of assisted reproduction (and consequent multiple gestations), and indicated preterm birth. Among other causes, coding of births at 22–24 weeks of gestation as preterm instead of miscarriages has undoubtedly increased the incidence in the United States. From its peak of 12.8% in 2006, the incidence of spontaneous preterm birth has decreased over 10% to about 11.5% in 2012. Implementation of preventive strategies

Table 42.2   Suggested prevention strategies to avoid preterm births

Preconception	Avoid extremes of age
	Aim for desirable interpregnancy interval (highest risk of PTB with interval less than 6 months)
	Avoid multiple gestations, with an emphasis on responsible ART
	Folate supplementation
	Vaccinations (especially varicella, rubella, hepatitis B)
	Balanced diet
	Exercise
	Avoid less than 120 lb maternal weight or BMI less than 19 kg/m^2
	Avoid illicit drug use and alcohol use
	Avoid sexually transmitted infections
	Optimize any medical disease (e.g., diabetes, hypertension, hypothyroidism, hyperthyroidism, asthma, lupus, HIV)
	Stop or substitute with safer medications any teratogenic drug
Prenatal care	Early ultrasound
	Screen for and treat asymptomatic bacteriuria
	Balanced diet
	Proper weight gain (at least 15 kg over 40 weeks for nonobese women)
	Avoid smoking, illicit drug use and alcohol
	Avoid prolonged standing more than 3 hours/day
	Avoid long work hours more than 39 hours/week
	Avoid shift work
	Avoid vaginal douching
	Screen for domestic violence and provide resources
	Screen for and treat sexually transmitted infections

PTB, preterm birth; ART, assisted reproductive technologies; BMI, body mass index.

(as shown in Table 42.2) will help continue to decrease this incidence, which is still one of the highest in the world.

Suggested reading

American College of Obstetricians and Gynecologists. Magnesium sulfate before anticipated preterm birth for neuroprotection. Committee Opinion No. 455. *Obstet Gynecol* 2010;115:669–71.

Doyle LW, Crowther CA, Middleton P, Marret S, Rouse D. Magnesium sulphate for women at risk of preterm birth for neuroprotection of the fetus. *Cochrane Database Syst Rev* 2009 Jan 21;(1):CD004661.

Ness A, Visintine J, Ricci E, Berghella V. Does knowledge of cervical length and fetal fibronectin affect management of women with threatened preterm labor? A randomized trial. *Am J Obstet Gynecol* 2007;197:426e1–426e7.

Spong CY. Prediction and prevention of recurrent spontaneous preterm birth. *Obstet Gynecol* 2007;110:405–15.

Premature Rupture of the Membranes

Brian Mercer
Department of Obstetrics & Gynecology, Case Western University-MetroHealth Medical Center, Cleveland, OH, USA

Overview

Premature rupture of the membranes (PROM), membrane rupture before the onset of contractions, complicates approximately 10% of pregnancies and is responsible for one-third of preterm deliveries.

Pathophysiology

Spontaneous membrane rupture occurs physiologically at term either before or after the onset of symptomatic contractions. This is believed to be related to progressive weakening of the membranes seen with advancing gestation, largely due to collagen remodeling and cellular apoptosis. When PROM occurs before term, the process of membrane weakening may be accelerated by a number of factors such as stretch, infection, inflammation and local hypoxia. Some clinical risk factors for preterm PROM are shown in Table 43.1. In asymptomatic women, a short cervix on transvaginal ultrasound (relative risk 3.2) and a positive cervico-vaginal fetal fibronectin (fFN) screen (relative risk 2.5) are also associated with increased risks of preterm birth due to PROM. While some recommend progesterone therapy for asymptomatic women with a short cervix, routine fFN screening is not recommended as an evidence-based intervention for those with a positive test is unavailable and such testing fails to identify the majority of women delivering preterm due to PROM.

Protocols for High-Risk Pregnancies: An Evidence-Based Approach, Sixth Edition.
Edited by John T. Queenan, Catherine Y. Spong and Charles J. Lockwood.
© 2015 John Wiley & Sons, Ltd. Published 2015 by John Wiley & Sons, Ltd.

Table 43.1 Clinical risk factors for preterm premature rupture of membranes

Risk factor	Odds ratio
Previous preterm PROM	3.3–6.3
Previous preterm delivery	1.9–2.8
Cigarette smoking	2.1
Bleeding during pregnancy	
• During first trimester	2.4
• During second trimester	4.4
• During third trimester	6.4
• More than one trimester	7.4
Acute pulmonary disease	1.8
Bacterial vaginosis	1.5

Source: Data from Harger et al., 1990; Naeye, 1992; Mercer et al., 2000.

Clinical implications

Hallmarks of PROM include brief latency from membrane rupture to delivery, increased risk of intrauterine and neonatal infection, and oligohydramnios.

At term, 95% of expectantly managed women will deliver within approximately 1 day of membrane rupture, but when women with preterm PROM are managed conservatively to prolong gestation, approximately half will deliver within 1 week. With PROM near the limit of viability, approximately one in four women will remain undelivered at least 1 month after membrane rupture. Because the benefits of conservative management include time for acceleration of fetal maturity with antenatal corticosteroids (24–48 hours latency required) and administration of magnesium sulfate for neuroprotection, as well as reduction of gestational age-dependent morbidity (extended latency approximately 1 week or more required), serious consideration should be given to expeditious delivery if the fetus is considered to be at low risk for gestational age-dependent morbidity in the late preterm and early term periods, or if adequate time to accrue corticosteroid and magnesium sulfate benefit and/or extended latency for fetal maturation are not anticipated.

Clinical chorioamnionitis is common after preterm PROM and increases with decreasing gestational age at membrane rupture. With PROM remote from term, clinical chorioamnionitis and endometritis can complicate 13–60% and 2–13% of pregnancies, respectively. Positive amniotic fluid cultures are obtained from amniocentesis specimens in 25–35% of women with preterm PROM. Maternal sepsis is a rare but serious complication of conservatively managed PROM affecting approximately 1% of women with PROM remote from term.

Fetal death complicates approximately 1–2% of conservatively managed cases of preterm PROM. This risk increases in the face of chorioamnionitis, and when PROM occurs near the limit of potential viability. It is believed that demise results from umbilical cord compression in most cases, though loss due to fetal infection and placental abruption can occur. Cord prolapse is an uncommon complication of PROM, but is more likely to occur with fetal malpresentation such as transverse lie or breech presentation.

Abruptio placentae is estimated to complicate about 4–12% of patients with preterm PROM. The onset of placental bleeding may occur before or after membrane rupture. The risks and benefits of conservative management to the fetus and mother should be reassessed if placental abruption is suspected. Attempts at extended latency should be reserved only for those with minimal bleeding, stable maternal cardiovascular status, and whose fetus is at high risk for death due to extreme prematurity with immediate delivery.

Diagnosis

Diagnosis of PROM can usually be made clinically based on a suggestive history combined with a sterile speculum examination. Demonstration of fluid passing per os is diagnostic of membrane rupture. Ancillary testing of vaginal fluid for an alkaline pH (greater than 6.0–6.5) with nitrazine paper is supportive, but can be falsely positive (17%) due to the presence of blood, semen, alkaline antiseptics or bacterial vaginosis, and can be falsely negative (9%) with prolonged leakage. The presence of a ferning pattern on microscopic examination of dried vaginal secretions can also be confirmatory and is less commonly falsely positive (6%) due to the presence of cervical mucus within the specimen (false negative rate 13%). Repeat speculum examination after prolonged recumbency may be helpful if the diagnosis is suspected but initial examination is not confirmatory.

Ultrasonographic evidence of oligohydramnios is supportive of a clinical diagnosis of membrane rupture but is not diagnostic as low amniotic fluid can occur for other reasons (e.g., fetal growth restriction, urinary tract anomalies), and the amniotic fluid volume may be within normal limits despite membrane rupture. The diagnosis can be confirmed unequivocally through ultrasound-guided amnioinfusion of indigo carmine (1 mL in 9 mL of sterile normal saline) followed by observation for passage of blue dye per vaginum. Testing with additional biomarkers for PROM is not needed and incurs unnecessary expense when the diagnosis is evident clinically. A number of biochemical markers have been found to be present in the vagina after PROM, and some of these are placental alpha microglobulin-1 (PAMG-1), insulin-like growth factor-binding protein-1 (IGFBP-1), fFN, alpha-fetoprotein, diamino-oxydase, total T4 and free T4, prolactin, human chorionic gonadotropin and interleukin-6. While there may be potential benefit of testing with these markers when the diagnosis of membrane rupture is unclear clinically, many are unavailable for bedside clinical use, and it is important to recognize that false-positive results can occur.

Evaluation

Women presenting with PROM at term or in the late preterm period (34–36 weeks) generally do not require additional specific evaluations once the diagnosis is made, unless other complicating circumstances are present, or in the unlikely event that conservative management is being considered.

Initial evaluation of the woman presenting with preterm PROM includes:

1 Ano-vaginal culture for group B streptococcus (GBS) if not performed within 6 weeks, and urinalysis with urine culture as appropriate. Consider cervical cultures for *Neisseria gonorrhoea* and *Chlamydia trachomatis*.

2 Digital cervical examinations should be avoided until the diagnosis of PROM has been excluded. Digital vaginal examinations after PROM can shorten the latent period from membrane rupture to delivery and increase the risk of chorioamnionitis, while adding little information regarding cervical dilatation and effacement over that available by visual inspection.

3 Initial maternal uterine activity and fetal heart rate monitoring to evaluate for evidence of labor, umbilical cord compression, and for fetal well-being if the limit of potential fetal viability has been reached. If conservative management is being considered, initial extended monitoring for approximately 6–12 hours followed by intermittent monitoring at least daily is appropriate.

4 Clinical assessment for chorioamnionitis including assessment of maternal and fetal heart rates, maternal temperature, uterine tenderness, and vaginal discharge. The combination of fever (38.0°C or 100.4°F, or more) with uterine tenderness and/or maternal or fetal tachycardia in the absence of another evident source for infection is suggestive of chorioamnionitis and is an indication for delivery regardless of gestational age.

5 A maternal white blood cell (WBC) count above $16,000 \times 10^9/L$ is supportive of suspicious clinical findings for chorioamnionitis. This test should not be used in isolation as there is significant variation in WBC count between patients and the WBC count is elevated in pregnancy and for 5–7 days after administration of antenatal corticosteroids.

It is helpful to obtain an initial baseline WBC count for subsequent comparison, if needed, when conservative management is considered.

6 Ultrasonographic examination to determine fetal position and presentation, exclude fetal malformations associated with PROM (e.g., hydrops fetalis, intestinal obstruction, diaphragmatic hernia may cause uterine stretch due to polyhydramnios), estimate fetal weight, assess amniotic fluid volume, and assess fetal well-being by biophysical profile if initial fetal heart rate testing is nonreactive.

7 Consider ultrasound-guided amniocentesis if intraamniotic infection is suspected clinically, but the diagnosis is not clear. Care should be paid to avoid the umbilical cord, which can be mistaken for a small amniotic fluid pocket if there is oligohydramnios. Amniotic fluid can be sent for Gram's stain, WBC count (30 cells/mm^3 or more considered abnormal), glucose (less than 16–20 mg/dL considered abnormal), and culture for aerobic and anaerobic bacteria. *Mycoplasma* is a common microorganism identified from amniotic fluid after PROM but it is not visible on Gram's stain.

Management

Conditions that mandate delivery after preterm or term PROM include clinical chorioamnionitis, nonreassuring fetal testing, significant vaginal bleeding, progressive labor and concurrent pregnancy complications indicating delivery (e.g., severe preeclampsia). In the absence of chorioamnionitis, placental abruption, fetal distress or labor, conservative management of women with preterm PROM may be appropriate. A gestational age-based approach to conservative management should be considered. The patient should be appraised of available current data regarding neonatal morbidity and mortality according to gestational age at delivery, in order to make appropriate decisions regarding the potential benefits of conservative management as opposed to expeditious delivery. It is important to recognize that regional factors may impact the risks and potential benefits of conservative management after PROM occurs. In some populations, the risk of intrauterine infection is higher and the potential for extended latency without complications is lower. In this setting, the tendency would be to focus on acceleration of fetal maturation, prevention of infection, and expeditious delivery when fetal benefit from prolonged latency is not anticipated. In other settings – particularly in populations at low risk for intrauterine infection – conservative management may be considered at a more advanced gestational age as extended latency without infection is more likely.

Term (37 weeks or more)

While labor will spontaneously ensue within 12 hours in 50%, and by 24 hours in 70% of women with PROM at term, the risk of chorioamnionitis increases with the duration of membrane rupture (2% 12 hours, 6% 12–24 hours, and 24% by 48 hours). Because of this, and because current evidence does not suggest an increased risk of infection or operative delivery with early induction, women with PROM at term are best served by labor induction/augmentation as needed, with cesarean delivery reserved for clinical indications. PROM is not a contraindication for pre-induction cervical priming with prostaglandin E_2 gel. GBS prophylaxis should be administered to those with positive ano-vaginal cultures within 6 weeks, positive urine cultures in the current pregnancy, or a previously affected child. GBS prophylaxis should also be initiated for those without a recent negative culture (within 6 weeks). Women with intrapartum fever should receive broad-spectrum antimicrobial therapy, including agents effective against gram-positive and gram-negative organisms, regardless of GBS culture status.

Preterm (34 weeks–36 weeks 6 days)

Newborns of women with PROM near term (34–36 weeks) are at relatively low risk of serious acute morbidity, and this risk is not likely to be reduced with the relatively brief anticipated latency. Although there are risks of newborn morbidity at this gestation, the risks of infection and umbilical cord compression outweigh the potential benefits of conservative management. Antenatal steroids for fetal maturation and magnesium for neuro-protection are not generally recommended at this gestation. While some studies have advocated for conservative management because newborn complications were not reduced with expectant management, the power of these to exclude fetal risk was low, chorioamnionitis was increased, and no newborn benefits with conservative management were demonstrated (Roberts and Dalziel, 2006). Therefore, it is recommended that these women be managed similarly to the term patient with PROM.

Preterm (32 weeks–33 weeks 6 days)

In the absence of an indication for delivery, evaluate fetal lung maturity status on amniotic fluid collected from the vaginal pool or by amniocentesis [phosphatidyl glycerol (PG) positive, or lecithin sphingomyelin (L/S) ratio 2:1 or more, or lamellar body count of 50,000/μL or more considered mature]. If there is blood or meconium-stained amniotic fluid, vaginal pool specimens for L/S ratio or lamellar body count may be falsely immature and should not be relied upon. However, delivery should be considered in these women because of the potential for fetal compromise.

If testing reveals a mature fetal pulmonary profile, expeditious delivery according to the recommendations for PROM at 34–36 weeks is recommended.

If testing reveals an immature lung profile or if fluid cannot be obtained:

1 Induction of fetal pulmonary maturation with antenatal corticosteroids followed by delivery in 24–48 hours or at 34 weeks of gestation is recommended.

2 If conservative management is pursued, broad-spectrum antibiotic treatment should be administered to reduce maternal and neonatal infections, to prolong latency in order to enhance steroid induced and spontaneous maturation.

3 Consideration should be given to delivery before infection or other complications ensue, if antenatal corticosteroids and antibiotics are not given in this setting.

4 Once antenatal corticosteroid benefit has been achieved, the patient should be assessed regarding the potential for extended latency (1 week or more) before 34 weeks. If the patient is more than 33 weeks 0 days of gestation at this time, it is unlikely that further delay of delivery to 34 weeks will result in substantial spontaneous fetal maturation, and delivery is recommended before complications ensue.

5 During conservative management, regular maternal and fetal assessment, as delineated below for PROM at 23–31 weeks, should be initiated.

Preterm (23 weeks–31 weeks 6 days)

Because the risks of neonatal morbidity and mortality due to prematurity is high with immediate delivery at 23–31 weeks of gestation, these women are generally best served by in-hospital conservative management to prolong pregnancy and reduce gestational age-dependent morbidity in the absence of evident infection, abruption, labor, vaginal bleeding, or fetal compromise. Should the patient be initially admitted to a facility without resources for emergent care of the mother and a very premature newborn, she should be transferred to a facility capable of providing care for these patients after initial assessment, and before acute complications occur, if possible.

During conservative management, the following should be considered:

1 Initial extended continuous fetal and maternal monitoring (approximately 6–12 hours) for contractions, nonreassuring fetal heart rate patterns, including umbilical cord compression.

2 At least daily clinical assessment for evidence of labor, chorioamnionitis, placental abruption. In addition, vital signs (temperature, pulse and blood pressure) should be documented at least each shift.

3 Antenatal corticosteroids for fetal maturation are recommended unless a full course has previously been given. Either two doses of betamethasone, 12 mg intramuscularly 24 hours apart, or four doses of dexamethasone, 6 mg intramuscularly 12 hours apart are appropriate.

4 Magnesium sulfate for neuroprotection is recommended: Several approaches to this intervention have been published. A recommended approach includes an initial 6-g bolus followed by 2 g per hour for 12 hours if undelivered (and continued if delivery is considered imminent), with retreatment if delivery before 34 weeks is subsequently considered imminent (Rouse et al., 2008).

5 Broad-spectrum antibiotic therapy should be administered during initial conservative management of preterm PROM to treat or prevent ascending subclinical decidual infection in order to prolong pregnancy, and to reduce neonatal infectious and gestational age-dependent morbidity. Intravenous therapy (48 hours) with ampicillin (2 g IV every 6 hours) and erythromycin (250 mg IV every 6 hours) followed by limited duration oral therapy (5 days) with amoxicillin (250 mg orally every 8 hours) and enteric-coated erythromycin base (333 mg orally every 8 hours) is recommended (Mercer et al., NICHD Maternal-Fetal Medicine Units network, 1997). Shorter duration therapy has not been shown to offer similar neonatal benefits, and is not recommended. Although not specifically studied, recent shortages in antibiotic availability have led to the need for substitution of alternative antibiotic treatments. Oral ampicillin, erythromycin, and azithromycin are likely appropriate substitutions for the above agents, as needed. Although a large multicenter study has suggested that broad-spectrum antibiotic therapy (oral amoxicillin-clavulonic acid) might increase the risk of necrotizing enterocolitis (Kenyon et al., ORACLE I Network, 2001), this finding is at variance with those of an NICHD funded Maternal-Fetal Medicine Units trial finding of reduced stage 2–3 necrotizing enterocolitis with broad-spectrum antibiotic therapy in a higher risk population, and this risk has not been confirmed in a meta-analysis of studies regarding this issue. Regardless, it is prudent to not treat these women with oral amoxicillin-clavulonic acid.

Management of the known GBS carrier after the initial 7 days of antibiotic therapy has not been well defined. In the absence of any studies addressing this issue, options include:

a. No further antepartum therapy, with intrapartum GBS prophylaxis of all known carriers.

b. Continued narrow-spectrum GBS prophylaxis of all known carriers from completion of the initial 7-day course through delivery.

c. Follow-up ano-vaginal culture after completion of the 7-day course, with continued narrow-spectrum therapy against GBS until delivery.

    d. Follow-up ano-vaginal culture of those having extended latency after initial antibiotic treatment, with repeat treatment of women with subsequently positive cultures (as well as intrapartum prophylaxis for all known carriers).

6 At least daily nonstress fetal heart rate and contraction monitoring to observe for evidence of subclinical contractions, fetal heart rate decelerations due to umbilical cord compression, sustained fetal tachycardia, or evidence of fetal compromise. Biophysical profile testing may be helpful when the fetal heart rate pattern is not reactive. A fetal heart rate pattern that is reactive initially but becomes nonreactive on follow-up testing, or a worsening biophysical profile score, should raise suspicion regarding the possibility of developing intrauterine infection or fetal compromise. Under such circumstances, prolonged monitoring and repeat biophysical profile testing should be considered.

7 WBC count monitoring can be helpful, but an elevated WBC count alone is not an indication for delivery. We perform an initial baseline WBC count for reference before administration of antenatal corticosteroids, and repeat testing if the initial result is elevated, or if equivocal clinical findings for intrauterine infection ensue. Repeat testing is not needed if the diagnosis of intrauterine infection is clear.

8 Treat specific cervico-vaginal pathogens and urinary tract infections.

9 Ultrasound should be performed every 3–4 weeks to assess fetal growth. It is not necessary to repeat amniotic fluid volume estimates frequently as persistent or worsening oligohydramnios is not an indication for delivery. Initial severe oligohydramnios has been associated with briefer latency to delivery, but this finding is an inaccurate predictor of latency or neonatal outcomes.

10 Current data do not suggest any long-term benefits of administering tocolysis to women with preterm PROM. Tocolytic therapy should not be administered after preterm PROM if there is suspicion of intrauterine infection, fetal compromise or placental abruption, and is unlikely to offer any potential benefit beyond delaying delivery while corticosteroids are being administered.

11 Because pregnancy and inactivity are risk factors for thromboembolic complications, preventative measures such as leg exercises, anti-embolic stockings, and/or prophylactic doses of subcutaneous heparin may be of value in preventing this outcome during conservative management with bed rest.

12 The patient who remains stable without evidence of infection, abruption or fetal compromise should generally be delivered at 34 weeks of gestation because of the ongoing but low risk of fetal death with conservative management and the high likelihood of survival without long-term sequelae with delivery at this gestational age. Assessment of fetal pulmonary maturity at 34 weeks, with continued conservative management of those with immature studies after further discussion of the risks and benefits of further conservative management, is acceptable.

13 Amnioinfusion has not been shown to be of benefit in preventing fetal compromise, or extending latency after preterm PROM. During labor, routine amnioinfusion is not recommended, and this treatment should be reserved for ameliorating significant umbilical cord compression (variable heart rate decelerations) that is unresponsive to maternal repositioning.

Preterm (prior to 23 weeks)

When PROM occurs prior to the limit of viability, the patient should be counseled with a realistic appraisal of potential fetal and neonatal outcomes. Regarding maternal morbidity, conservative management of mid-trimester PROM is associated with a high risk of chorioamnionitis (39%), endometritis (14%), abruptio placentae (3%) and retained placenta with postpartum hemorrhage requiring curettage (12%). The risk of stillbirth during conservative management of mid-trimester PROM is approximately 15%. Most of these pregnancies will deliver before or near the limit of viability, where neonatal death is either assured or common. The risk of long-term sequelae will depend on the gestational age at delivery. Persistent oligohydramnios is a poor prognostic indicator after PROM before 20 weeks, placing the fetus at high risk of lethal pulmonary hypoplasia regardless of extended latency.

Management options for women with PROM before 23 weeks include:

1 Labor induction with the following according to individual clinical circumstances and local regulations
   a. high-dose intravenous oxytocin
   b. intravaginal prostaglandin E_2
   c. oral or intravaginal prostaglandin E_1 (misoprostol)
2 Dilatation and evacuation. Intracervical laminaria placement prior to labor induction or dilatation and evacuation may be helpful.
3 Conservative management. Should conservative management be pursued, the following should be considered:
   a. The patient should be monitored initially for the development of infection, labor or placental abruption.
   b. Strict pelvic rest and initial modified bed rest with bathroom privileges should be encouraged to enhance the potential for membrane resealing, and to reduce the potential for ascending infection. Given the absence of data regarding the superiority of either, initial inpatient or outpatient monitoring may be appropriate according to individual clinical circumstances.

c. Serial ultrasound is recommended to evaluate for fetal pulmonary growth and for persistent oligohydramnios. Fetal pulmonary growth can be easily estimated by ultrasound measurement of the thoracic/abdominal circumference ratio or chest circumference. A low thoracic/abdominal circumference ratio in the setting of persistent oligohydramnios is highly predictive of lethal pulmonary hypoplasia after PROM. Other evaluations, such as lung length and 3-D lung volume determinations have similar predictive accuracies. When identified before the limit of viability, the diagnosis of suspected fetal pulmonary hypoplasia may help the patient regarding the decision between continued conservative management and delivery.

d. Women with PROM before 23 weeks gestation have been included in some studies of antibiotic therapy after PROM. Treatment as described above for women at 23–31 weeks is appropriate. However, this population has not been studied separately, and it is not known if treatment is beneficial.

e. Once the pregnancy reaches the limit of viability, many physicians will admit the patient to hospital for ongoing bed rest and continue treatment in a similar manner to that described above for those with PROM at 23–31 weeks of gestation. The purpose of admission at this time is to allow for early diagnosis and intervention for infection, abruption, labor and nonreassuring fetal heart rate patterns. Because these women remain at high risk for early delivery, administration of antenatal corticosteroids for fetal maturation and magnesium for neuroprotection is appropriate. It is unlikely that delayed administration of broad-spectrum antibiotics for pregnancy prolongation at this time will assist this population.

f. Novel treatments for membrane sealing after pre-viable PROM, including serial amnioinfusion, membrane plugging with Gelfoam or fibrin-platelet-cryoprecipitate plugs, and indwelling transcervical infusion catheter have been studied. Further research regarding the maternal and fetal risks and benefits of these interventions is needed before membrane sealing is incorporated in clinical practice.

Special circumstances

Cervical cerclage

When the cervical stitch is removed on admission after preterm PROM, the risk of adverse perinatal outcomes is not higher than for those women with preterm PROM and no cervical stitch in-situ. Studies comparing cervical stitch retention or removal after preterm PROM have suggested trends toward increased maternal infection with retained cervical stitch; however, no individual study has reached statistical significance. Alternatively, no study has found a significant reduction in the infant morbidity with cervical stitch retention subsequent to preterm PROM, and one study found increased neonatal death due to infection with cervical stitch retention. As such, the cervical stitch should generally be removed when PROM occurs. Should the cervical stitch be retained during attempts to enhance fetal benefit with antenatal corticosteroids and magnesium sulfate for neuroprotection, concurrent antibiotic administration should be considered to reduce the risk of infection and it is recommended that the stitch be removed after antenatal steroid and magnesium sulfate benefit have been achieved (24–48 hours).

Herpes simplex virus

A history of herpes simplex virus infection is not a contraindication for expectant management of PROM remote from term. If herpetic lesions are present at the onset of labor, cesarean delivery is indicated. Alternatively, with PROM at 30 weeks or thereafter, the presence of primary or secondary herpetic lesions should lead to consideration of expeditious cesarean delivery.

Human immunodeficiency virus

Intrapartum vertical transmission of HIV increases with increasing duration of membrane rupture. Given the poor prognosis of perinatally acquired HIV infection, expeditious abdominal delivery after PROM at any gestational age after the limit of fetal viability is recommended. Vaginal delivery may be appropriate for women with HIV, if the viral titer is low (see Protocol 30). If conservative management of the patient with PROM at or before the limit of viability is undertaken, multi-agent antiretroviral therapy with serial monitoring of maternal viral load and CD4 counts should be initiated.

Resealing of the membranes

A small number of women with PROM at 23–31 weeks of gestation will experience cessation of leakage with resealing of the membranes. Under this rare circumstance, our general approach is to continue monitoring in hospital for approximately 1 week after cessation of leakage and normalization of the amniotic fluid index to encourage healing of the membrane rupture site. These women are subsequently discharged to modified bed rest and pelvic rest, with frequent reevaluation.

Prevention of recurrent preterm PROM

Women with a history of preterm birth, especially that due to preterm PROM, are at increased risk for recurrent preterm birth due to PROM. Women with a prior preterm birth due to PROM have a 3.3-fold higher risk of recurrence, and a 13.5-fold higher risk of preterm PROM before 28 weeks of gestation. In addition to general guidance regarding adequate nutrition, smoking cessation, avoidance of heavy lifting and prolonged standing without breaks, weekly intramuscular injections with 17-hydroxyprogesterone caproate (250 mg) has been shown to reduce the risk of a recurrence (Meis *et al.*, 2003). Daily vaginal progesterone suppositories (100 mg) have also been shown to prevent preterm birth in high-risk women, but progesterone vaginal gel (90 mg) has not. Though vitamin C deficiency could potentially result in preterm PROM, vitamin C supplementation is not helpful and may be harmful.

Suggested reading

Alexander JM, Mercer BM, Miodovnik M, *et al.* The impact of digital cervical examination on expectantly managed preterm rupture of membranes. *Am J Obstet Gynecol* 2000;183:1003–7.

American College of Obstetricians and Gynecologists. Prevention of early-onset group B streptococcal disease in newborns. Committee Opinion No. 485. *Obstet Gynecol* 2011;117:1019–27.

Belady PH, Farhouh LJ, Gibbs RS. Intra-amniotic infection and premature rupture of the membranes. *Clin Perinatol* 1997;24:43–57.

Casanueva E, Ripoll C, Tolentino M, Morales RM, Pfeffer F, Vilchis P, Vadillo-Ortega F. Vitamin C supplementation to prevent premature rupture of the chorioamniotic membranes: a randomized trial. *Am J Clin Nutr* 2005;81:859–63.

Chen FC, Dudenhausen JW. Comparison of two rapid strip tests based on IGFBP-1 and PAMG-1 for the detection of amniotic fluid. *Am J Perinatol* 2008;25:243–6.

D'Alton M, Mercer B, Riddick E, Dudley D. Serial thoracic versus abdominal circumference ratios for the prediction of pulmonary hypoplasia in premature rupture of the membranes remote from term. *Am J Obstet Gynecol* 1992;166:658–63.

Doyle LW, Crowther CA, Middleton P, Marret S, Rouse D. Magnesium sulphate for women at risk of preterm birth for neuroprotection of the fetus. *Cochrane Database Syst Rev* 2009;1:CD004661.

Eriksen NL, Parisi VM, Daoust S, Flamm B, Garite TJ, Cox SM. Fetal fibronectin: a method for detecting the presence of amniotic fluid. *Obstet Gynecol* 1992;80:451–4.

Hannah ME, Ohlsson A, Farine D, *et al.* Induction of labor compared with expectant management for prelabor rupture of the membranes at term. TERMPROM Study Group. *N Engl J Med* 1996;334:1005–10.

Harger JH, Hsing AW, Tuomala RE, *et al.* Risk factors for preterm premature rupture of fetal membranes: a multicenter case-control study. *Am J Obstet Gynecol* 1990;163:130.

Kenyon SL, Taylor DJ, Tarnow-Mordi W, Oracle Collaborative Group. Broad spectrum antibiotics for preterm, prelabor rupture of fetal membranes: the ORACLE I randomized trial. *Lancet* 2001;357:979–88.

Lee SM, Lee J, Seong HS, Lee SE, Park JS, Romero R, Yoon BH. The clinical significance of a positive Amnisure test in women with term labor with intact membranes. *J Matern Fetal Neonat Med* 2009;22:305–10.

Meis PJ, Klebanoff M, Thom E, Dombrowski MP, Sibai B, Moawad AH, Spong CY, Hauth JC, Miodovnik M, Varner MW, Leveno KJ, Caritis SN, Iams JD, Wapner RJ,

Conway D, O'Sullivan MJ, Carpenter M, Mercer B, Ramin SM, Thorp JM, Peaceman AM, Gabbe S, National Institute of Child Health and Human Development Maternal-Fetal Medicine Units Network. Prevention of recurrent preterm delivery by 17 alpha-hydroxyprogesterone caproate. *N Engl J Med* 2003;348:2379–85.

Mercer BM. Preterm premature rupture of the membranes. *Obstet Gynecol* 2003;101(1):178–93.

Mercer BM, Goldenberg RL, Meis PJ, Moawad AH, Shellhaas C, Das A, Menard MK, Caritis SN, Thurnau GR, Dombrowski MP, Miodovnik M, Roberts JM, McNellis D. and the NICHD-MFMU Network. The preterm prediction study: Prediction of preterm premature rupture of the membranes using clinical findings and ancillary testing. *Am J Obstet Gynecol* 2000;183:738–45.

Mercer B, Miodovnik M, Thurnau G, Goldenberg R, Das A, Merenstein G, Ramsey R, Rabello Y, Thom E, Roberts J, McNellis D, The NICHD-MFMU Network. Antibiotic therapy for reduction of infant morbidity after preterm premature rupture of the membranes: a randomized controlled trial. *JAMA* 1997;278:989–95.

Naeye RL. Factors that predispose to premature rupture of the fetal membranes. *Obstet Gynecol* 1992;60:93.

Roberts D, Dalziel S. Antenatal corticosteroids for accelerating fetal lung maturation for women at risk of preterm birth. *Cochrane Database Syst Rev* 2006;(3):CD004454.

Romero R, Yoon BH, Mazor M, *et al.* A comparative study of the diagnostic performance of amniotic fluid glucose, white blood cell count, interleukin-6, and Gram stain in the detection of microbial invasion in patients with preterm premature rupture of membranes. *Am J Obstet Gynecol* 1993;169:839–51.

Rouse DJ, Hirtz DG, Thom E, Varner MW, Spong CY, Mercer BM, Iams JD, Wapner RJ, Sorokin Y, Alexander JM, Harper M, Thorp JM Jr,, Ramin SM, Malone FD, Carpenter M, Miodovnik M, Moawad A, O'Sullivan MJ, Peaceman AM, Hankins GD, Langer O, Caritis SN, Roberts JM, Eunice Kennedy Shriver NICHD Maternal-Fetal Medicine Units Network. A randomized, controlled trial of magnesium sulfate for the prevention of cerebral palsy. *N Engl J Med* 2008;359:895–905.

Spinnato JA 2nd,, Freire S, Pinto e Silva JL, *et al.* Antioxidant supplementation and premature rupture of the membranes: a planned secondary analysis. *Am J Obstet Gynecol* 2008;199:433.e1–8.

van der Ham DP, Vijgen SM, Nijhuis JG, van Beek JJ, Opmeer BC, Mulder AL, Moonen R, Groenewout M, van Pampus MG, Mantel GD, Bloemenkamp KW, van Wijngaarden WJ, Sikkema M, Haak MC, Pernet PJ, Porath M, Molkenboer JF, Kuppens S, Kwee A, Kars ME, Woiski M, Weinans MJ, Wildschut HI, Akerboom BM, Mol BW, Willekes C, PPROMEXIL trial group. Induction of labor versus expectant management in women with preterm prelabor rupture of membranes between 34 and 37 weeks: a randomized controlled trial. *PLoS Med* 2012;9:e1001208.

PROTOCOL 44

Indicated Late-Preterm and Early-Term Deliveries

Catherine Y. Spong
Bethesda, MD, USA

Clinical significance

Preterm birth is associated with significant short-term and long-term morbidity and mortality with implications beyond the neonatal period. Given that over 70% of preterm infants are born in the late preterm period (34–37 weeks) and the recent work highlighting morbidities and mortality for infants electively born in the early term period, numerous public health efforts have been appropriately undertaken to reduce preterm births emphasizing these groups. However, in certain situations, indicated preterm birth or early term birth will result in the best outcome for mother, baby or both. This protocol outlines a number of these situations, identifying the optimal timing of delivery based on available evidence and expert opinion.

Pathophysiology

The pathophysiology underlying conditions that are indications for an indicated birth before 39 weeks can be loosely grouped into four areas: placenta/uterus, fetal, maternal, and obstetric conditions.

Placental conditions include those that increase the risk of bleeding such as placenta previa, accreta, increta, percreta and those that increase the risk of uterine rupture such as a prior classical cesarean delivery and myomectomy involving the myometrium. Fetal conditions include fetal anomalies, multifetal gestations, fetal growth abnormalities, and oligohydramnios. Maternal conditions include diabetes and hypertension. Obstetric conditions include preterm rupture of membranes and preterm labor.

Protocols for High-Risk Pregnancies: An Evidence-Based Approach, Sixth Edition.
Edited by John T. Queenan, Catherine Y. Spong and Charles J. Lockwood.
© 2015 John Wiley & Sons, Ltd. Published 2015 by John Wiley & Sons, Ltd.

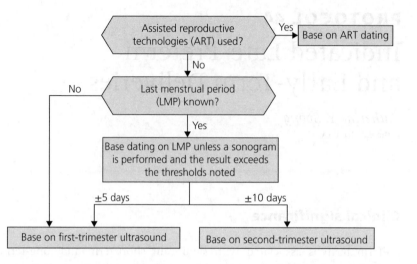

Figure 44.1 Proposed approach for determination of gestational age.   Source: Spong, 2013. Reproduced with permission of American Medical Association.

Diagnosis

When considering early delivery due to any of these indications, there are several important considerations. First and foremost is the accuracy of dating. It is extremely important to have confidence in the dating of the pregnancy when making decisions based on specific days. There are many algorithms for dating. In pregnancies using artificial reproductive technologies, those dates should be used. If not, algorithms based on sonography and last menstrual period, and then confirmed by physical examination or subsequent ultrasounds, are necessary (see Fig. 44.1).

In addition, when early delivery is recommended due to one of these indications in a well-dated pregnancy, amniocentesis for evaluation of fetal lung maturity generally should not be performed to guide the timing of delivery. The timing of delivery is based on balancing the maternal and fetal risks of early delivery with the risks for both of continuing the pregnancy.

Management

When one of these conditions is present it is important to consider what is the optimal timing of delivery for the pregnancy. Based on the available evidence and expert opinion, recommendations for delivery timing were outlined in several publications and are summarized in Table 44.1. These are recommendations, and are based on the anticipation that the problem described is the only one present. However it is important to appreciate that

Table 44.1   Timing of indicated deliveries in the late-preterm and early-term period

Placental/uterine issues	
Placenta previa	36.0–37 6/7 weeks
Placenta previa with suspected accreta/increta/percreta	34.0–35 6/7 weeks
Prior classical (upper uterine segment) cesarean	36.0–37 6/7 weeks
Prior myomectomy (through uterine muscle)	37.0–38 6/7 weeks
Fetal issues	
Fetal growth restriction (singleton): uncomplicated	38.0–39 6/7 weeks
Fetal growth restriction (singleton) with complications	34.0–37 6/7 weeks
Multifetal gestation (dichorionic diamniotic)	38.0–38 6/7 weeks
Multifetal gestation (monochorionic diamniotic)	34.0–37 6/7 weeks
Multifetal gestation (dichorionic diamniotic) + FGR	36.0–37 6/7 weeks
Multifetal gestation (monochorionic diamniotic) + FGR	32.0–34 6/7 weeks
Oligohydramnios	36.0–37 6/7 weeks
Maternal issues	
Chronic hypertension: controlled, no medications	38.0–39 6/7 weeks
Chronic hypertension: controlled, on medications	37.0–39 6/7 weeks
Chronic hypertension: difficult to control	36.0–37 6/7 weeks
Gestational hypertension	37.0–38 6/7 weeks
Severe preeclampsia	At diagnosis (>34.0 weeks)
Mild preeclampsia	At diagnosis (>37.0 weeks)
Diabetes: pregestational with vascular disease	37.0–39 6/7 weeks
Obstetrical issues	
Spontaneous preterm rupture of membranes after 34 weeks	At diagnosis (>34 weeks)
Spontaneous active preterm labor	At diagnosis if progressive labor or additional maternal or fetal indication

Note, all assume the issue is the only one present; if there are superimposed conditions such as fetal growth restriction, oligohydramnios, etc in addition to the issue such as placenta previa, the timing of delivery may need to be altered based on clinical judgment.
FGR, fetal growth restriction.
Source: Adapted from Spong CY, Mercer BM, D'alton M, Kilpatrick S, Blackwell S, Saade G. Timing of indicated late-preterm and early-term birth. Obstet Gynecol. 2011; 118:323–33.

most patients have more than one of these conditions, such as diabetes and fetal growth restriction. In these situations, both should be considered in the decision and the timing may need to be different from what is recommended in the text to optimize outcome.

Complications

Preterm birth is associated with a number of complications and risks for both the mother and the child. For the preterm newborn, risks of early delivery include the gestational age-dependent morbidities of respiratory distress syndrome, intraventricular hemorrhage, necrotizing enterocolitis, hyperbilirubinemia, feeding difficulties and temperature instability. Maternal risks include complications from labor induction, cesarean delivery, hemorrhage, and infection.

Follow up and prevention

For many of these conditions, additional consideration in a subsequent pregnancy will be important. As examples, in the case of prior classical cesarean or myomectomy, these will persist for subsequent pregnancies. Women should be counseled on the implications including the risks of multiple cesareans in this situation. Women with preeclampsia may benefit from low dose aspirin therapy in a subsequent pregnancy to prevent recurrence. If spontaneous preterm labor or premature rupture of the membranes and preterm birth complicated the pregnancy, progesterone supplementation in a subsequent pregnancy should be considered to prevent recurrence. Women with diabetes should be counseled on the importance of glycemic control prior to conception.

Conclusion

Although preterm birth is associated with significant morbidity and mortality, in some specific conditions such as placenta previa and multifetal gestation, preterm birth or early-term birth is optimal for the mother, baby or both, because of maternal and/or fetal risks with continued pregnancy. The timing of these deliveries should be individualized to optimize the outcome based on evidence and expert opinion, as well as the specific clinical situation.

Suggested reading

American College of Obstetricians and Gynecologists. Medically indicated late-preterm and early-term deliveries. Committee Opinion No. 560. *Obstet Gynecol* 2013;121:908–10.

Spong CY. Defining term pregnancy. Recommendations from the defining "term" pregnancy workgroup. *JAMA* 2013;309:2445–6.

Spong CY, Mercer BM, D'alton M, Kilpatrick S, Blackwell S, Saade G. Timing of indicated late-preterm and early-term birth. *Obstet Gynecol* 2011;118:323–33.

Tita AT, Lai Y, Landon MB, Spong CY, Leveno KJ, Varner MW, Caritis SN, Meis PJ, Wapner RJ, Sorokin Y, Peaceman AM, O'Sullivan MJ, Sibai BM, Thorp JM, Ramin SM, Mercer BM, Eunice Kennedy Shriver National Institute of Child Health and Human

Development (NICHD) Maternal-Fetal Medicine Units Network (MFMU). Timing of elective repeat cesarean delivery at term and maternal perioperative outcomes. *Obstet Gynecol* 2011;117:280–6.

Tita AT, Landon MB, Spong CY, Lai Y, Leveno KJ, Varner MW, Moawad AH, Caritis SN, Meis PJ, Wapner RJ, Sorokin Y, Miodovnik M, Carpenter M, Peaceman AM, O'Sullivan MJ, Sibai BM, Langer O, Thorp JM, Ramin SM, Mercer BM, Eunice Kennedy Shriver NICHD Maternal-Fetal Medicine Units Network. Timing of elective repeat cesarean delivery at term and neonatal outcomes. *N Engl J Med* 2009;360:111–20.

Prevention of Cerebral Palsy

Dwight J. Rouse[1, 2]
[1] Maternal-Fetal Medicine Division, Women & Infants Hospital of Rhode Island, Providence, RI, USA
[2] Department of Obstetrics and Gynecology, Warren Alpert School of Medicine at Brown University, Providence, RI, USA

Clinical significance

Cerebral palsy is a related group of disorders characterized by abnormal control of movement or posture that arise due to nonprogressive damage or dysfunction of the developing fetal or infant brain. Cerebral palsy is a leading cause of chronic childhood disability and affects 200,000 American children between the ages of 3 and 13 years. Preterm birth is a major risk factor for cerebral palsy – infants born at the extreme of viability face up to a 50-fold increased risk compared with those born at term. In fact, half of all cerebral palsy is associated with prematurity.

Pathophysiology

The pathophysiology of cerebral palsy is poorly understood. Associated factors include genetic disorders, thrombophilias and maternal infection or fever in the antepartum period. Intrapartum asphyxiating events give rise to a minority of cases. The preterm fetal brain is especially vulnerable to the damaging effects of cytokines and excitatory amino acids that characterize the inflammatory milieu of early spontaneous preterm birth. Approximately half of cerebral palsy cases in preterm infants are presaged by severe neonatal cranial ultrasound abnormalities, e.g., cystic periventricular leukomalacia or grade III or IV intraventricular hemorrhage.

Diagnosis

In its more severe forms, a diagnosis of cerebral palsy can be made in the first year of life. Milder forms of what appears to be cerebral palsy may not

Protocols for High-Risk Pregnancies: An Evidence-Based Approach, Sixth Edition.
Edited by John T. Queenan, Catherine Y. Spong and Charles J. Lockwood.
© 2015 John Wiley & Sons, Ltd. Published 2015 by John Wiley & Sons, Ltd.

persist, and thus a definitive diagnosis should be delayed until the age of at least 2 years.

Cerebral palsy should be diagnosed on the basis of the following three factors by a clinician trained and experienced in the diagnosis: (1) minimum 30% delay in gross motor developmental milestones; (2) abnormalities in muscle tone such as scissoring, 4+ or absent deep tendon reflexes, or movement abnormality such as posturing or gait asymmetry; and (3) persistence of primitive, or absence of protective, reflexes. Findings in at least two of these three categories must be present. When cerebral palsy is diagnosed, the Gross Motor Function Classification Scale can be used to assess its severity.

Prevention

That magnesium sulfate ($MgSO_4$) administered to mothers delivering prematurely could prevent cerebral palsy in their offspring was first suggested by a case–control study performed by Karin Nelson and Judy Grether.

Since the report of Nelson and Grether, three large, randomized placebo-controlled trials of antenatal $MgSO_4$ for fetal neuroprotection have been conducted and reported. Alone and in combination, the results of these trials support the use of $MgSO_4$ to lower the risk of cerebral palsy among the survivors of early preterm birth. The three trials used differing treatment regimens: 6 gm loading dose of $MgSO_4$ followed by 2 g/hour (Table 45.1), 4 g loading dose followed by 1 g/hour (Crowther) or simply a 4 g loading dose (Marret).

These three trials and two more have been incorporated into a Cochrane Systematic Review. $MgSO_4$ was associated with a significant reduction in cerebral palsy (RR 0.68, 95% CI 0.54–0.87) without an effect on fetal or infant mortality (RR 1.04, 95% CI 0.92–1.17). In four trials (4446 children) neuroprotection was the specific outcome. In these trials, not only was $MgSO_4$ associated with a reduction in cerebral palsy, but also with a reduction in the combined outcome of cerebral palsy or fetal/infant death (RR 0.85, 95% CI 0.74–0.98).

Gibbins and colleagues reported their hospital's experience with the implementation of a $MgSO_4$ protocol for neuroprotection. Uptake was rapid, a high percentage of eligible women were treated, and there were no maternal or perinatal complications attributed to the protocol.

The number needed to treat with $MgSO_4$ to prevent cerebral palsy is in line with the current use of $MgSO_4$ for the prevention of eclamptic convulsions: treating 63 women threatening to deliver prior to 32 weeks of gestation will prevent one case of moderate or severe cerebral palsy. In contrast, approximately 100 women with preeclampsia need to be treated to

Table 45.1   Protocol: magnesium sulfate ($MgSO_4$) for the prevention of cerebral palsy

---

Eligible candidates
Gestational age: 24–31 weeks
At risk of immediate delivery
Preterm premature rupture of membranes
Advanced preterm labor (cervix 4 cm or more)
Indicated (severe fetal growth restriction)

Magnesium administration
Initial therapy
6 g intravenous load over 20–30 minutes
2 g/hour constant infusion until delivery
If delivery not imminent, infusion discontinued
Retreatment
When delivery again threatens prior to 34 weeks*
If less than 6 hours from discontinuation, no $MgSO_4$ bolus
Monitor
Deep tendon reflexes
Urine output
Serum Mg^{++} concentrations (e.g., renal dysfunction)

---

*For pragmatic reasons, the practice at many institutions, including Women and Infants Hospital of Rhode Island, is to not retreat after 31 weeks, 6 days of gestation.
Source: Rouse *et al.*, 2008. Reproduced with permission of the Massachusetts Medical Society.

prevent one eclamptic convulsion. If treatment were limited to 28 weeks of gestation or below, the NINDS/NICHD MFMU Network trial suggests that treating only 29 women would prevent one case of moderate or severe cerebral palsy.

Complications

Although $MgSO_4$ has a high margin of safety, and was associated with no life-threatening events in the over 3000 maternal exposures in the Cochrane review, it should be utilized only with close monitoring of maternal reflexes (neuromuscular depression occurs at Mg^{++} concentrations of 10 mEq/L and above) and urine output (Mg^{++} is renally excreted). The administration of $MgSO_4$ in the face of renal dysfunction requires especial vigilance. Suspicion of significant hypermagnesiumenia should be evaluated by measurement of serum Mg^{++} concentration and in many cases by discontinuation of the $MgSO_4$ infusion. Frank respiratory depression (and the even rarer cardiopulmonary arrest) is treated by administration of 1 g of intravenous calcium gluconate, discontinuation of the $MgSO_4$ infusion, and ventilatory support as necessary. To facilitate the safe use of $MgSO_4$ for fetal neuroprotection, the American College of Obstetricians and Gynecologists have developed a patient safety checklist.

Conclusion

Antenatal $MgSO_4$ offers an opportunity to improve the neurodevelopmental prognosis of fetuses destined to deliver at early gestational ages. In the United States, 2% of women deliver prior to 32 weeks of gestation. If they all received $MgSO_4$ for fetal neuroprotection, over 1000 children a year in the United States alone could be spared from handicapping cerebral palsy.

Suggested reading

American College of Obstetricians and Gynecologists. Magnesium sulfate before anticipated preterm birth for neuroprotection. Patient Safety Checklist No. 7. *Obstet Gynecol* 2012;120:432–3.

Crowther CA, Hiller JE, Doyle LW, Haslam RR. Effect of magnesium sulfate given for neuroprotection before preterm birth: a randomized controlled trial. *JAMA* 2003;290:2669–76.

Doyle LW, Crowther CA, Middleton P, Marret S, Rouse D. Magnesium sulphate for women at risk of preterm birth for neuroprotection of the fetus. *Cochrane Database Syst Rev* 2009;1:CD004661. DOI: 10.1002/14651858.CD004661.pub3.

Gibbins KJ, Browning KR, Lopes VV, Anderson BL, Rouse DJ. Evaluation of the clinical use of magnesium sulphate for cerebral palsy prevention. *Obstet Gynecol* 2013;121:235–40.

Hirtz DG, Nelson KN. Magnesium sulfate and cerebral palsy in premature infants. *Curr Opin Pediatr* 1998;10:131–7.

Lucas MJ, Leveno KJ, Cunningham FG. A comparison of magnesium sulfate with phenytoin for the prevention of eclampsia. *N Engl J Med* 1995;333:201–5.

Marret S, Maroeau L, Follet-Bouhamed C, *et al.* Effect of magnesium sulphate on mortality and neurologic morbidity of the very preterm newborn with two-year neurological outcome: results of the prospective PREAMAG trial. *Gynecologie Obstetrique & Fertilite* 2008;36:278–88.

Nelson KB, Grether JK. Can magnesium sulfate reduce the risk of cerebral palsy in very low birthweight infants? *Pediatrics* 1995;95:263–9.

Rouse DJ, Hirtz DG, Thom E, *et al.* A randomized, controlled trial of magnesium sulfate for the prevention of cerebral palsy. *N Engl J Med* 2008;359:895–905.

PROTOCOL 46

Amnionitis

George A. Macones

Department of Obstetrics & Gynecology, Washington University School of Medicine, St Louis, MO, USA

Overview

Amnionitis (chorioamnionitis, intraamniotic infection) is common, occurring in 1–5% of term deliveries and up to 25% of preterm deliveries. Amnionitis may be a causative factor in preterm births due to preterm labor or preterm premature rupture of membranes (PPROM).

Depending on the type and severity of the infection as well as the gestational age at which it occurs, amnionitis may lead to a variety of outcomes including spontaneous abortion, stillbirth, prematurity (and the various complications that might result from prematurity), neonatal sepsis, cerebral palsy, infectious maternal morbidity and even sepsis and shock.

Pathophysiology

It is believed that amnionitis results from an ascending infection from the lower genital tract into the amniotic cavity, although hematogenous and transplacental etiologies have also been proposed. In the early stages of an ascending bacterial invasion of the choriodecidual interface, there may be no maternal symptomatology (subclinical intrauterine infection). However, as the infection ascends and continues, clinical manifestations may become apparent.

Amnionitis is a polymicrobial infection and most commonly involves bacteria that are part of the normal vaginal flora. These bacteria include: *Bacteroides* (25%), *Gardnerella* (25%), *streptococcus* species (25%), *E. coli* and other gram-negative rods (20%) and mycoplasmas.

In term patients, amnionitis seems to occur more as a consequence of multiple risk factors such as prolonged rupture of membranes or multiple vaginal examinations. However, in preterm patients it is believed that

Protocols for High-Risk Pregnancies: An Evidence-Based Approach, Sixth Edition.
Edited by John T. Queenan, Catherine Y. Spong and Charles J. Lockwood.
© 2015 John Wiley & Sons, Ltd. Published 2015 by John Wiley & Sons, Ltd.

amnionitis might incite preterm labor or PPROM. There are multiple hypotheses regarding how amnionitis may trigger PPROM or premature labor. One theory is that the infection may trigger prostaglandin synthesis and release from amniotic membranes, which may lead to preterm labor or PPROM. A second hypothesis is that there is bacterial lipopolysaccharide (endotoxin) release causing release of cytokines (IL-1, IL-6, tumor necrosis factor, etc.) which then increase the production of collagenases and matrix metalloproteinases (which can lead to membrane weakening and PPROM).

Risk factors

Many factors have been associated with amnionitis. Established risk factors include long labor, nulliparity, low socioeconomic status, multiple vaginal examinations, internal fetal monitoring, length of internal monitoring and maternal bacterial vaginosis infection as well as other lower-genital tract infections such as *Chlamydia trachomatis, Neisseria gonorrheae,* and *Ureoplasma urealyticum*. Other associated risk factors are cigarette smoking and history of prior preterm delivery or PPROM.

Clinical presentation

There are two main categories of patients in which amnionitis should be suspected.

1 Term pregnancies, in which there are clinical symptoms suggestive of infection. In this scenario, amnionitis is defined as: maternal fever (greater than 100.4°F or 38°C) and one of the following additional findings:

   a. maternal tachycardia (greater than 100 beats/minute)

   b. fetal tachycardia (greater than 160 beats/minute)

   c. uterine tenderness

   d. leukocytosis (greater than 18,000 white blood cell (WBC) count)

   e. foul-smelling vaginal discharge.

Other conditions in the differential diagnosis include pyelonephritis or urinary tract infection, appendicitis, viral illnesses and respiratory infections.

2 Patients presenting with preterm labor or PPROM.

Some patients who present with preterm labor or PPROM may also have clinical symptoms that strongly suggest amnionitis (same criteria as above). In subjects with preterm labor or PPROM who do not exhibit any of these classic signs or symptoms, physicians must still be concerned about a subclinical intrauterine infection. For women in preterm labor, amnionitis is common in those who are failing first-line tocolytic therapy.

Diagnosis and management

1 In patients at term, amnionitis is primarily a clinical diagnosis: maternal fever with one of the following additional signs: maternal tachycardia, fetal tachycardia, uterine tenderness, leukocytosis, or foul-smelling vaginal discharge.
   a. Delivery is indicated when the diagnosis of amnionitis is made at term in order to minimize infectious morbidity to both the mother and fetus.
   b. If fetal heart monitoring is reassuring, labor should be induced and an attempt should be made at a vaginal delivery.
   c. If a nonreassuring fetal heart rate pattern is detected, a cesarean delivery should be performed (note that indications for cesarean delivery are standard obstetrical indications. Amnionitis in itself is not an indication for cesarean delivery).
   d. Once the diagnosis of amnionitis is made, broad-spectrum antibiotics should be started immediately (i.e., ampicillin 2 g IV every 6 hours and gentamicin 1.5 mg/kg every 8 hours, or other broad-spectrum regimens).

2 Patients who present with PPROM or preterm labor should be considered at high risk for having amnionitis. Overall, the management of patients with PPROM or preterm labor depends on gestational age at presentation and the presence or absence of clinical symptoms.
   a. *Preterm labor/PPROM with symptoms of amnionitis*
      • Once diagnosis of chorioamnionitis is made, delivery is indicated regardless of gestational age.
      • Broad-spectrum antibiotics should be utilized.
      • Vaginal delivery is preferred, with cesarean reserved for standard obstetrical indications.
   b. *Preterm labor/PPROM without clinical symptoms*
      • This group is at risk of having amnionitis of chorioamnionitis.
      • Monitor closely for maternal symptoms (fever, uterine tenderness) or fetal symptoms (tachycardia, nonreactive nonstress test) of infection.
      • Consider amniocentesis for diagnosis if vague/unclear clinical symptoms.
      • If an amniocentesis is needed, send the transabdominally obtained fluid for culture (aerobic, anaerobic) and for the following tests: Gram stain, glucose concentration, and WBC count. In some

Table 46.1   Abnormal results in diagnosing amnionitis

Amniotic fluid glucose: less than 15 mg/dL

Amniotic fluid WBC: greater than 30 cells/mL

Amniotic fluid IL-6: 7.9 ng/mL or higher

Amniotic fluid leukocyte esterase: 1 or
   higher; positive reaction

Amniotic fluid Gram stain: any organism on
   an oil immersion field

Amniotic fluid: any positive growth of an
   aerobic or anaerobic microorganism

institutions, IL-6 and leukocyte esterase may also be obtained. The gold standard for diagnosis is a positive amniotic fluid culture. Delivery should be strongly considered if bacteria are seen on Gram stain or if the amniotic fluid culture is positive.

   If any of the other parameters listed in Table 46.1 are abnormal, the entire clinical picture should be taken into account and delivery should not be pursued based on a single abnormal value.

- If amnionitis is diagnosed via amniocentesis results or based on high level of clinical suspicion, broad-spectrum antibiotics should be initiated and a move toward delivery should be undertaken.

3 Patients who present with fever without a clear source. These cases can be challenging to manage. Take care to entertain a wide differential diagnosis of which amnionitis should be considered. Other diagnoses include pyelonephritis, appendicitis, gastroenteritis, etc. The other clinical manifestations will help to distinguish between these diagnoses. If the diagnosis is uncertain, an amniocentesis may be appropriate to rule out amnionitis since the presence of an intrauterine infection would warrant delivery.

Table 46.1 contains laboratory values used in diagnosing amnionitis.

Treatment

Once the diagnosis of amnionitis is made either clinically or by amniocentesis, preparations for delivery should be undertaken. Additionally, given that amnionitis is polymicrobial in nature, broad-spectrum antibiotics should be initiated. The most common recommended regimen is ampicillin 2 g every 6 hours and gentamicin 1.5 mg/kg every 8 hours although other regimens that offer similar coverage may be utilized. If the patient undergoes a cesarean delivery, clindamycin may be added. Further, antibiotics should be used after cesarean delivery until the patient has been afebrile for 24–48 hours.

Complications

In patients with amnionitis, an increased cesarean delivery rate (30–40%) is seen, mostly secondary to arrest disorders. Patients with amnionitis are also at increased risk of postpartum hemorrhage, endometritis and post cesarean delivery wound infection.

Prevention

Several risk factors have been identified for amnionitis and care should be taken to avoid these when possible. These include extended duration of labor, prolonged rupture of membranes (more than 18 hours), multiple vaginal examinations and internal monitoring. Other risk factors associated with amnionitis that are not preventable include young maternal age, low socioeconomic status and nulliparity.

Additionally, some infection control measures have been evaluated such as chlorhexidine vaginal washes, and have been found to be ineffective in preventing amnionitis. Antepartum treatment of bacterial vaginosis has also not been shown to prevent amnionitis. The effective preventive strategies that have been proven to decrease the incidence of amnionitis are active labor management, induction of labor after PROM at term and the use of antibiotics in selected patients.

Conclusion

The diagnosis of amnionitis is typically clinical and based upon the presence of maternal fever (greater than 100.4°F or 38°C) and one of the following additional criteria: maternal tachycardia (greater than 100 beats/minute), fetal tachycardia (greater than 160 beats/minute), uterine tenderness, leukocytosis (greater than 18,000 WBC count) or foul-smelling vaginal discharge.

Amniocentesis for amniotic fluid culture is the best diagnostic test for subclinical amnionitis or in uncertain clinical presentations.

Maternal complications include bacteremia, labor abnormalities (mainly arrest disorders), and hemorrhage. In addition, cesarean delivery in the presence of amnionitis increases risk of hemorrhage and wound infection.

Amnionitis has been linked to long-term neurodevelopmental delay and cerebral palsy in children. Continuous intrapartum fetal monitoring is recommended for cases of amnionitis in order to observe evidence of fetal compromise.

Immediate delivery has not been shown to improve outcome in cases of amnionitis where there is reassuring intrapartum testing and antibiotic administration. However, the true cure for amnionitis is delivery, so induction should be expeditious and cesarean delivery should be performed for standard obstetric indications. Amnionitis in itself is not an indication for cesarean delivery.

Amnionitis is polymicrobial in nature. Broad-spectrum antibiotics should be initiated once the diagnosis is made to minimize maternal and neonatal morbidity. Antibiotics are recommended postpartum after a cesarean delivery until the patient has been afebrile for 24 hours.

Suggested reading

Creasy RK, Resnick R, Iams JD, editors. *Creasy & Resnik's Maternal-Fetal Medicine: Principles and Practice*. 6th ed. Philadelphia: Saunders Elsevier; 2009.

Gibbs RS, Duff P. Progress in pathogenesis and management of clinical intra-amniotic infection. *Am J Obstet Gynecol* 1991;164:1317.

Newton ER. Preterm labor, preterm premature rupture of membranes, and chorioamnionitis. *Clin Perinatol* 2005;32:571–600.

Romero R, Espinoza J, Goncalves LF, Kusanovic JP, Friel L, Hassan S. The role of inflammation and infection in preterm birth. *Semin Reprod Med* 2007;25:21–39.

Romero R, Sirtori M, Oyarzun E, *et al*. Infection and Labor V. Prevalence, microbiology and clinical significance of intra-amniotic infection in women with preterm labor and intact membranes. *Am J Obstet Gynecol* 1989;161:817.

Yoon BH, Romero R, Moon JB, *et al*. Clinical significance of intra-amniotic inflammation in patients with preterm labor and intact membranes. *Am J Obstet Gynecol* 2001;185:1130–6.

PROTOCOL 47
Third Trimester Bleeding

Yinka Oyelese
Atlantic Health System, Morristown, NJ, USA

Third trimester bleeding complicates approximately 3% of pregnancies. Bleeding can be associated with major perinatal and maternal morbidity and mortality. Bleeding in the third trimester warrants prompt and thorough evaluation and management.

Pathophysiology

In about one-half of cases of third trimester bleeding, especially that of a minor degree, no etiology is found. It is assumed that the majority of these result from small separations of the placental edge. However, the two most common identifiable causes of significant vaginal bleeding in the third trimester are placental abruption, which refers to premature separation of the normally implanted placenta before delivery of the baby, and placenta previa, where the placenta is implanted over the cervix or in close proximity to it. In the former condition, the fetus is in jeopardy, and there is potential for severe maternal hemorrhage, while in the latter, bleeding during labor is inevitable, and if untreated, often becomes life-threatening to the mother. Another cause of bleeding is from the rupture of exposed fetal vessels, known as vasa previa, where fetal vessels are in the membranes over the cervix, unsupported by placental tissue or umbilical cord. This may result in fetal shock or death. Third trimester bleeding may also be caused by the cervical changes associated with preterm labor, infections of the lower genital tract, trauma, foreign bodies, and neoplasms. Much less frequently, the urinary tract or lower gastrointestinal tract may be the source of bleeding that may be mistaken for vaginal bleeding.

Placenta previa refers to a placenta that is abnormally located in the lower uterine segment, either overlying or in close proximity to the internal os.

Protocols for High-Risk Pregnancies: An Evidence-Based Approach, Sixth Edition.
Edited by John T. Queenan, Catherine Y. Spong and Charles J. Lockwood.
© 2015 John Wiley & Sons, Ltd. Published 2015 by John Wiley & Sons, Ltd.

It complicates approximately 1 in 250 pregnancies. When labor starts, and the cervix dilates, placental separation occurs, resulting in heavy bleeding. Consequently, these patients usually require cesarean delivery. Lesser degrees of placental separation occur with development of the lower uterine segment in the early third trimester, leading to painless bleeding, which is usually self-limiting. It has been observed that over 90% of cases of placenta previa diagnosed by ultrasonography in the second trimester will resolve prior to term. This is because of the development of the lower uterine segment with advancing gestation, leading to the placenta appearing to move away from the cervix.

The main risk factor for placenta previa is prior cesarean delivery. Other risk factors include any surgery that disrupts the endometrial lining, such as myomectomy or curettage of the uterine cavity. Smoking, multiparity, multifetal pregnancies, maternal age, and cocaine use have also been shown to be associated with increased risk of placenta previa. Patients who have a placenta previa and a prior cesarean are at increased risk of placenta accreta, a condition in which the placenta abnormally adheres to the myometrium or actually invades it. In placenta accreta, it is not possible to separate the placenta at delivery, and these women typically suffer massive postpartum hemorrhage. More recent data suggest that placenta accreta can result from implantation of the embryo in a cesarean scar. Thus, it is thought that placenta accreta may start off as a cesarean scar pregnancy which then grows into the fundus of the uterus. Hence, it is likely that rather than the placenta invading the myometrium as the pregnancy progresses, it was implanted in the myometrium. The risk of placenta accreta increases with the number of prior cesareans. The risk may be as high as 67% with three prior cesareans if there is also a placenta previa.

Placental abruption refers to placental separation before the birth of the baby. Abruption may be revealed, when blood escapes through the cervix into the vagina, or concealed, with blood accumulating behind the placenta, with no obvious vaginal bleeding. The effects of abruption depend on the degree of placental separation, and the gestational age at which it occurs. The vast majority of abruptions involve only small degrees of placental separation and have few clinical consequences. However, abruption, even in minor cases, carries an increased risk of preterm labor and birth, preterm premature rupture of the membranes, intrauterine growth restriction, perinatal death, and other adverse perinatal outcomes. Thus, all cases of suspected abruption must be taken seriously. When over 50% of the placenta separates, fetal death often results. Placental abruption may result from acute events such as direct or indirect abdominal trauma and cocaine use. It may also be associated with longstanding pathological processes such as hypertension, intrauterine growth restriction, and placental dysfunction. Risk factors for abruption include smoking, trauma, hypertension and preeclampsia, cocaine use, intrauterine infection, oligohydramnios and preterm premature rupture of the membranes. The rapid uterine decompression that occurs when the membranes rupture in patients with polyhydramnios may also lead to abruption. Patients with abruption may present in shock that is out of proportion to the apparent blood loss, especially when the abruption is concealed. Similarly, concealed abruption may be associated with disseminated intravascular coagulopathy, especially when fetal death occurs. There is consumption of coagulation factors and fibrinogen, with resultant failure of coagulation.

Vasa previa refers to exposed fetal vessels running over the cervix and under the presenting part. In this condition, the umbilical cord inserts into the membranes rather than into the placenta. These vessels are unsupported by umbilical cord or placental tissue and can rupture when the membranes rupture, resulting in fetal hemorrhage, exsanguination, and, in the majority of cases, death. Unfortunately, fetal death is not uncommon due to the condition not being recognized before the membranes rupture. Risk factors include a second trimester low-lying placenta (even when the low-lying placenta has apparently resolved by the time of birth), multifetal gestations, pregnancies with bilobed placentas and those resulting from in vitro fertilization. Vasa previa can be diagnosed prenatally with ultrasonography and color Doppler. A high index of suspicion is crucial to making the diagnosis. Prenatal diagnosis and cesarean delivery prior to rupture of the membranes are essential to achieving good perinatal outcomes. In the absence of prenatal diagnosis, perinatal mortality exceeds 50%.

Diagnosis

The main differential diagnosis in third trimester bleeding is between placenta previa and placental abruption. A carefully taken history is essential, and will generally help distinguish between the two. If an ultrasound was previously performed, it is likely that if there was a placenta previa, it would have been noted and the patient may be aware of such a history. History of recent intercourse, trauma, drug use or hypertension may aid in the diagnosis. Generally, the bleeding associated with placenta previa is painless, while pain frequently occurs with placental abruption. However, there are exceptions to this rule. Placenta previa may be associated with painful contractions in cases in which there is preterm labor. Conversely, abruption may be painless. In fact, when abruption occurs with a posterior placenta, backache may be the only symptom. In any patient who presents with third trimester bleeding, an ultrasound should be performed to evaluate for placenta previa before a digital vaginal examination, since a digital examination in the presence of placenta previa may result in torrential hemorrhage. When the lower uterine segment and the lower placental edge cannot be adequately visualized by transabdominal sonography (TAS), transvaginal sonography (TVS) should be performed. TVS is more accurate for diagnosing placenta previa than TAS, and is safe, not associated with increased bleeding, and is well tolerated. Recent guidelines recommend using the term "placenta previa" to describe any placenta that covers the internal os to any degree, and using the term "low-lying placenta" to describe a placenta that lies within 2 cm of the internal os. The uterus is generally soft and nontender to palpation in cases of bleeding with placenta previa, and the absence of pain and tenderness suggests a placenta previa.

The diagnosis of placental abruption is clinical, and based on a high index of suspicion, as well as recognition of the symptoms and signs associated with abruption – typically abdominal pain, uterine contractions, uterine tenderness, and occasionally an abnormal fetal heart rate tracing or fetal death. The uterus may feel hard on palpation and have a "woody" feel in cases of severe abruption. Fetal heart rate monitoring in abruption may reveal variable or late decelerations, bradycardia, reduced variability, or a sinusoidal pattern. Tocography typically shows high frequency, low-amplitude contractions. Sonography is of limited utility in the diagnosis of placental abruption. In cases of acute revealed abruption, blood frequently does not have time to accumulate behind the placenta. Thus the absence of any sonographic findings does not rule out placental abruption. However, when sonographic evidence of abruption is seen, it virtually confirms the diagnosis. Findings of retroplacental hematoma, free clot floating in the amniotic cavity, a thickened heterogenous placenta, or a subchorionic hematoma all have a good positive predictive value for abruption, especially when there is a history suggestive of abruption.

In patients with placenta previa and prior cesareans, a high index of suspicion for placenta accreta is essential. Perhaps the most reliable sonographic sign of placenta accreta is the presence of large vascular lacunae in the placenta in the lower uterine segment, giving a "moth-eaten" appearance.

When there is third trimester vaginal bleeding, it is important to attempt to rule out vasa previa. If possible, sonographic examination of the region over the cervix with color Doppler should be performed in order to rule out a vasa previa. Recent guidelines have recommended that all patients who have a second trimester placenta previa or low-lying placenta should have an evaluation in the third trimester to rule out vasa previa, since most cases occur in patients with "resolved" placenta previa. Fetal vessels may have the appearance of linear echolucent structures on gray-scale sonography. Pulsed Doppler may reveal a fetal vessel waveform. In cases in which the fetal vessels have ruptured, fetal heart rate abnormalities such as a sinusoidal pattern, fetal heart rate decelerations, or bradycardia may occur.

Tests for fetal blood in the vaginal blood such as the Apt test were previously used to rule out a ruptured vasa previa, but are no longer in wide use.

When placenta previa and abruption have been ruled out, a speculum examination should be performed. This may reveal other causes of bleeding such as vaginal infections, cervical ectropion, lacerations of the vagina or cervix (that may occasionally follow intercourse), foreign bodies, polyps, or more rarely, neoplasms of the lower genital tract.

Management

The management of women who present with third trimester bleeding depends on the gestational age, the suspected cause and degree of bleeding and the stability of the mother and fetus. In all cases, the first step is evaluation and stabilization of the mother and fetus. However, in cases with heavy bleeding resulting in maternal or fetal compromise, regardless of the cause, expeditious delivery, usually by cesarean, with simultaneous maternal resuscitation is warranted. Similarly, a suspicion of a ruptured vasa previa should lead to immediate cesarean delivery.

Intravenous access with wide-bore catheters should be established. Blood should be assessed for complete blood count, type and screen. In cases of abruption, coagulation studies should be performed. Blood may be taken in a tube without anticoagulant and inverted every few minutes. Failure to clot within 10 minutes suggests coagulopathy. In cases of placenta previa, when there is coagulopathy, or when blood loss is in excess of 500 mL, blood should be cross-matched. Restoration of intravascular volume should be performed promptly. This may initially be with crystalloid, however cases with significant blood loss should have blood replacement as required. Coagulopathy should be corrected. This is typically done using fresh frozen plasma, although cryoprecipitate may be used.

The fetus should be monitored continuously until it is clear that the fetal status is both stable and reassuring. If the fetus is stable and the gestational age is less than 34 weeks, antenatal corticosteroids should be considered to promote fetal lung maturation. Rh immune globulin should be administered to women who are Rh-negative. Generally, any significant bleeding after 37 weeks warrants delivery. Delivery should be by the safest route for mother and fetus. In cases of placenta previa where the placental edge covers or lies within 1 cm of the internal os, delivery should be by cesarean. When the placental edge is more than 1 cm from the internal os, vaginal birth is considered safe as long as there are no other contraindications. Women with placenta previa who have active bleeding after 34 weeks should be delivered promptly by cesarean. In those cases where there is no bleeding, elective cesarean delivery at 37 weeks is recommended.

This will allow the patient to be delivered in a controlled situation, rather than as an emergency if severe bleeding were to occur. However, it must be emphasized that these pregnancies should be managed on a case-by-case basis.

When placenta previa presents with bleeding in the third trimester prior to 34 weeks, the patient should be admitted for at least 48 hours. If bleeding continues, the patient should remain in hospital. However, if she has not bled for 48 hours, consideration may be given to management as an outpatient provided the patient is reliable, and has good and quick access to the hospital. Women who have low-lying placentas who have a vaginal delivery are still at risk of postpartum hemorrhage since the lower uterine segment is noncontractile.

In cases of minor abruption at term where the fetus and mother are stable, the mother may be allowed to labor as long as both mother and fetus are monitored, and emergent cesarean can be performed quickly. In cases of fetal compromise, cesarean is the safest option for the fetus. When fetal death has occurred, the patient is often in advanced labor, and if labor progresses rapidly, and the mother is stable, a vaginal delivery is desirable. Coagulopathy is a particular problem, and the patient should be monitored for evidence of impaired clotting, and clotting factors should be replaced aggressively.

In cases of abruption prior to 34 weeks, if the mother and fetus are both stable, conservative management in hospital may help achieve an increased gestational age at delivery. However, these pregnancies should be monitored closely, since there is a significant risk of sudden worsening abruption with fetal death. Only in cases in which the fetus and mother have been shown to be stable on prolonged monitoring, and in which there is no bleeding, should outpatient management be considered. Tocolytics may be used with extreme caution in women with abruption who are stable and experiencing uterine contractions, since inhibiting contractions may prevent further abruption and bleeding. In addition, women with suspected abruption between 24 and 34 weeks of gestation should receive corticosteroids to promote fetal lung maturation.

Vasa previa carries a risk of rupture of the exposed vessels when the membranes rupture. Therefore, these cases should be delivered by elective cesarean at 35–36 weeks, or earlier should bleeding, evidence of a non-reassuring fetal heart rate tracing, labor or rupture of the membranes occur. In patients known to have a vasa previa, consideration should be given to hospital admission at about 32 weeks to provide rapid access to the operating room should the membranes rupture. However, in carefully selected cases in which the cervix is long and closed on transvaginal ultrasound, with no symptoms of contractions, and with a negative fetal fibronectin, consideration may be given to outpatient management. If not previously administered, steroids should be given at about 32 weeks to promote fetal lung maturation since these pregnancies are at risk for preterm birth. It is important to deliver these pregnancies in centers with adequate neonatal care.

The risk of placenta accreta is high in women who have both a placenta previa and a prior cesarean delivery and increases with the number of prior cesareans. There is evidence that outcomes with placenta accreta are optimized when the condition is diagnosed prenatally, and delivery occurs in a scheduled manner, and delivery management is by a multidisciplinary approach, involving specialties such as anesthesiology, neonatology, blood bank, urology, maternal fetal medicine, interventional radiology and gynecologic oncology.

Complications

Perhaps the most important complication of third trimester bleeding is hypovolemic shock, which may be severe and life-threatening. There may be severe morbidity or even death of the fetus or the mother. Disseminated intravascular coagulopathy may occur in abruption, and sometimes with placenta previa when there has been massive blood loss with volume replacement deficient in coagulation factors. Hypovolemia may result in renal failure. Abruption may also be associated with acute renal cortical necrosis. Sheehan syndrome or postpartum pituitary infarction is rarely seen in the Western world, but may result from severe hemorrhage. Finally, the patient is at risk from anesthetic and surgical complications. However, the majority of these complications are preventable by accurate prenatal diagnosis and prompt appropriate management.

Conclusion

Bleeding in the third trimester is often a serious complication of pregnancy that carries a significant risk of perinatal death and severe maternal morbidity. It should always be treated seriously and with a high index of suspicion. Careful evaluation should be performed; ultrasonography is an important tool to assist in the diagnosis. Accurate diagnosis and appropriate treatment will optimize outcomes for mother and fetus in most cases.

Suggested reading

Bhide A, Thalinganathan B. Recent advances in the management of placenta previa. *Curr Opin Obstet Gynecol* 2004;16:447–51.

Comstock CH, Bronsteen RA. The antenatal diagnosis of placenta accreta. *BJOG* 2014;121:171–182.

Oyelese Y, Ananth CV. Placental abruption. *Obstet Gynecol* 2006;108(4):1005–16.

Oyelese Y, Smulian JC. Placenta previa, placenta accreta, and vasa previa. *Obstet Gynecol* 2006;107(4):927–41.

Reddy UM, Abuhamad AZ, Levine D. Saade G for the Fetal Imaging Workshop Invited Participants. Fetal imaging: Executive summary of a Joint Eunice Kennedy Shriver National Institute of Child Health and Human Development, Society for Maternal-Fetal Medicine, American Institute of Ultrasound in Medicine, American College of Obstetricians and Gynecologists, American College of Radiology, Society for Pediatric Radiology, and Society of Radiologists in Ultrasound Fetal Imaging Workshop. *Am J Obstet Gynecol* 2014;210:387–397.

PROTOCOL 48

Amniotic Fluid Embolus

Robert Resnik
Department of Reproductive Medicine, UCSD School of Medicine, La Jolla, CA, USA

Since the entity was first described by Meyer, amniotic fluid embolism (AFE) has come to be recognized as a dramatic and dire event. Although rare, with an incidence of approximately 1:40,000 live births, it remains a significant cause of maternal mortality. Accurate figures are difficult to obtain due to varying reporting methods and accuracy of diagnosis. The clinical presentation is that of a term or near-term patient, more frequently multiparous, in whom the sudden onset of dyspnea, loss of consciousness and cardiorespiratory arrest develops during labor, delivery or in the first few hours postpartum. Early publications suggested a mortality rate of 50% or higher, but more recent studies report lower death rates, ranging from 21% to 30%. This is likely due to more rapid recognition and aggressive cardiopulmonary support. Among those who survive the acute event, left ventricular failure may develop in a clinical picture consistent with adult respiratory distress syndrome as well as disseminated intravascular coagulation.

Pathophysiology

The pathophysiology of AFE remains elusive. However, data from Romero et al would suggest it is the consequence of activation of inflammatory mediators similar to the systemic inflammatory response syndrome. This results initially in pulmonary and systemic hypertension, followed by a profound decrease in left ventricular function and alterations in ventilation-perfusion. Data obtained by Clark et al from patients presumed to have AFE, monitored with pulmonary artery catheters, reveal a severe reduction in left ventricular systolic work index and secondary increase in pulmonary wedge and diastolic pressures. This is followed by a coagulopathy. Information collected from the National AFE Registry suggests that the syndrome is similar to anaphylaxis and septic shock, conditions although the triggering event is only speculative.

Protocols for High-Risk Pregnancies: An Evidence-Based Approach, Sixth Edition.
Edited by John T. Queenan, Catherine Y. Spong and Charles J. Lockwood.
© 2015 John Wiley & Sons, Ltd. Published 2015 by John Wiley & Sons, Ltd.

Management

Given this clinical picture, it is clear that immediate recognition of the cardiorespiratory collapse is required with urgent initiation of Basic and Advanced Cardiac Life Support methodology:

1 Maintenance of oxygen flow rates dictated by monitoring arterial blood gases. Endotracheal intubation will frequently be necessary.

2 Cardiac resuscitative measures may be needed. Crystalloids should be administered to maintain intravascular volume and cardiac output. Inotropic agents may be required to treat hypotension and heart failure. The appropriate use of these agents necessitates continuous intensive care cardiopulmonary monitoring. Use of a triple-lumen pulmonary catheter may be required.

3 Careful attention should be paid to blood loss following delivery and measurement of clotting factors. Blood should be obtained for measurement of clotting factors, partial thromboplastin time, platelets, fibrin split products, and fibrinogen. In addition, while awaiting these results, one should observe the time required for blood to form a solid clot in a red-top tube (normal, less than 8 min). In the presence of disseminated intravascular clotting, component therapy should be initiated with fresh frozen plasma or platelets, or both. (Fresh frozen plasma contains approximately 1 g fibrinogen/unit; each unit of platelets raises the platelet count by approximately 8000/mL.). The use of recombinant factor VIIa may be considered, although extensive experience is lacking.

Patients who survive the cardiopulmonary event may have a 2-day to 5-day course of mild to substantial respiratory insufficiency, probably due to adult respiratory distress syndrome, and complicated by pulmonary edema, secondary to diminished left ventricular function. A detailed review of AFE in 2014 by Clark may be of interest to readers.

Suggested reading

Abenhaim HA, Azoulay L, Kraner MS, *et al.* Incidence and risk factors of amniotic fluid embolisms: a population-based study on 3 million births in the United States. *Am J Obstet Gynecol* 2008;199:49.e1–49.e8.

Clark SL, Montz FJ, Phelan JP. Hemodynamic alterations associated with amniotic fluid embolism: a reappraisal. *Am J Obstet Gynecol* 1985;151:617.

Clark SL, Cotton DB, Gonik B, Greenspoon J, Phelan JP. Central hemodynamic alterations in amniotic fluid embolism. *Am J Obstet Gynecol* 1988;158:1124.

Clark SL, Hankins GDV, Dudley DA, *et al.* Amniotic fluid embolism: analysis of a national registry. *Am J Obstet Gynecol* 1995;172:1158.

Clark SL. Amniotic fluid embolism. *Obstet Gynecol* 2014;123:337–48.

Gilbert WM, Danielsen B. Amniotic fluid embolism: decreased mortality in a population-based study. *Obstet Gynecol* 1999;93:973.

Meyer JR. Embolia pulmonar amnio-casiosa. *Brazil Med* 1926;2:301.

Romero R, Kadar N, Vaisbuch E, Hassan SS. Maternal death following cardiopulmonary collapse after delivery: amniotic fluid embolism or septic shock due to intrauterine infection? *Am J Reprod Immunol* 2010;64:113–25.

Tuffnell DJ. United Kingdom amniotic fluid embolism register. *Br J Obstet Gynecol* 2005;112:1625.

Labor and Delivery

PROTOCOL 49

Induction of Labor

Deborah A. Wing
Department of Obstetrics and Gynecology, Division of Maternal-Fetal Medicine, University of California, Irvine, CA, USA

Overview

Induction of labor is the artificial stimulation of uterine contractions for the purpose of vaginal birth. It is one of the most commonly practiced procedures in obstetrics, occurring in over 22% of pregnancies. Labor induction is indicated when the maternal or fetal benefits from delivery outweigh the risks of prolonging the pregnancy. Indications for induction vary in acuity and may be for medical, obstetrical or elective reasons (Table 49.1). If an elective induction for reasons such as distance from hospital or risk of precipitous labor is undertaken, the criteria for term gestation should be met including: (1) ultrasound measurements at less than 20 weeks of gestation confirms gestational age of 39 weeks or more; (2) fetal heart tones have been documented to be present for more than 30 weeks by Doppler ultrasonography; (3) it has been 36 weeks or more since a positive serum or urine human chorionic gonadotropin pregnancy test. Morbidity and mortality rates are greater among infants delivered in the early term and late preterm than those delivered between 39 and 40 weeks of gestation, thus nonmedically indicated delivery prior to 39 completed weeks should be avoided.

Risks associated with labor induction include prolonged labors, uterine contractile abnormalities, fetal heart rate abnormalities, and an increased propensity for cesarean birth. Some of these cesareans may be performed for failed inductions. Although there have been many historical definitions of failed induction, a more standardized contemporary definition was established following a joint *Eunice Kennedy Shriver* National Institute of Child Health and Human Development, Society for Maternal-Fetal Medicine, and American College of Obstetricians and Gynecologists Workshop. The diagnosis of a failed induction should only be used when there is failure to generate regular contractions and cervical change for

Protocols for High-Risk Pregnancies: An Evidence-Based Approach, Sixth Edition.
Edited by John T. Queenan, Catherine Y. Spong and Charles J. Lockwood.
© 2015 John Wiley & Sons, Ltd. Published 2015 by John Wiley & Sons, Ltd.

Table 49.1   Selection criteria for induction of labor

Indications	Gestational hypertension
	Preeclampsia, eclampsia
	Maternal medical problems (e.g., diabetes mellitus, renal disease, chronic hypertension, antiphospholipid syndrome)
	Abruptio placentae
	Chorioamnionitis
	Post-term gestation
	Fetal compromise (e.g., severe fetal growth restriction, isoimmunization, oligohydramnios)
	Fetal demise
	Logistic factors (e.g., risk of rapid labor, distance from hospital, psychosocial reasons)
Contraindications	Complete placenta previa or vasa previa
	Transverse fetal lie
	Umbilical cord prolapse
	Prior classical uterine incision
	Active genital herpes infection
	Previous myomectomy with entry into the endometrial cavity

Source: adapted from Induction of Labor. ACOG Practice Bulletin No. 107. American College of Obstetricians and Gynecologists. Obstet Gynecol 2009;114: 386–97. (Reaffirmed 2013).

at least 24 hours of oxytocin administration with artificial rupture of membranes if feasible. These criteria are used after cervical ripening in the cases where ripening is indicated. The presence or absence of cervical "ripening," can influence the probability of induction success. An assessment of cervical readiness for labor induction can be communicated by using the modified Bishop score (Table 49.2). A Bishop score less than 6 indicates an unfavorable cervix, which may require a prelabor cervical ripening agent. The higher the Bishop score, the greater is the likelihood of induction success, with a Bishop score of more than 8 generally conferring the same likelihood of vaginal delivery as a woman entering spontaneous labor. Choices of induction agents include some mechanical and others pharmacological. The indication for induction, modified Bishop score, and following summaries can be employed to determine appropriate management algorithms for patients.

Consideration of maternal, fetal, and logistic factors should always occur prior to opting for induction. Generally, induction of labor is reasonable with stable maternal and fetal status and should be undertaken in a facility with the ability to intervene rapidly for any change in status. Specific mention should be made regarding preterm induction of labor in cases such as preeclampsia with severe features. Although the success rate of preterm induction of labor ranges from 30% to 60% increasing with gestational age, there is a moderate rate of nonreassuring fetal heart rate abnormalities

Table 49.2 Bishop pelvic scoring system

	0	1	2	3
Dilation (cm)	0	1–2	3–4	5–6
Effacement (%)	0–30	40–50	60–70	80
Station	–3	–2	–1 to 0	+1 to +2
Cervical consistency	Firm	Medium	Soft	–
Position of cervix	Posterior	Mid	Anterior	–

Source: adapted from Induction of Labor. ACOG Practice Bulletin No. 107. American College of Obstetricians and Gynecologists. Obstet Gynecol 2009;114: 386–97. (Reaffirmed 2013).

during these inductions. Judicious decision-making and the ability to intervene appropriately are prerequisites in these cases.

Cervical ripening agents

Mechanical agents

Membrane stripping
Cervical ripening by "stripping" the amniotic membranes is performed by manually separating the membranes from the lower uterine segment during a cervical examination, resulting in an increase in phospholipase A_2 and endogenous prostaglandin $F_{2\alpha}$ release, which are known to precede the spontaneous onset of labor. Most studies have reported membrane stripping to be safe and, when performed as a general policy at term, it is associated with a reduction in pregnancies extending to 41 and 42 weeks of gestation. Group B strep colonization is not a contraindication to membrane stripping, though there is a relative paucity of reliable data on this scenario. Membrane stripping may be offered at 39 or more weeks after consideration of the risks and benefits of the procedure.

Intracervical balloon catheter placement
There are currently multiple available devices for mechanical dilation of the cervix including intracervical Foley balloon (14–26 F) and the Atad double balloon device. These devices work by applying local pressure on the cervix by filling the balloon (or balloons) after placement in the endocervical canal. This pressure facilitates cervical ripening most likely by stimulating the release of local prostaglandins. Multiple studies have attempted to assess if intracervical Foley or prostaglandin is more efficacious. A meta-analysis of randomized trials demonstrated a similar rate of caesarean delivery between the two methods but also

demonstrated a higher rate of oxytocin augmentation when balloons were used and a higher rate of tachysytole with fetal heart rate changes when prostaglandins were used. Advantages of these balloons are that they can be placed in the face of regular uterine contractions precluding prostaglandin placement as well as in women with previous caesarean birth where misoprostol administration is contraindicated. Although these balloons do stimulate some uterine activity, it is less than that provoked by prostaglandin preparations. Thus, this method may also be considered when inducing women with intrauterine fetal growth restriction (IUGR) or oligohydramnios where there is concern about possible intrapartum fetal heart rate abnormalities associated with uterine tachysystole in early labor. Continuous fetal monitoring should be utilized when women with IUGR are undergoing induction due to the increased prevalence of oligohydramnios and chronic hypoxia among these fetuses. There may be a benefit to obtaining some cervical dilation prior to initiation of regular contractions in order to facilitate interventions such as amnioinfusion or more direct monitoring of fetal status.

Pharmacological agents

Prostaglandins cause dissolution of collagen bundles and an increase in the submucosal water content of the cervix and attempt to mimic the changes of spontaneous labor.

Prostaglandin E$_1$

Prostaglandin E$_1$ has been found to be safe and effective in numerous clinical trials for cervical ripening and induction of labor. It has numerous advantages over other prostaglandin compounds including temperature stability and low cost. The dose most commonly recommended for a term pregnancy induction is 25 µg every 3–6 hours placed in the posterior fornix. Repeat dosing is not recommended if there are more than three contractions in 10 minutes. The clinical efficacy of vaginally administered misoprostol includes a decrease in cesarean rate, higher incidence of vaginal delivery within 24 hours of initiation, and a decreased need for oxytocin. An important consideration in the use of misoprostol for labor induction is the reported increased occurrence of uterine tachysystole with or without fetal heart rate abnormalities, and the potential for disruption of the uterine scar in women with a previous cesarean delivery. If oxytocin is necessary after misoprostol treatment for cervical ripening, it should be started no sooner than 4 hours after the last dose of misoprostol. A misoprostol vaginal insert consisting of a controlled-release, retrievable polymer chip for gradual delivery of 200 µg of misoprostol into the vagina is under investigation but is currently not commercially available in the United States.

Prostaglandin E$_2$

There are two prostaglandin E$_2$ compounds that have been approved by the U.S. Food and Drug Administration for cervical ripening for medically indicated inductions of labor. One is Prepidil (Pfizer, Inc.), a dinoprostone intracervical gel; the other is Cervidil (Forest Laboratories), a dinoprostone timed-release vaginal insert. Prepidil is 0.5 mg of PGE$_2$, which is to be placed intracervically. It may be redosed as necessary in 6 hours if regular contractions are not present and the fetal heart rate is reassuring. Cervidil is 10 mg of dinoprostone in a mesh polymer; after placement in the posterior vaginal fornix, the polymer insert releases PGE$_2$ at a rate of 0.3 mg/hour. The manufacturer recommends a maximum exposure of 12 hours to Cervidil. Vaginal prostaglandins used for cervical ripening compared with placebo or oxytocin alone increase the likelihood of delivery within 24 hours, although increase the risk of uterine tachysystole with associated fetal heart rate changes.

Recommendations for fetal surveillance after prostaglandin use

Labor inductions using prostaglandin compounds should only occur in settings in which continuous uterine activity and fetal heart rate monitoring can occur for the initial observation period. Further monitoring may ensue as dictated by the clinical condition or the institutional policy. After placement of any prostaglandin, the woman should remain recumbent for 30 minutes. There is evidence that the onset of uterine activity occurs within the first hour and peaks at 4 hours after prostaglandin administration, so that it seems prudent in most circumstances to continue monitoring for at least this period of time. If regular contractions begin, continuous cardiotocographic monitoring should be applied as well as monitoring of the mother's vital signs.

Prostaglandins should not be used for induction of labor in the setting of frequent fetal heart rate abnormalities because of the limited ability to quickly terminate the effects on uterine contractility.

Labor-inducing procedures and agents

Amniotomy

Amniotomy can safely and effectively induce or augment labor, particularly in women with favorable Bishop scores (8 or higher).[1] The combination of oxytocin plus amniotomy for labor induction appears to shorten the time interval from start of induction to delivery compared to amniotomy alone.

When performing amniotomy, care should be taken to ensure the fetal head is well applied to the cervix and the umbilical cord is not presenting. The fetal heart rate should be recorded immediately following amniotomy.

Oxytocin

Oxytocin is one of the most widely used medications in obstetrical practice and may be used for induction or augmentation of labor, although it has proven inferior as a cervical ripening agent when the cervix is unfavorable. There are many different dosing regimens, none of which have been scientifically tested against each other. It is recommended that hospitals initiate a standard protocol in order to minimize error and improve patient safety. Examples of protocols for oxytocin delivery can be found in Tables 49.3 and 49.4. Higher dose protocols have demonstrated a shorter time to delivery and fewer failed inductions but are often associated with uterine tachysystole and fetal heart rate abnormalities.

Conclusion

Labor inductions have become increasingly more common. In the United States there has been a doubling of the induction rate in the past two

Table 49.3 Examples of low- and high-dose oxytocin infusion protocols for labor stimulation

Regimen	Starting dose (mU/minute)	Incremental increase (mU/minute)	Maximum dose (mU/minute)
Low-dose	0.5–2.0	1–2	15–40
High-dose	6	3–6*	15–40

*The dose is reduced to 3 mU/minute in the face of uterine tachysystole with fetal heart rate abnormalities, and reduced further to 1 mU/minute if the uterine tachysystole with fetal heart rate abnormalities is persistent.
Source: adapted from Induction of Labor. ACOG Practice Bulletin No. 107. American College of Obstetricians and Gynecologists. Obstet Gynecol 2009;114: 386–97. (Reaffirmed 2013).

Table 49.4 Oxytocin checklist example

1	Dilution: 10 U oxytocin in 1000 mL normal saline for resultant concentration of 10 mU oxytocin/mL
2	Infusion rate: 2 mU/minute or 12 mL/hour
3	Incremental increase: 2 mU/minute or 12 mL/hour every 45 minutes until contraction frequency adequate
4	Maximum dose: 16 mU/minute or 96 mL/hour

Source: Alfirevic Z, Kelly AJ, Dowswell T. Intravenous oxytocin alone for cervical ripening and induction of labour. Cochrane Database Syst Rev. 2009 Oct 7;(4):CD003246.

decades, and the upward trend is continuing. Despite therapeutic advances and continued research into the initiation of human parturition, the clinical features which are most critical for determining induction management and predicting success are the cervical condition at the start of the induction, and gestational age, among other maternal demographic characteristics such as multiparity and normal weight.

Acknowledgement

The author would like to acknowledge the contributions of Megan Stephenson, MD, to this protocol.

Suggested reading

Alfirevic Z, Kelly AJ, Dowswell T. Intravenous oxytocin alone for cervical ripening and induction of labour. *Cochrane Database Syst Rev* 2009 Oct 7;(4):CD003246.

American College of Obstetricians and Gynecologists. Induction of Labor. ACOG Practice Bulletin No. 107. *Obstet Gynecol* 2009;114:386–97. (Reaffirmed 2013).

American College of Obstetricians and Gynecologists. Vaginal birth after previous cesarean delivery. Practice Bulletin No. 115. *Obstet Gynecol* 2010;116:450–63 (Reaffirmed 2013).

American College of Obstetricians and Gynecologists. Nonmedically indicated early-term deliveries. Committee Opinion No. 561. *Obstet Gynecol* 2013;121:911–5.

Boulvain M, Stan C, Irion O. Membrane sweeping for induction of labour. *Cochrane Database Syst Rev* 2005:CD000451.

Bricker L, Luckas M. Amniotomy alone for induction of labour. *Cochrane Database Syst Rev* 2000;(4):CD002862.

Hofmeyr GJ, Gulmexoglu AM. Vaginal misoprostol for cervical ripening and labour induction at term. *Cochrane Database Syst Rev* 2003;(1):CD000941.

Jozwiak M, Bloemenkamp KW, Kelly AJ, Mol BW, Irion O, Boulvain M. Mechanical methods for induction of labour. *Cochrane Database Syst Rev* 2012;(3):CD001233.

Nassar AH, Adra AM, Chakhtoura N, Gómez-Marín O, Beydoun S. Severe preeclampsia remote from term: labor induction or elective cesarean delivery? *Am J Obstet Gynecol* 1998;179(5):1210.

Spong CY, Berghella V, Wenstrom KD, Mercer BM, Saade GR. Preventing the first cesarean delivery: summary of a joint Eunice Kennedy Shriver National Institute of Child Health and Human Development, Society for Maternal-Fetal Medicine, and American College of Obstetricians and Gynecologists Workshop. *Obstet Gynecol* 2012;120(5):1181.

Wing DA. Misoprostol Vaginal Insert Consortium. Misoprostol vaginal insert compared to dinoprostone vaginal insert: a randomized, controlled trial. *Obstet Gynecol* 2008 Oct;112(4):801–12.

PROTOCOL 50

Intrapartum Fetal Heart Rate Monitoring

Roger K. Freeman

Long Beach Memorial Medical Center, University of California Irvine, Long Beach, CA, USA

Rationale

Intrapartum fetal heart rate monitoring was developed in the mid-1960s after patterns of heart rate change in relation to uterine contractions had been described by Hon, Caldero-Barcia and Hammacher. At the time of development of fetal heart rate monitoring it was believed that most cases of congenital neurological abnormalities were due to fetal hypoxia proximate to birth. When the method was first developed, there were numerous non-randomized studies comparing electronically monitored patients to either historical controls or low-risk patients who were monitored by auscultation which was not rigorous. It was clear early on that the intrapartum fetal death rate was significantly less in electronically monitored patients than in the non-randomized controls, even if the controls were low risk and the electronically monitored patients were high risk.

In the mid-1970s Haverkamp [1] did the first prospectively randomized controlled study where the study group was openly electronically monitored and the control group had the electronic fetal monitor covered up so the caregivers could not use the information in patient management. The control group was monitored by auscultation with a rigorous protocol of listening every 15 minutes in the first stage of labor and every 5 minutes in the second stage by a dedicated one-on-one nurse assigned to each patient. The results of this study and of several more randomized prospective trials revealed no benefit to electronic fetal heart rate monitoring during the intrapartum period when compared to intensive auscultation [2]. Several of the studies also found higher cesarean delivery rates in the electronically monitored group. The only statistically significant benefit was shown in the large Dublin trial where the electronically monitored patients had neonates with fewer seizures but on follow-up the incidence of cerebral

Protocols for High-Risk Pregnancies: An Evidence-Based Approach, Sixth Edition.
Edited by John T. Queenan, Catherine Y. Spong and Charles J. Lockwood.
© 2015 John Wiley & Sons, Ltd. Published 2015 by John Wiley & Sons, Ltd.

palsy was not different between the electronically monitored patients and those with intensive auscultation [3].

Today as we look back it has been pointed out that, even with the introduction of electronic fetal monitoring in the majority of laboring patients, there has been no reduction in the incidence of cerebral palsy [4]. This finding has indicated to some that the technique has no benefit. However, if we accept the reduction in term intrapartum deaths in electronically monitored patients compared to those with non-intensive auscultation from the original non-randomized trials [5], and also compare the marked increase in perinatal survival over the past 30 years, we must conclude that some fetuses that used to die intrapartum now survive damaged and some that used to survive damaged now survive intact. Thus electronic intrapartum fetal monitoring probably has been valuable. Nevertheless, it is clear that the vast majority of non-reassuring patterns do not result in neurological damage and to the epidemiologist this high false-positive rate makes the technique invalid [6]. However, if the technique were perfect, intervention based on the fetal monitor pattern would prevent all cases of cerebral palsy due to intrapartum hypoxia and there would be zero correlation with neurological outcome, rendering the technique not predictive of future outcome, which is the standard used by epidemiologists.

Pattern interpretation

Baseline fetal heart rate characteristics [7] include rate with tachycardia defined as >160 bpm (beats per minute) and bradycardia defined as <110 bpm. Variability is classified as absent, minimal (1 to 5 bpm), moderate (5–25 bpm) and increased (>25 bpm).

There are five periodic fetal heart rate patterns [7] that have been described.

1 Fetal heart rate acceleration with an amplitude of >15 bpm and a duration of >15 seconds from onset to offset is seen in most patients beyond 32 weeks' gestation and signifies good fetal oxygenation and an umbilical arterial pH of >7.20. If accelerations are not present spontaneously, one can evoke fetal heart rate accelerations with fetal scalp stimulation after membrane rupture or with vibroacoustic stimulation before membrane rupture. This technique can be useful when following a problematic fetal heart rate pattern where spontaneous or evoked accelerations may allow one to avoid intervention [8].

2 Early deceleration is a uniform pattern with slow onset and offset that is a mirror image of the contraction. This is believed to be due to fetal head compression and is mediated as a vagal reflex. It is not associated with fetal hypoxia or acid–base change and requires no intervention.

3 Variable deceleration is a pattern characterized by rapid onset and rapid offset and usually has an amplitude of 30 to 40 bpm or more. It is believed to be due to umbilical cord compression giving rise to a vagal response. Unless the deceleration is prolonged beyond 40 to 60 seconds on a repetitive basis, is associated with a rising baseline rate or decreased fetal heart rate variability, it is considered evidence of good oxygenation and does not require intervention. However, if cord compression is sufficient to produce more than transient fetal hypoxia, the finding of absent variability (category III) indicates that hypoxia and acidosis may be more than transient and intervention may be indicated.

4 Late deceleration is characterized as a uniform decrease in fetal heart rate beginning after the peak of a contraction of normal duration and with a return to baseline after the contraction is over. The onset and offset are gradual. It is believed to be due to decreased oxygen transfer across the placenta, which may be due to decreased uteroplacental blood flow or maternal hypoxemia. Initially late deceleration is usually associated with moderate fetal heart rate variability and may be due to a vagal reflex but, as hypoxia increases and the fetus develops metabolic acidosis, the variability decreases and at this point the mechanism for the late deceleration is believed to be due to myocardial depression. Recurrent late deceleration with absent variability is category III and requires prompt intervention and or delivery.

5 The last periodic change that is described is prolonged deceleration which lasts more than 2 minutes by definition. Its onset may be similar to a late deceleration or a variable deceleration. This pattern may be seen with a sentinel event such as a prolapsed cord, ruptured uterus or sudden complete abruption. The clinical management of a pattern of prolonged deceleration includes application of intrauterine resuscitation techniques (position change, oxygen administration, stopping oxytocin, vaginal exam to rule out prolapsed cord and if not successful, moving toward operative vaginal delivery or caesarean section.

The National Institute of Child Health and Human Development (NICHD) conducted workshops in 1997 [9] and 2008 [10] designed to address issues of definitions and recommendations for future research in electronic fetal monitoring. In the 2008 conference the terms reassuring and non-reassuring fetal heart rate tracings were abandoned due to the lack of precision and agreement attributed to these terms. At this meeting fetal heart rate patterns were subdivided into three categories with category I indicating good oxygenation and no need for intervention. Category III indicated patterns consistent with ongoing hypoxic damage and or death. While there was good agreement among the participants on these two categories, category II includes all patterns between categories I and III and it remains unclear what the significance of category II patterns are and management recommendations were sought from the American College of Obstetricians and Gynecologists[*,†]. Within category II it appears that, if moderate variability is preserved, significant ongoing hypoxia is unlikely but further research is necessary for specific management recommendations. A recent publicationproposes an algorhythm for the management of category II patterns and may serve as the basis for studies to evaluate this approach.[‡]

Finally, inter and intra observer variation in fetal heart rate pattern interpretation is significant [11, 12] and it is hoped that the new three-category classification will improve this problem.

Fetal inflammatory response to maternal chorioamnionitis

Many reports have indicated that fetal inflammatory response to maternal infection may result in the elaboration of proinflammatory cytokines that may be responsible for damage in the periventricular areas of the premature fetal brain resulting in spastic diplegia. In term infants this fetal inflammatory response may result in damage to the same cortical and subcortical watershed areas of the motor cortex that are affected by prolonged intermittent hypoxia resulting in spastic quadriplegia. Fetal heart rate patterns have not been described in these situations but in this author's anecdotal experience there are commonly findings of tachycardia with decreased variability, usually in association with maternal fever, and inconsistent deceleration patterns may be present. While antibiotics are advisable when maternal chorioamnionitis is suspected, there have been no strategies that have proven effective in preventing neurological damage due to the fetal inflammatory response [13, 14].

Medical-legal implications

While there may be disagreement on the overall value of intrapartum fetal heart rate monitoring, in the courtroom, the fetal monitor strip is usually the main focus when a lawsuit alleges negligence in cases of cerebral palsy

---

[*] ACOG Practice Bulletin # 106, Intrapartum Fetal Heart Rate Monitoring: Nomenclature, Interpretation, and General Management Principles. July 2009.
[†] ACOG Practice Bulletin #116 Management of Intrapartum Fetal Heart Rate Tracings. November 2010.
[‡] Intrapartum management of category II fetal heart rate tracings: towards standardization of care. Steven L. Clark, Michael P. Nageotte, Thomas J. Garite, Roger K. Freeman et al. *Am J. Ob Gyn*, August 2013.

believed to be due to intrapartum fetal asphyxia. Thus there are important considerations for the obstetrician when there is concern at the time
of birth about the neonatal condition. The determination of a cord arterial
pH of greater than 7.0 and a Base deficit <12.0 mm/liter indicates that fetal
hypoxia proximate to birth cannot be implicated as a cause of later neurological damage. The presence of chorioamnionitis and funisitis may indicate
that the cause of later neurological damage could be due to a fetal inflammatory response to maternal infection. Thus when delivery of a depressed
infant occurs or when fetal heart rate patterns have been of concern it is
often helpful to get fetal cord arterial blood gases and to save the placenta in
order to later determine the likely cause of any neurological developmental
problems.

References

[1] Haverkamp AD, Thompson HE, McFee JG, *et al.* The evaluation of continuous fetal
    heart rate monitoring in high risk pregnancy. *Am J Obstet Gynecol* 1976;125:310.
[2] Freeman RK. Intrapartum fetal monitoring – a disappointing story. *N Eng J Med*
    1990;322:624–6.
[3] Grant A, O'Brien N, Joy MT, Hennessy E, MacDonald D. Cerebral palsy among
    children born during the Dublin randomized trial of intrapartum monitoring. *Lancet*
    1989;2:1233–6.
[4] Stanley FJ, Watson L. The cerebral palsies in western Australia: trends 1968–1981.
    Am J Obstet Gynecol 1988;158:89.
[5] *Antenatal Diagnosis. Report of a Consensus Development Conference.* NIH Publication
    #79-1973. Bethesda, MD: April 1979.
[6] Nelson KB, Dambrosia DM, Ting TY, Grether JK. Uncertain value of electronic fetal
    monitoring in predicting cerebral palsy. *N Eng J Med* 1996;334:613–18.
[7] Freeman RK, Garite TJ, Nageotte MP, Miller L., *Fetal Heart Rate Monitoring*, 4th edn.
    Philadelphia, PA: Lippincott Williams & Wilkins, 2012.
[8] Clark SL, Gimovsky ML, Miller FC. Fetal heart rate response to scalp blood sampling.
    Am J Obstet Gynecol 1982;44:706.
[9] National Institute of Child Health and Human Development. Electronic fetal
    heart rate monitoring: research guidelines for interpretation. *Am J Obstet Gynecol*
    1997;177:1385–90.
[10] Macones G, Hankins G, Spong C, Hauth J, & Moore T. The 2008 National Institute
    of Child Health and Human Development Report on Electronic Fetal Monitoring.
    Obstet Gynecol 2008;112:661–6.
[11] Beaulieu M, Fabia J, Leduc B, *et al.* The reproducibility of intrapartum
    cardiotocogram interpretation. *Can Med Assoc J* 1982:127:214–16.
[12] Chauhan S, Klauser C, Woodring T, *et al.* Intrapartum nonreassuring fetal heart rate
    tracing and prediction of adverse outcomes: interobserver variability. *Am J Obstet
    Gynecol* 2008;199:623e1–623e5.
[13] Royal College of Obstetricians and Gynecologists. *Intrauterine infection and perinatal
    brain injury.* Scientific Advisory Committee Opinion Paper #3. November 2002.
[14] American College of Obstetricians and Gynecologists and American Academy of
    Pediatrics. *Neonatal encephalopathy and cerebral palsy: defining the pathogenesis and
    pathophysiology.* January 2003.

PROTOCOL 51

Breech Delivery

G. Justus Hofmeyr

Department of Obstetrics and Gynecology, Frere Maternity Hospital/University of the Witwatersrand/University of Fort Hare/Eastern Cape Department of Health, South Africa

Overview

By term, 96% to 97% of babies actively turn to a cephalic presentation. Failure to do so before birth may be due to prematurity, multiple pregnancy, abnormalities of the uterus, amniotic volume or the baby, or otherwise benign factors such as cornual placental locations. Breech presentation may be a marker for subtle fetal abnormalities, as apparently healthy breech babies have on average poorer long-term neurodevelopmental scores than cephalic babies, irrespective of the mode of delivery.

Diagnosis

The clinical diagnosis of breech presentation is made by abdominal palpation. A cephalic fetal pole in the upper abdomen is characteristically "ballottable" because of free movement of the head, compared with more sluggish movement of the breech, which moves together with the rest of the baby's body. The presenting breech lacks the sulcus between the shoulders and head. Vaginal examination may be useful for confirmation. However, up to 20% of breech presentations are missed clinically.

By 28 weeks of gestation the incidence of breech presentation is down to 25%, and the diagnosis warrants ultrasound examination checking for clinically relevant associated features such as fetal anomalies, placenta previa, abnormalities of amniotic fluid volume and (very rarely) extra-uterine pregnancy. At 36 weeks of gestation, careful routine clinical assessment of the baby's presentation is important so that breech presentation can be managed appropriately.

Protocols for High-Risk Pregnancies: An Evidence-Based Approach, Sixth Edition.
Edited by John T. Queenan, Catherine Y. Spong and Charles J. Lockwood.
© 2015 John Wiley & Sons, Ltd. Published 2015 by John Wiley & Sons, Ltd.

Management

External cephalic version

Before 36 weeks of gestation, we reassure women that most breech presentations will turn spontaneously before term. Relaxing in a knee-chest
posture from time to time has been suggested to enhance the chance of
spontaneous version, though randomized trials have not confirmed this.
For breech presentation at or beyond 36 weeks of gestation we evaluate
the pregnancy carefully, including ultrasound assessment as mentioned
above, to counsel the woman and her family about the option of external
cephalic version (ECV). If not contraindicated, for example by a condition
requiring caesarean delivery such as placenta previa, we offer ECV based
on high-quality evidence that it reduces both the risk of breech birth and
of cesarean delivery, and because complications are very rare. Neither HIV
infection nor previous cesarean is an absolute contraindication. We emphasize that the procedure is not always successful.

If the mother requests ECV, we confirm the baby's wellbeing with
cardiotocography. To relax the uterus, we use a beta-sympathomimitic
agent while monitoring for maternal tachycardia (greater than 120
beats/minute), immediately prior to the procedure. We position the
woman with about 45 degrees lateral tilt on a narrow examination couch
positioned against a wall, her back supported against the wall with a
cushion. We position the baby's back initially toward the operator. We
use corn powder or ultrasound gel to reduce friction on the skin. We lift
the breech from the pelvis with the fingertips of both hands, then use
the edge of an open hand to push the breech away from the pelvis and
toward the upper flank (a backward somersault). If this maneuver alone
is not successful, we use the other hand to gently push the baby's head
toward the other flank and inferiorly. If this is not successful, we turn
the mother so that the baby's back is away from the operator. We use the
same maneuvers, this time for a forward somersault.

Whether the ECV was successful or not, we check the baby's condition
again with cardiotocography. It is common for the baby to be in a quiet
sleep state with nonreactive heart rate pattern for about 20 minutes after
ECV attempt.

Delivery

If ECV is contraindicated, declined or unsuccessful, a plan needs to be
made for the birth of the baby. This involves careful discussion of benefits
and risks in the context of the parents' priorities and preferences. In many
settings cesarean delivery has become routine for breech births, based
primarily on the findings of the Term Breech Trial conducted by Hannah
et al. In that trial, women with clinical features considered suitable for

vaginal breech birth were randomly allocated to planned cesarean delivery (of whom about 10% gave birth vaginally) and planned vaginal birth (of whom about half gave birth by cesarean). In the group allocated to planned caesarean, fewer babies died (3/1039 compared with 13/1039), and there were fewer cases of death or severe morbidity (17/1039 compared with 52/1039). In settings where there were low perinatal mortality rates, the number of deaths was too few for meaningful comparison (0/514 compared with 3/511). In settings (mainly well-resourced) where follow up to 2 years was possible, the rate of death or neurodevelopmental delay was similar between groups (14/457 for planned cesarean compared with 13/463 for vaginal delivery). There was thus no evidence of long-term disability despite the increase morbidity at birth. Subsequent large cohort studies in Europe have shown very low morbidity from planned vaginal breech birth. Other factors to take into account are the increased current and future morbidity from cesarean delivery and the importance the mother attaches to the experience of giving birth without cesarean.

Certain clinical criteria are considered necessary for safe vaginal birth, including: an estimated fetal weight of 2000–3500 g; no hyperextension of the fetal neck; no pelvic contracture on clinical or CT pelvimetry (antero-posterior diameter at the pelvic inlet 11 cm or more, transverse diameter at the pelvic inlet 12 cm or more and interspinous diameter at the midpelvis 10 cm or more); and a frank or complete breech presentation. Fetal condition is monitored closely during labor. Other precautions include an intravenous line, oxytocin available and a beta-sympathomimetic tocolytic available in case progress is poor and the decision is taken to deliver by cesarean.

If labor progresses well according to partograph plotting and the combined cross-sectional area of the baby's body and thighs pass easily through the pelvis, difficulty with the after-coming head is most unlikely. In the rare event of absolute obstruction to the birth of the after-coming head, symphysiotomy with local analgesia has been reported to be effective as an emergency life-saving procedure. However, in many settings symphysiotomy is not available. Another salvage procedure for absolute obstruction to the after-coming head is tocolysis followed by cesarean delivery.

The delivery is best managed in or close to an operating room, with anesthetist and pediatrician on standby. During the second stage, we encourage the mother to bear down (usually in the dorsal semi-sitting position with legs in obstetric stirrups) to expel the baby in a flexed position. If the breech delivers easily and spontaneously, we start an oxytocin infusion to expedite the rest of the delivery. If not, we opt for cesarean delivery. We resist the temptation to assist by pulling downward on the baby. Any traction encourages the arms and head to extend. In the case of a frank breech, gentle flexion of the knees may be needed to release the legs, which tend to splint the baby's body. Once the cord is visible, we pull down a small loop to prevent stretching of the cord. If the baby's back is tending to rotate posteriorly, we gently rotate the back anteriorly with downward traction, holding the baby around the pelvis with a dry towel. Ideally, the arms and shoulders should deliver spontaneously. If not we deliver each arm by passing two fingers up the baby's back to the level of the elbow, and sweeping the baby's arm in front of his or her face and downwards. If this is not successful, we hold the baby around the pelvis with a warm towel and rotate the shoulders through 180°, keeping the back upwards, deliver what was the posterior shoulder under the symphysis pubis, then repeat in the other direction (Lovset maneuver). To deliver the after-coming head, we use either the Mauriceau-Smellie-Veit maneuver or Piper forceps.

During cesarean delivery, similar maneuvers are used for delivery of the arms and shoulders, with fundal pressure replacing the mother's bearing down efforts to keep the after-coming head flexed during delivery. For preterm breech cesarean, the lower uterine segment may be too narrow to allow an adequate transverse incision. In this case, a midline lower segment incision may be needed, which can be extended into the upper segment as a classical incision if the lower segment is inadequate for gentle delivery of the baby.

Conclusion

It is important for those who care for women during labour to maintain the skills necessary for safe vaginal breech delivery. Even when routine cesarean delivery is the practice, situations will arise where precipitate labor leaves no option other than vaginal birth. Teaching videos are available on ECV (https://www.youtube.com/watch?v=fKaNZfUno50), and breech delivery and symphysiotomy (https://www.youtube.com/watch?v=G5c4GAxmEgE) on the World Health Organization Reproductive Health Library.

Suggested reading

Alarab M, Regan C, O'Connell M, Keane D, O'Herlihy C, Foley M. Singleton vaginal delivery at term: still a safe option. *Obstet Gynecol* 2004;103:407–12.

Albertson S, Rasmussen S, Reigstad H. Evaluation of a protocol for selecting fetuses in breech presentations for vaginal delivery or cesarean section. *Am J Obstet Gynecol* 1997;177:586–92.

American College of Obstetricians and Gynecologists. Mode of term singleton breech delivery. ACOG Committee Opinion No. 340. *Obstet Gynecol* 2006;108:235–7. (Reaffirmed 2012).

Deering S, Brown J, Hodor J, Satin A. Simulation training and resident performance of singleton breech delivery. *Obstet Gynecol* 2006;107:86–90.

Gimovsky M. Breech presentation. In: O'Grady J, Gimovsky M, Bayer-Zwirello L, Giordano K, editors. *Operative Obstetrics*. 2nd ed. New York: Cambridge University Press; 2008.

Hannah M, Hannath W, Hewson S, Hodnett E, Saigai S, Willan A. Planned cesarean section versus planned vaginal birth for breech presentation at term: a randomized multicentre trial. *Lancet* 2000;356:1375–83.

Hofmeyr GJ, Hannah M, Lawrie TA. Planned caesarean section for term breech delivery. *Cochrane Database Syst Rev* 2003;(2. Art. No.):CD000166. doi: 10.1002/14651858.

Hofmeyr GJ, Kulier R. External cephalic version for breech presentation at term. *Cochrane Database of Systematic Reviews* 2012;(10. Art. No.):CD000083.

Mostello D, Chang JJ, Bai F, Wang J, Guild C, Stamps K, Leet TL. Breech presentation at delivery: a marker for congenital anomaly? *J Perinatol* 2014 Jan;34(1):11–5. DOI: 10.1038/jp.2013.132. Epub 2013 Oct 24.

Whyte H, Hannah M, Saigal S, *et al*. Outcomes of children at 2 years after planned caesarean birth versus planned vaginal birth for breech presentation at term: The International Randomized Term Breech Trial. *Am J Obstet Gynecol* 2004;191:864–71.

Vaginal Birth After Cesarean

James R. Scott

Department of Obstetrics and Gynecology, University of Utah Medical Center, Salt Lake City, UT, USA

The cesarean delivery rate in the United States has dramatically risen from 5% in 1970 to 33% in 2012. Many believe the current cesarean rate and rising rates in other countries are too high, and vaginal birth after cesarean (VBAC) has long been promoted as one way to lower them. Despite more than 1000 citations in the literature and the current emphasis on evidence-based medicine, there are only two small, randomized trials and neither proved definitively that maternal and neonatal outcomes are better with either a trial of labor (TOL) after cesarean or repeat cesarean delivery. Contemporary issues that affect VBAC rates include the right for women to have a cesarean with no medical indication ("on request"), the possibility of future pelvic support disorders after vaginal delivery, and substantial medical legal risks should uterine rupture occur during a TOL to achieve VBAC. Consequently, deciding between TOL and repeat cesarean delivery is an ongoing challenge for both physicians and patients. The purpose of this protocol is to outline a careful and safe approach to VBAC.

Prelabor counseling

The decision for a trial of labor after a previous cesarean (TOLAC) involves balancing risks versus benefits (Fig. 52.1). TOL in a carefully selected patient with a low transverse cesarean scar is usually desirable, but physicians and patients need to know about potential adverse outcomes. Most studies on VBAC have been conducted in university or tertiary level centers under ideal conditions with 24-hour staff coverage and in-house anesthesia. Although patients were carefully selected in initial studies, the list of obstetric conditions reportedly appropriate for VBAC rapidly expanded. Usually derived from small series, they included unknown uterine scar, twins, post-term pregnancy, and suspected macrosomia.

Protocols for High-Risk Pregnancies: An Evidence-Based Approach, Sixth Edition.
Edited by John T. Queenan, Catherine Y. Spong and Charles J. Lockwood.
© 2015 John Wiley & Sons, Ltd. Published 2015 by John Wiley & Sons, Ltd.

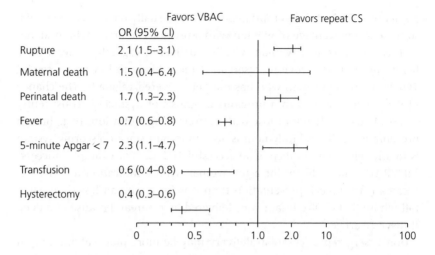

Figure 52.1   Odds ratio graph comparing morbidity of trial of labor with elective repeat cesarean delivery.   Source: American College of Obstetricians and Gynecologists, 2010 [*Obstet Gynecol* 2010;116:450–63]. Reproduced with permission of Lippincott Williams & Wilkins.

Understanding limitations of this literature and preparation for the possibility of an emergency cesarean delivery is important when attempting VBAC in these situations. Common sense should prevail.

Many women in the United States deliver in smaller rural and community hospitals where obstetricians and anesthesiologists may not be available in-house on nights and weekends. Largely because of this lack of provider availability and the current liability climate, one-third of hospitals and physicians have stopped offering TOLAC, and others vary in what they provide. This dilemma requires a careful evaluation and discussion of benefits of VBAC compared with the risks. Counseling includes taking into account the patient's wishes and her risk tolerance for the rare uterine rupture and its potential adverse outcome. Options include a plan for attempted VBAC at the hospital, delivery by repeat cesarean, or referral to another hospital that can provide 24-hour in-house services for a TOLAC attempt.

It is reasonable to encourage appropriately selected women to undertake TOLAC in a safe setting, but potential complications should be discussed. Thorough, impartial, and fact-based counseling beginning early in pregnancy provides the best preparation for TOLAC. Medical records should be obtained to review the circumstances surrounding the indication for the previous cesarean(s) and to confirm the type of uterine incision.

Vaginal delivery is associated with fewer complications, is less expensive, has a faster recovery, and for many women there is an important satisfaction factor. Published series indicate that about 60–80% of TOLACs result in successful vaginal births. However, these rates often represent a selected population. Patients inappropriate for TOLAC usually have been excluded, so the exact percentage of women with a previous cesarean who undergo TOL is not known. A woman who has delivered vaginally at least once before or after her previous cesarean is more likely to have a successful TOLAC than the woman who has not yet delivered vaginally. The chance of success for those with a previous diagnosis of dystocia is consistently lower (40–70%) than for those with nonrecurring indications (e.g., breech presentation). Clinical judgment is also important since no scoring system is totally reliable in predicting a successful TOLAC. For example, successful VBAC is more likely for a tall woman whose indication for the first cesarean was breech presentation than it is for a woman less than 5 feet tall whose first 4300 g infant was delivered by cesarean because of a deep transverse arrest.

Conversely, repeat cesarean delivery may be more practical and safe in certain settings, particularly in women who plan to have only one or two children. It can be scheduled; is predictable; avoids a failed TOLAC attempt with its attendant frustration and morbidity; and essentially eliminates uterine rupture with its potential catastrophic outcome and litigation. However, elective cesarean delivery carries with it a likelihood of more cesareans with their additive future risks. Placenta previa and accreta have become serious problems associated with multiple cesarean deliveries. Taken together, previa and accreta occur in less than 5% of women with no prior cesarean, but when they occur together the prevalence progressively increases to as high as 67% with four or more previous cesareans. Severe bleeding associated with these conditions now account for over half of peripartum hysterectomies. These are difficult cases, often requiring extensive preoperative preparation, and associated with extensive surgery, bladder and ureter injury, excessive blood loss, and even maternal death.

Criteria most predictive of a safe and successful TOLAC

1 One (or two) prior low segment transverse cesarean deliveries
2 Clinically adequate pelvis and normal fetal size
3 No other uterine scars, anomalies or previous rupture
4 Patient enthusiasm and consent
5 Spontaneous labor
6 Physician available capable of monitoring labor, the fetus, and performing a cesarean delivery
7 Anesthesia, blood bank and personnel available, and prior simulation training for emergency cesarean deliveries.

Potential contraindications

1 Prior classical or T-shaped incision or previous uterine surgery
2 Contracted pelvis and/or macrosomia
3 Medical or obstetric condition precluding vaginal delivery
4 Patient refusal
5 Unripe cervix, induction and augmentation
6 Inability to perform emergency cesarean delivery because of unavailable obstetrician or anesthesiologist, nursing and other staff or inadequate facility.

The final decision for TOLAC versus repeat cesarean delivery should be made by the patient and her physician after careful consideration and discussion (Fig. 52.2). A plan of management should then be outlined and documented in the prenatal record. Once the decision for TOLAC is made, the patient deserves support and encouragement. This does not mean that the plan cannot be altered if the situation changes.

Management of labor and delivery

Each hospital should develop a protocol for management of VBAC patients. Epidural anesthesia is not contraindicated. In fact, adequate pain relief may allow more women to choose TOLAC. The safety of induction of labor with prostaglandin gel and augmentation with oxytocin remains controversial, and misoprostol is contraindicated. Once labor has begun, the patient should be promptly evaluated and monitored; continuous electronic monitoring is usually preferable. It is important for personnel to be familiar with the potential complications of VBAC and to watch closely for fetal heart rate (FHR) abnormalities and inadequate progress of labor. These women are at risk for labor problems in view of the 20–40% rate of unsuccessful TOLAC. Timely diagnosis and prompt management of labor abnormalities are essential in any woman with a uterine scar to avoid the added risk of obstructed labor. Prospective simulation training that allows for a prompt and organized response to any maternal or fetal emergency is highly desirable.

There is nothing particularly unique about delivery of the infant after TOLAC. The necessity for routine exploration of the uterus after successful VBAC is controversial. If there is excessive vaginal bleeding or signs of hypovolemia, immediate assessment of the scar and entire genital tract is necessary. There is an increased incidence of infection and morbidity in patients who require cesarean because of a failed TOL.

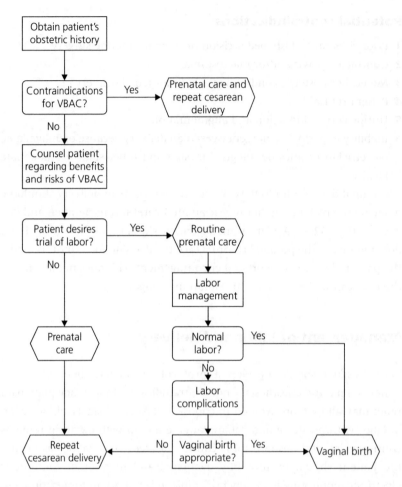

Figure 52.2   Flow sheet showing one management scheme for vaginal birth after cesarean.   Reproduced with permission from Porter TF, Scott JR. Cesarean Delivery in. In Scott JR, Gibbs RS, Karlan BY, Haney AF, eds. Obstetrics and Gynecology. 9th ed. Philadelphia: Lippincott Williams & Wilkins, 2003:449–60.

Uterine rupture

Rupture of the uterine scar is the most serious complication of VBAC, and it can be life-threatening for both mother and baby. During labor, the rupture usually involves the previous scar and lower uterine segment, but it may be stellate and extend intraperitoneally or retroperitoneally. Associated factors include excessive amounts of oxytocin, dysfunctional labor, more than one cesarean delivery, multiparity and even a previous nonpregnant uterine perforation. However, in most cases the reason rupture occurs is unclear, and adverse outcomes can occur even in appropriate VBAC candidates. The rate of rupture is related to the type and location of the previous incision. The risk of uterine rupture with a classical or T-incision is 4–9%, with a low transverse incision it is 0.5–1.0%, and the risk with a low vertical incision is estimated to be between 1% and 4%.

Diagnosis

Uterine rupture is sometimes difficult to diagnose, and close surveillance is necessary. Signs and symptoms may progress gradually or rapidly. The most common presenting signs are FHR abnormalities. A FHR pattern with subtle variable decelerations may rapidly evolve into late decelerations, bradycardia, and undetectable fetal heart activity. Uterine or abdominal pain most commonly occurs in the area of the previous incision but may range from mild to "tearing" in nature. Uterine contractions often diminish in intensity and frequency. Vaginal or intraabdominal bleeding produces anxiety, restlessness, weakness, dizziness, gross hematuria, shoulder pain and shock. This clinical picture has sometimes been mistaken for abruption. Loss of station of the presenting part on vaginal examination is diagnostic.

Management

These findings in a patient undergoing TOLAC warrant immediate exploratory laparotomy. The condition of the infant is dependent on the severity of the rupture and relationship to the placenta and umbilical cord. The outcome is usually, but not always, favorable even when delivery occurs within 30 minutes. The combined rate of fetal death and severe long-term neurologic impairment when rupture occurs has been estimated to be between 1% and 20%. Repair of the uterus is possible in the majority of patients. In others, hemorrhage from extension of the rupture into the broad ligament or extensive damage to the uterus requires hysterectomy.

Summary

VBAC was enthusiastically supported by many groups during the past three decades. With more experience, it became apparent that there are rare but significant risks to the mother and infant. Poor perinatal outcome associated with uterine rupture is a common cause of litigation. Most problems occur when the patient is not under direct observation or the diagnosis and management of uterine rupture is delayed. The latest ACOG Practice Bulletin (Bulletin 115, August 2010) still recommends that a physician capable of performing a cesarean should be "immediately available" but that patients should be allowed to attempt TOLAC under less than optimum circumstances if they understand the risks involved. Although outcomes from TOLAC and elective repeat cesarean delivery are relatively equivalent, one may be better than the other for an individual case. With careful selection and close attention during labor, the majority of women can successfully deliver vaginally.

Suggested reading

American College of Obstetricians and Gynecologists. Vaginal birth after previous cesarean delivery. Practice Bulletin No. 115. *Obstet Gynecol* 2010;116:450–63.

Cahill AG, Macones GA. Vaginal birth after cesarean delivery: evidence-based practice. *Clin Obstet Gynecol* 2007;50(2):518–25.

Dodd JM, Crowther CA, Huertas E, Guise J-M, Horey D. Planned elective repeat caesarean section versus planned vaginal birth for women with a previous caesarean birth. *Cochrane Database of Systematic Reviews* 2013 Dec 10;12:CD004224.

Fineberg A, Tilton ZA. VBAC in the Trenches: a community perspective. *Clin Obstet Gynecol* 2012;55(4):997–1003.

Hamilton BE. Martin JA, Ventura SJ. Births preliminary data for 2010: Natl Vital Stat Rep. 2011. January 9, 2012. www.cdc.gov/nchs/data/nvsr/nvsr60/nvsr

Holmgren C, Scott JR, Porter TF, Esplin MS, Bardsley T. Uterine rupture with attempted vaginal birth after cesarean delivery. *Obstet Gynecol* 2012;119:725–31.

Landon MB. Vaginal birth after cesarean delivery. *Clin Perinatol* 2008;35:491–504.

Landon MB, Hauth JC, Leveno KJ, *et al.* Maternal and perinatal outcomes associated with a trial of labor after prior cesarean delivery. *N Engl J Med* 2004;351:2581–9.

Lauria MR, Flanagan V, Capeless E. Why VBAC in Northern New England is still viable: the Northern New England perinatal quality improvement network. *Clin Obstet Gynecol* 2012;55(4):1021–5.

Lavin JR Jr., Dipasquale L, Crane S, Stewart J Jr,. A statewide assessment of the obstetric, anesthesia, and operative team personnel who are available to manage the labors and deliveries and to treat the complications of women who attempt vaginal birth after cesarean delivery. *Am J Obstet Gynecol* 2002;187:611–4.

Scott JR. Intrapartum management of trial of labour after caesearean delivery: evidence and experience. *BJOG* 2014;120:157–62.

Scott JR. Vaginal birth after cesarean delivery: a common sense approach. *Obstet Gynecol* 2011;118:342–50.

Srinivas SK, Stamillo DM, Stevens EJ, *et al.* Predicting failure of a vaginal birth attempt after cesarean delivery. *Obstet Gynecol* 2007;109:800–5.

Silver RM, Landon MB, Rouse DJ, *et al.* Maternal morbidity associated with multiple repeat cesarean deliveries. *Obstet Gynecol* 2006;107:1226–32.

PROTOCOL 53

Placenta Accreta

Robert M. Silver
Department of Obstetrics & Gynecology, Division of Maternal-Fetal Medicine, University of Utah Health Sciences Center, Salt Lake City, UT, USA

Overview and clinical significance

Placenta accreta occurs when the placenta becomes abnormally adherent to the myometrium rather than the uterine decidua. After delivery, the placenta does not easily separate from the uterus, leading to potentially life-threatening hemorrhage. If the placenta actually invades the myometrium it is termed placenta increta. If it invades through the uterine serosa or into organs adjacent to the uterus it is termed placenta percreta. In many circumstances and within this protocol, the term placenta accreta is used to describe accretas, percretas and incretas interchangeably as a single disease spectrum.

Placenta accreta is associated with considerable maternal morbidity including the common need for large volume blood transfusion, need for hysterectomy, intensive care unit (ICU) admission, infection, and prolonged hospitalization. Hemorrhage may be fatal and can lead to disseminated intravascular coagulation (DIC) and multi-organ failure. Fetal risks are similar to those for placenta previa and mostly consist of the complications of preterm birth.

Rates of placenta accreta are dramatically increasing, primarily due to the increase in the rate of cesarean delivery (see Pathophysiology and risk factors section below). The incidence has increased from a reported 1 in 30,000 in the 1960s to 1 in 533 in 2002. It may even be higher now. Every practitioner of obstetrics should be familiar with the risk factors, diagnosis and management of this increasingly common and life-threatening condition.

Pathophysiology and risk factors

The pathophysiology of placenta accreta remains somewhat uncertain. Under normal circumstances, trophoblast invades into the decidua,

Protocols for High-Risk Pregnancies: An Evidence-Based Approach, Sixth Edition.
Edited by John T. Queenan, Catherine Y. Spong and Charles J. Lockwood.
© 2015 John Wiley & Sons, Ltd. Published 2015 by John Wiley & Sons, Ltd.

behaving somewhat like a cancer. Once the cytotrophoblast cells reach a certain level, termed Nitabuch's layer (or spongiosus layer of the decidua), they stop invading and differentiate. After cesarean delivery there may be a failure to reconstitute the endometrium or decidua basalis. Thus, if the placenta implants over the uterine scar from a prior cesarean, cytotrophoblast does not receive the normal "stop" signal and keeps invading to an abnormal degree. Histology reveals trophoblast invading into myometrium without intervening decidua.

Relative hypoxia in the cesarean scar also may play a role in the development of accreta. Hypoxia stimulates cytotrophoblast invasion; these cells differentiate once they reach the spiral arterioles and increased oxygen tension. However, the cesarean scar is relatively avascular, acellular and hypoxic, promoting further invasion. In fact, the relative hypoxia of the scar may actually preferentially allow for the development of the early embryo, perhaps explaining why previas and accretas are more common in women with multiple cesareans.

Regardless of the pathophysiology, it is clear that the overwhelming risk factor for placenta accreta is *multiple prior cesarean* deliveries. The vast majority of women with accreta have had at least one prior cesarean delivery and the risk increases with the number of cesarean deliveries. Women having their fourth or fifth cesarean have over a 2% chance of accreta and the risk increases to almost 7% in those having their sixth or greater cesarean. The combination of placenta previa and prior cesarean dramatically increases the risk since the placenta overlies the uterine scar. A recent large cohort study estimates the risk of accreta in women with previa to be 3%, 11%, 40%, 61%, and 67% for first, second, third, fourth and fifth or more cesarean deliveries, respectively. Indeed, women with two or more prior cesareans and a placenta previa are at extreme risk for placenta accreta. Since the rate of cesarean deliveries continues to escalate, the rate of placenta accreta will increase as well.

Prior uterine surgery such as uterine curettage, myomectomy, or hysteroscopic surgery is another risk factor for placenta accreta. Patients who develop Asherman syndrome after uterine curettage (or for any reason) are at especially high risk for accreta. Other risk factors include prior endometrial ablation, uterine artery or fibroid embolization, prior accreta and pelvic irradiation. In short, anything that might affect the normal architecture of the endometerial cavity increases the odds of accreta. Demographic risk factors include advanced maternal age and increasing parity. Also, placenta previa alone, even without prior cesarean, is a risk factor for accreta.

Diagnosis

The gold standard for the diagnosis of placenta accreta is histological examination of the placenta and uterus. Of course, this is only possible when a hysterectomy is performed. Although it is controversial, a clinical diagnosis of accreta may be made in cases of abnormally adherent placenta if a hysterectomy is not performed.

In order to optimize outcomes, it is highly desirable to diagnose placenta accreta prior to delivery. The best-studied modality for antenatal diagnosis is ultrasonography. The sensitivity of ultrasonography for the diagnosis of accreta has been reported to be 80–90% and the specificity for excluding the condition is 98%. It is important to note that almost all published studies have been conducted in women wherein there was a high index of suspicion (and major risk factors) for accreta. Thus, ultrasound may be less accurate for the identification of accreta in low-risk populations. Also, reported studies have been conducted in tertiary care centers with expertise in obstetric sonogram. Results may not be widely reproducible and there is evidence that prediction of accreta based on sonogram is considerably worse in "real world" circumstances. Also, there is considerable inter-observer variability with regard to the interpretation of ultrasound images for the prediction of accreta.

The single most helpful finding on sonogram is to determine whether or not there is a placenta previa (Protocol 48 "Third trimester bleeding" covers this topic in more detail). If there is no previa, the risk for accreta is substantially less. In cases of normal placentation, there is a very uniform, homogenous appearance to the placenta and the bladder wall. In addition, there is a distinct echolucent zone (termed the myometrial zone) between the placenta and the bladder wall. In cases of accreta, there is a loss or disruption in the continuity of the echolucent myometrial zone. Also, there may be a disruption in the continuity of the bladder wall and sometimes the placenta will actually protrude into the bladder. The placenta may have irregularly shaped vascular spaces, termed lacunae, giving the placenta a "Swiss cheese" appearance. Finally, there may be increased vascularity in the placenta–bladder interface or turbulence within the lacunae that can be demonstrated with Doppler velocimetry. Lacunae and turbulent flow are the findings most consistently associated with accreta.

Magnetic resonance imaging (MRI) also has been used for the antenatal diagnosis of accreta. In centers with an interest and expertise, MRI has been reported to have a sensitivity of over 90% and a specificity of 99% for the diagnosis of accreta. Also, MRI may delineate the extent of placental invasion into adjacent organs more clearly than ultrasonography. However, performance has been substantially worse in centers without such expertise. At present, it is probably best to consider MRI as an adjunctive tool for the diagnosis of accreta unless there is expertise in your center.

Several maternal blood tests have the potential to diagnose accreta. For the most part these are markers of placental damage or abnormal placental development. Examples include elevated levels of alpha-fetoprotein, free fetal DNA, placental mRNA, beta-human chorionic gonadotropin and creatinine kinase. Although of interest, none of these tests are recommended for clinical use at present.

Complications

The primary risk of placenta accreta is hemorrhage and associated complications such as DIC and multi-organ failure. In one recent series of 76 cases, blood transfusion was required in over 80% of cases and transfusion of 4 units or more of packed red blood cells in over 40% of cases. Twenty-eight percent had DIC. Another series reported an average blood loss of 3000 mL and an average transfusion of 10 units of packed red blood cells.

The most common surgical complication is cystotomy. True rates are hard to ascertain since many reports include cases of intentional cystotomy. Ureteral injury has been reported in 10–15% of cases. Less common injuries occur to bowel, large vessels and pelvic nerves. Other relatively frequent morbidities include wound, abdominal and vaginal cuff infections and the need for a second operation (most often to control bleeding or treat infection).

Between one-quarter to one-half of patients require admission to the ICU. Rates of associated complications such as pyelonephritis, pneumonia, and thromboembolism are increased. Maternal deaths may occur and have been reported in up to 7% of cases. Outcomes are influenced by the severity of the case (e.g., percreta) and the expertise of the center caring for the patient. There assuredly is under-reporting of this complication from centers seeing a low volume of the condition. Vesicovaginal fistula is an important late complication of cesarean hysterectomy for accreta.

Finally, perinatal morbidity is increased. This is primarily due to prematurity. However, maternal hemorrhage may lead to compromised fetal oxygenation/perfusion and associated complications. One series reported a perinatal death rate of 9%, although fetal outcomes are better in more recent cohorts.

Management

The most important consideration for the management of accreta is prenatal diagnosis. This allows for the most advantageous obstetric management and a reduction in morbidity. In turn, antenatal diagnosis requires a high index of suspicion based on risk factors. This is especially true for women with multiple prior cesareans, placenta previa, and Asherman syndrome.

There are no randomized clinical trials delineating the optimal obstetric management of accreta. The following recommendations are based on retrospective studies and expert opinion. Ideally, delivery should be accomplished in a hospital with a state-of-the-art blood bank, anesthesiologists experienced in critically ill patients and surgeons with experience in treating accreta and the ability to perform retroperitoneal dissection and bladder, ureteral and bowel surgery. Indeed, outcomes are improved in cases managed by a multidisciplinary team in tertiary care centers with appropriate expertise and experience. In some cases, hemorrhage is life-threatening in spite of the most optimal planning, surgeons and facilities. Placenta accretas are among the most difficult obstetric conditions to treat and require the utmost respect and preparation.

The optimal timing of delivery for patients with placenta accreta also is uncertain. Outcomes are better when delivery is scheduled under optimal circumstances. The later the gestational age, the more likely a woman with accreta is to have vaginal bleeding, labor, or both. Accordingly, medically indicated late preterm birth prior to the onset of labor or bleeding is indicated. However, the optimal gestational age that balances the risks of prematurity with preterm birth versus the chances of bleeding or labor prompting an emergency delivery under suboptimal circumstances is unknown. A decision analysis estimates the best timing of delivery to be 34 weeks of gestation. Ideally, it will be possible to individualize the optimal timing of delivery in each case. For example, women with bleeding and or labor should deliver a bit earlier while those without bleeding or labor may deliver later in gestation.

Antepartum obstetric care (suspected accreta)

1 Obstetric sonogram to assess the probability of accreta.
2 Consideration of MRI to assess the probability of accreta.
3 Pelvic rest.
4 Consideration of bed rest and/or hospitalization in cases of antepartum bleeding.
5 Administration of corticosteroids to enhance fetal pulmonary maturity in cases of antepartum bleeding at the time of hospital admission.
6 If there is no antepartum bleeding, empiric administration of corticosteroids to enhance fetal pulmonary maturity at 34 weeks of gestation.
7 Consultation with the patient and her family to discuss delivery options, risks of the disease, potential complications, and impact of treatment on fertility.
8 Consultation with a multidisciplinary team to plan the delivery (see below).
9 In cases without antepartum bleeding, delivery at 34–35 weeks of gestation is advised. It is not necessary to assess fetal pulmonary maturity with amniocentesis.

10 In cases with episodic bleeding, delivery between 32 and 34 weeks of gestation is advised, depending upon the severity of bleeding.

11 Heavy bleeding may require earlier delivery.

Surgical (suspected accreta)

1 Care should be provided with a multidisciplinary team. This should include surgeons with experience in accreta, critical care specialists, anesthesiologists, and blood bank specialists. Gynecological oncologists are ideal because of their experience with bladder and ureteral surgery in addition to difficult pelvic surgery. Interventional radiologists and vascular surgeons should be available.

2 If all of the requirements under (1) are not available, consider transfer to a center with appropriate expertise.

3 If possible, the case should be performed in the "main" operating room rather than in the labor and delivery unit. In most centers the staff in the "main" operating room is considerably more experienced with the care of critically ill patients than labor and delivery personnel.

4 Adequate blood products should be available. Ideally, this should include 20 units of packed red blood cells and fresh frozen plasma and 12 units of platelets. Additional blood products should be available in reserve. Recombinant activated factor VII also should be available.

5 A vertical skin incision should be made, regardless of prior abdominal or pelvic scars. A Cherney incision is a reasonable alternative.

6 General anesthesia should be used. It is reasonable to use a regional anesthetic for the delivery of the infant, followed by general anesthetic for the hysterectomy in stable patients.

7 The patient should be kept warm and a (relatively) normal pH maintained.

8 Strong consideration should be given to preoperative placement of ureteral stents. Our group has found this to be extremely helpful with minimal risk.

9 Consideration should be given to using an autologous blood salvage device. Although there are theoretical risks of contamination with amniotic fluid, blood obtained with a cell saver at time of cesarean delivery appears to be safe for maternal transfusion.

10 Consideration should be given to preoperative placement of either regular or balloon catheters in the uterine arteries. These can be infused with material for embolization or the balloons inflated after the delivery of the fetus. In turn, this may decrease blood loss at the time of hysterectomy or allow for the avoidance of hysterectomy (see below). Alternatively, catheters can be placed and only used if needed. This practice is controversial and serious adverse events with balloon placement have been reported.

11 Ideally, in cases of strongly suspected accreta, planned cesarean hysterectomy should be accomplished. A classical hysterotomy that does not compromise the placenta should be used to deliver the infant. *No attempt should be made to remove the placenta.* Placental removal has the potential to dramatically increase the risk of life-threatening hemorrhage. The hysterotomy should be quickly sutured to achieve some measure of hemostasis, followed by hysterectomy. If the case is difficult to accomplish or if the patient is unstable, consideration should be given to supracervical hysterectomy.

12 Umbrella packs or other tamponade devices such as a Bakri balloon should be available.

13 Consideration may be given to hypogastric artery ligation. Our group has not found this to be helpful.

14 Consideration may be given to leaving the placenta in situ, closing the hysterotomy, and planning a "delayed" hysterectomy in 6 weeks. In theory, this may allow some of the enhanced vascularity associated with pregnancy to regress, facilitating the hysterectomy. This approach has been advocated in women with percretas to avoid bladder resection. Our group has not found this to be helpful.

Surgical (unsuspected accreta)

1 Once an accreta is recognized, help should be summoned. This should include surgeons with experience in accreta, critical care specialists, anesthesiologists, and blood bank specialists. Gynecological oncologists are ideal because of their experience with bladder and ureteral surgery in addition to difficult pelvic surgery. Interventional radiologists and vascular surgeons should be considered.

2 If the surgeon or medical center is not capable of caring for the patient, consideration should be given to performing a stabilizing procedure and transferring the patient to an appropriate center for definitive therapy. This may require packing the abdomen to control bleeding, transfusion, and medical stabilization of the patient. This is not always possible.

3 If labor and delivery personnel are uncomfortable with the case, personnel from the main operating room should be recruited. Instruments and equipment may need to be obtained from the main operating room as well.

4 The blood bank should be alerted to the need for adequate blood products. Many hospitals have a massive transfusion protocol. If so, this should be activated. Recombinant activated factor VII also should be available.

5 If a Pfannenstiel incision is used, a Mallard or Cherney incision can be used to allow better pelvic access.

6 The patient should be kept warm and a (relatively) normal pH maintained.

7 Consideration should be given to converting to general anesthesia.

8 Consideration should be given to using an autologous blood salvage device. Although there are theoretical risks of contamination with amniotic fluid, blood obtained with a cell saver at the time of cesarean delivery appears to be safe for maternal transfusion.

9 The hysterotomy should be quickly sutured to achieve some measure of hemostasis, followed by hysterectomy. If the case is difficult to accomplish or if the patient is unstable, consideration should be given to supracervical hysterectomy.

10 Umbrella packs or other tamponade devices such as a Bakri balloon should be available.

11 Consideration may be given to hypogastric artery ligation. Our group has not found this to be helpful.

12 Consideration may be given to leaving the placenta in situ, closing the hysterotomy, and planning a "delayed" hysterectomy in 6 weeks. In theory, this may allow some of the enhanced vascularity associated with pregnancy to regress, facilitating the hysterectomy. This approach has been advocated in women with percretas to avoid bladder resection. Our group has not found this to be helpful.

Conservative management

There is an obvious and understandable desire on the part of some families with placenta accreta to preserve fertility. Numerous strategies have been employed in an attempt to avoid hysterectomy in cases of accreta and several successful cases have been reported. These include leaving the placenta in situ after delivery, surgical uterine devascularization, embolization of the uterine vessels, uterine compression sutures, oversewing of the placental vascular bed and the use of methotrexate to inhibit trophoblast growth and hasten postpartum involution of the placenta. However, our experience with attempted conservative management has been poor. In many cases, attempted conservative management delays but does not prevent hysterectomy. However, the delay may result in increased morbidity. For example, cases wherein the placenta is left in situ have led to severe infection and uncontrolled hemorrhage. Also, it is likely that complications of attempts at conservative management are under-reported in published literature. Finally, the risk of obstetric complications including recurrent accreta in subsequent pregnancies is uncertain. In contrast, there are increasing numbers of accreta cases that have been managed conservatively with good reported success rates. In addition, some authorities advocate performing a delayed hysterectomy to decrease bleeding and associated complications. Hence, the issue remains a matter of debate. Women desiring preservation of fertility should be closely monitored and extensively counseled regarding the risks. Cases that may be relatively amenable to attempts at conservative management include posterior placenta previa/accreta, fundal accreta, and cases when the diagnosis of accreta is uncertain.

Prevention

The best strategy to avoid placenta accreta is to avoid multiple cesarean deliveries. In turn, the best strategy to avoid multiple cesarean deliveries is to avoid primary cesarean delivery. Also, vaginal birth after cesarean delivery should be available for appropriate candidates.

It is possible that alterations in the surgical technique for cesarean delivery may reduce the risk of accreta in subsequent pregnancies. For example, a two-layer versus one-layer closure of the hysterotomy may facilitate reconstitution of the decidua basalis. A variety of other surgical techniques and/or the use of topical agents may promote revascularization of the cesarean scar. As the cesarean rate continues to rise, this should be an active area of investigation.

Follow up

The patient should be offered a postpartum visit at 1–2 weeks to assess surgical complications and emotional well-being and to offer support. Patients often go through a difficult time trying to recover from a major surgery and illness while trying to care for their infant. Also, there is often a period of anger and mourning for their lost fertility and their inability to choose when this would occur. Counseling may be helpful and should be offered. Another visit should be scheduled at 6 weeks postpartum. Women who did not have a hysterectomy should be advised that the risk in subsequent pregnancies is uncertain. Close monitoring and careful preparation for possible recurrent accreta seems prudent in subsequent pregnancies.

Conclusion

Placenta accreta is an increasingly common cause of major maternal morbidity and mortality. The most important risk factor is multiple prior cesarean deliveries. Patients with identified risk factors should be evaluated with obstetric sonogram by a specialist familiar with the condition. In cases of suspected accreta, care should be delivered by a multidisciplinary team in a large center with a state-of-the-art blood bank. Planned cesarean hysterectomy should be scheduled under optimal circumstances prior to the onset of hemorrhage.

Suggested reading

Bowman ZS, Eller AG, Kennedy AM, Richards DS, Winter TC, Woodward PJ, Silver RM. Accuracy of ultrasound for the prediction of placenta accreta. *Am J Obstet Gynecol* 2014 Aug;211(2):177.e1–7. doi: 10.1016/j.ajog.2014.03.029. Epub 2014 Mar 14.

Bowman ZS, Manuck TA, Eller AG, Simons M, Silver RM. Risk factors for unscheduled delivery in patients with placenta accreta. *Am J Obstet Gynecol* 2013;210(3): 241.e1–241.e6.

Comstock CH, Bronsteen RA. The antenatal diagnosis of placenta accreta. *BJOG* 2014;121:171–82.

Eller AG, Bennett Michele A, Sharshiner R, Masheter C, Soisson AP, Dodson M, Silver RM. Maternal morbidity in cases of placenta accreta managed by a multidisciplinary care team compared to standard obstetrical care. *Obstet Gynecol* 2011;117:331–7.

Eller AG, Porter TF, Soisson P, Silver RM. Optimal management strategies for placenta accreta. *Br J Obstet Gynaecol* 2009;116:648–54.

Flood KM, Said S, Geary M, Robson M, Fitzpatrick C, Malone FD. Changing trends in peripartum hysterectomy over the past 4 decades. *Am J Obstet Gynecol* 2009;200:632.e1–632.e6.

Khan M, Sachdeva P, Arora R, Bhasin S. Conservative management of the morbidly adherent placenta – a case report and review of the literature. *Placenta* 2013;34:963–6.

Silver RM, Landon MB, Rouse DJ, Leveno KJ, Spong CY, Thim EA, *et al.* Maternal morbidity associated with multiple repeat cesarean deliveries. *Obstet Gynecol* 2006;107:1226–32.

Wright JD, Pri-Paz S, Herzog T, *et al.* Predictors of massive blood loss in women with placenta accreta. *Am J Obstet Gynecol* 2011;205:38.e1–6.

Wortman AC, Alexander JM. Placenta accreta, increta, and percreta. *Obstet Gynecol Clin N Am* 2013;40:137–54.

PROTOCOL 54

Shoulder Dystocia

Robert Gherman
Division of Maternal Fetal Medicine, Frannklin Square Medical Center, Baltimore, MD, USA

Overview

All healthcare providers attending vaginal deliveries must be prepared to handle this unpredictable obstetric emergency. Knowledge of the maneuvers employed for the alleviation of shoulder dystocia is relevant not only for obstetric residents and attending house staff, but also for family practitioners, nurses and nurse midwives. The reported incidence varies in the literature, ranging from 0.2% to 3.0%.

Pathophysiology and diagnosis

In a normal delivery after expulsion of the fetal head, external rotation occurs, returning the head to a right angle position in relation to the shoulder girdle. The fetal shoulder during descent is in an oblique pelvic diameter. After expulsion and restitution, the anterior fetal shoulder should emerge from the oblique axis under the pubic ramus.

Shoulder dystocia represents the failure of delivery of the fetal shoulder(s), whether it be the anterior, posterior or both. Shoulder dystocia results from a size discrepancy between the fetal shoulders and the pelvic inlet. A persistent anterior–posterior location of the fetal shoulders at the pelvic brim may occur with a large fetal chest relative to the biparietal diameter (e.g., an infant of a diabetic mother) or when truncal rotation does not occur (e.g., precipitous labor). Shoulder dystocia typically occurs when the descent of the anterior shoulder is obstructed by the pubic symphysis. It can also result from impaction of the posterior shoulder on the maternal sacral promontory.

The retraction of the fetal head against the maternal perineum accompanied by difficulty in accomplishing external rotation has been called the "turtle sign." Most authors have defined shoulder dystocia to include those

Protocols for High-Risk Pregnancies: An Evidence-Based Approach, Sixth Edition.
Edited by John T. Queenan, Catherine Y. Spong and Charles J. Lockwood.
© 2015 John Wiley & Sons, Ltd. Published 2015 by John Wiley & Sons, Ltd.

Table 54.1 Risk (%) for shoulder dystocia based on fetal weight, diabetic status, and method of delivery

Fetal weight (kg)	Nondiabetic	Diabetic: spontaneous delivery	Diabetic: assisted delivery
4–4.25	5	8	12
4.26–4.5	9	12	17
4.51–4.75	14	20	27
4.76–5	21	24	35

deliveries requiring maneuvers in addition to gentle downward traction on the fetal head to effect delivery. Several studies have proposed defining shoulder dystocia as a prolonged head-to-body delivery interval (60 seconds) and/or the use of ancillary obstetric maneuvers.

The risk of shoulder dystocia increases significantly as birth weight increases; it must be remembered, however, that approximately 50% to 60% of shoulder dystocias occur in infants weighing less than 4000 g. Even if the birth weight of the infant is over 4000 g, shoulder dystocia will only complicate 3.3% of the deliveries.

No single associated condition or combination of antenatal factors, however, allows for clinically useful positive predictive values for shoulder dystocia. Risks for shoulder dystocia based on known (but not estimated) fetal weight are listed in Table 54.1.

Management

There are no randomized clinical trials to guide physicians in the order of maneuvers that are to be performed. A single randomized trial assessing prophylactic usage of the McRoberts maneuver showed no difference in head-to-body delivery times. The best evidence available shows fetal injury to be associated with all described maneuvers to relieve shoulder dystocia.

The length of delay that results in permanent brain injury will depend on the condition of the fetus at the time that the shoulder dystocia is diagnosed. It may be as short as 3 to 4 minutes, or as long as 15 to 20 minutes. Most, if not all, of the commonly encountered shoulder dystocia episodes can be relieved within several minutes.

1 The patient should be instructed to stop pushing as soon as the shoulder dystocia is initially recognized.
2 Maternal expulsive efforts will need to be restarted after the fetal shoulders have been converted to the oblique diameter, in order to complete the delivery.

3 Additional assistance may be obtained by summoning other obstetricians, an anesthetist or anesthesiologist, additional nursing support, or a pediatrician.

4 Ask someone to note the time.

5 The McRoberts maneuver is typically used as the first technique for shoulder dystocia alleviation. This can be done by having the patient grasp her posterior thighs and flexing the legs against her abdomen or by having birth attendants (or family members) flex the patient's legs in a similar position. McRoberts' position causes cephalic rotation of the pubic symphysis and flattening of the sacrum. Care should be taken to avoid prolonged or overly aggressive application of McRoberts.

6 Suprapubic pressure, commonly administered by nursing personnel, is typically used immediately prior to or in direct conjunction with the McRoberts maneuver. This pressure is usually directed posteriorly, but other described techniques have included lateral application from either side of the maternal abdomen or alternating between sides using a rocking pressure.

7 If these techniques fail to accomplish delivery, attempt to deliver the posterior arm. Posterior arm extraction replaces the biacromial diameter with the axilloacromial diameter, thereby reducing the obstructing diameter in the pelvis. Pressure should be applied at the antecubital fossa in order to flex the fetal forearm. The arm is subsequently swept out over the infant's chest and delivered over the perineum. Rotation of the fetal trunk to bring the posterior arm anteriorly is sometimes required. Grasping and pulling directly on the fetal arm, as well as application of pressure onto the mid-humeral shaft, should be avoided as bone fracture may occur.

8 If after delivery of the posterior fetal arm, delivery of the baby cannot be accomplished, perform rotation of the posterior shoulder 180° to the anterior position while simultaneously rotating the anterior shoulder 180° to the posterior position. If the fetus is facing the mother's right side, rotation should be attempted in a counterclockwise direction as a first step.

9 Some physicians are more comfortable attempting fetal rotational maneuvers before attempting to deliver the posterior arm. In the Woods corkscrew maneuver, the practitioner attempts to abduct the posterior shoulder by exerting pressure onto its anterior surface. In the Rubin (reverse Woods) maneuver, pressure is applied to the posterior surface of the most accessible part of the fetal shoulder (either the anterior or posterior shoulder). If the anterior shoulder is tightly wedged underneath the symphysis pubis, it may be necessary to push the fetus slightly upward in order to facilitate the rotation.

10 Shoulder dystocia is considered to be a "bony dystocia" and therefore episiotomy alone will not release the impacted shoulder. The need for cutting a generous episiotomy or proctoepisiotomy must be based on clinical circumstances, such as a narrow vaginal fourchette in a nulliparous patient.

11 Attendants should refrain from applying fundal pressure as a maneuver for the alleviation of shoulder dystocia. Pushing on the fundus serves only to further impact the anterior shoulder behind the symphysis pubis. Fundal pressure can be employed to assist with delivery of the fetal body, but only if the shoulder dystocia has already been alleviated.

12 Providers should use downward axial traction, which is a pulling force (traction) applied in alignment with the fetal cervico-thoracic spine. This is typically along a 25–45° vector below the horizontal plane when the woman is in a lithotomy position. The provider should not attempt to rotate the fetal head.

Extraordinary maneuvers

If neither rotational maneuvers nor extraction of the posterior arm is possible, bilateral shoulder dystocia or posterior arm shoulder dystocia may be present. In this case, the anterior arm is lodged behind the symphysis pubis and/or the posterior shoulder is lodged high in the pelvis at or near the sacral promontory. Under these circumstances, consideration should be given to "heroic" maneuvers.

Gaskin maneuver

The mother's position is rotated 180° from the supine position to one in which the mother is positioned on her hands and knees, with the maternal back pointing toward the ceiling. This change in maternal position is thought to allow for a change in fetal position within the maternal pelvis. An attempt is now made to deliver the posterior shoulder by downward (toward the floor) traction followed by delivery of the anterior fetal shoulder by gentle upward traction.

Cephalic replacement (Zavanelli maneuver)

The fetal head is rotated back to a pre-restitution occiput anterior position and then gently flexed. Constant firm pressure is used to push the fetal head back into the vagina and cesarean delivery is subsequently performed. Halothane or other general anesthetics, in conjunction with tocolytic agents, may be administered. Oral or intravenous nitroglycerin may be used as well.

Abdominal rescue

A low transverse uterine incision can be performed, the anterior shoulder manually rotated into the oblique diameter by the surgeon doing the uterine incision, and vaginal delivery accomplished. This requires at least two skilled delivery attendants and should rarely be used.

Symphysiotomy

This should be performed only as a last-ditch effort to deliver a neurologically intact fetus. It is rarely used in the United States.

Documentation

Documentation of delivery maneuvers and the sequence of these maneuvers is an essential part of patient care and risk management. The use of a pre-printed form listing important elements is suggested for use in cases of shoulder dystocia, regardless of apparent fetal injury at the time of delivery.

Suggested documentation for shoulder dystocia

- When and how shoulder dystocia was diagnosed.
- Inform patient that shoulder dystocia has occurred.
- Position and rotation of infant's head.
- Which shoulder was anterior.
- Presence of episiotomy, if performed.
- Estimate of head-to-body time interval.
- Estimation of force of traction applied.
- Order, duration, and results of maneuvers employed.
- Additional medical personnel present for assistance.
- Birth weight.
- 1-minute and 5-minute Apgar scores.
- Venous and/or arterial umbilical cord blood gas evaluation.

Suggested reading

American College of Obstetricians and Gynecologists. Shoulder dystocia. ACOG Practice Bulletin No. 40. *Obstet Gynecol* 2002;100:1045–50 (Reaffirmed 2013).

American College of Obstetricians and Gynecologists. *Neonatal brachial plexus palsy*. Washington, DC: American College of Obstetricians and Gynecologists; 2014.

Crofts JF, Fox R, Ellis D, Winter C, Hinshaw K, Draycott TJ. Observations from 450 shoulder dystocia simulations: lessons for skills training. *Obstet Gynecol* 2008;112:906–12.

Gherman RB, Chauhan S, Ouzounian JG, Lerner H, Gonik B, Goodwin TM. Shoulder dystocia: the unpreventable obstetric emergency with empiric management guidelines. *Am J Obstet Gynecol* 2006;195:657–72.

Gherman RB, Ousounian JG, Goodwin TM. Obstetric maneuvers for shoulder dystocia and associated fetal morbidity. *Am J Obstet Gynecol* 1998;178:1126–30.

Hoffman MK, Bailit JL, *et al.* A comparison of obstetric maneuvers for the acute management of shoulder dystocia. *Obstet Gynecol* 2011;117:1272–78.

Hope P, Breslin S, Lamont L, *et al.* Fatal shoulder dystocia: a review of 56 cases reported to the Confidential Enquiry into Stillbirths and Deaths in Infancy. *Br J Obstet Gynaecol* 1998;105:1256–61.

MacKenzie IZ, Shah M, Lean K, Dutton S, Newdick H, Tucker DE. Management of shoulder dystocia: trends in incidence and maternal and neonatal morbidity. *Obstet Gynecol* 2007;110:1059–68.

Nesbitt TS, Gilbert WM, Herrchen B. Shoulder dystocia and associated risk factors with macrosomic infants born in California. *Am J Obstet Gynecol* 1998;179:476–80.

Ouzounian JG, Gherman RB. Shoulder dystocia: Are historic risk factors reliable predictors? *Am J Obstet Gynecol* 2005;192:1933–38.

Poggi SH, Spong CY, Allen RH. Prioritizing posterior arm delivery during severe shoulder dystocia. *Obstet Gynecol* 2003;101:1068–72.

Spong CY, Beall M, Rodrigues D, *et al.* An objective definition of shoulder dystocia: prolonged head-to-body delivery intervals and/or the use of ancillary obstetric maneuvers. *Obstet Gynecol* 1995;86:433–6.

PROTOCOL 55

Twins, Triplets and Beyond

Mary E. D'Alton
Department of Obstetrics and Gynecology, Columbia University College of Physicians and Surgeons, New York Presbyterian Hospital, New York, NY, USA

Clinical significance

Compared to singletons, multifetal pregnancies are associated with higher risks for both maternal and fetal complications. Women carrying multiples are at risk for a number of pregnancy complications in both the antepartum and postpartum period including preeclampsia, anemia, cholestasis and, although rare, acute fatty liver is also more common in multifetal pregnancies. It is unclear whether gestational diabetes occurs more commonly in multifetal pregnancies. Although multiple gestations represent only a fraction of all pregnancies in the United States, they account for a disproportionate amount of infant deaths. The increased risk of perinatal morbidity and mortality results largely from preterm delivery, intrauterine growth restriction (IUGR), and congenital anomalies. Given the maternal and fetal risks, patients carrying multiples require close monitoring and frequent follow up throughout pregnancy as well as careful planning of delivery.

Pathophysiology

Multiple gestations result either from the fertilization of multiple ova or from the division of a single fertilized ovum or early embryo into more than one fetus. The terms "monozygotic" and "dizygotic" refer to the number of ova responsible for a multiple gestation. A monozygotic pregnancy results from a single fertilized ovum that splits into two or more distinct fetuses. By definition, monozygotic pregnancies are genetically identical. In contrast, dizygotic pregnancies originate from the fertilization of two separate ova and are therefore genetically dissimilar.

The frequency of monozygotic twins is constant worldwide at 4 per 1000 births. In contrast, the frequency of dizygotic twins varies by maternal age,

Protocols for High-Risk Pregnancies: An Evidence-Based Approach, Sixth Edition.
Edited by John T. Queenan, Catherine Y. Spong and Charles J. Lockwood.
© 2015 John Wiley & Sons, Ltd. Published 2015 by John Wiley & Sons, Ltd.

parity, family history, maternal weight, nutritional state, race and the use of infertility drugs. In the United States, two-thirds of spontaneously occurring twins are dizygotic and one-third are monozygotic.

The frequency of dizygotic twinning is increased with increasing serum concentrations of follicle-stimulating hormone (FSH) and luteinizing hormone (LH). As a result of these higher gonadotropin levels, multiple ovulations can occur in a single menstrual cycle, increasing the likelihood of dizygotic twinning. Gonadotropin levels fluctuate depending on maternal age, weight, nutrition, parity, and heredity. For these reasons, both infertility treatments and advanced maternal age are associated with increased frequency of dizygotic twinning.

Placentation

It is clinically important to determine the placentation, chorionicity, and amnionicity of multiple pregnancies. Dizygotic pregnancies are by definition dichorionic–diamniotic. Chorionicity of monozygotic gestations is determined by the time at which division of the fertilized ovum/eralyembryo occurred and can be dichorionic–diamniotic, monochorionic–diamniotic or monochorionic–monoamniotic.

In the United States, 20% of twin pregnancies are monochorionic and approximately 80% are dichorionic. Determination of chorionicity in multiple gestations is essential for proper management of the pregnancy. Approximately 20% of monochorionic–diamniotic twin gestations are complicated by twin–twin transfusion syndrome, whereas monochorionic–monoamniotic gestations are at risk of conjoining or cord entanglement.

Diagnosis

Delayed diagnosis of multiple gestations can result in an increased risk of complications. Therefore, early diagnosis is essential.

1 *Clinical examination.* Multifetal gestations should be suspected if the uterine size is greater than expected or if multiple fetal heart tones are detected.
2 *Maternal serum alpha-fetoprotein.* Multiple gestations should be excluded if an elevated level of maternal serum alpha-fetoprotein is noted on second trimester serum screening.
3 *Ultrasonography.* Ultrasonography can be used to diagnose multiple gestations in the first trimester as well as later in gestation. In the first trimester, visualization of two distinct gestational sacs suggests a dichorionic twin gestation. Visualization of a single gestational sac with two fetal poles and two yolk sacs suggests a monochorionic–diamniotic twin

gestation. Visualization of a single gestational sac with two fetal poles but one yolk sac suggests a monochorionic–monoamniotic twin pregnancy. Later in gestation, ultrasonography can be used to determine the number of fetuses, the number of placentas, and fetal sex, and to assess the presence and thickness of a dividing membrane.

Determining chorionicity

1 *Placental number.* If two placental disks are seen, the pregnancy is dichorionic.
2 *Fetal sex.* If the fetuses are opposite sex, the pregnancy is dichorionic.
3 *Dividing membrane.* If the membrane is thick (greater than 2 mm) or has three to four visible layers, consider dichorionic–diamniotic as most likely. Visualization of a triangular projection of placenta between the layers of the dividing membrane (known as the twin peak or lambda sign) is also useful in diagnosis of dichorionicity, but its absence is not a reliable predictor of monochorionicity. If membrane is thin, consider monochorionic–diamniotic. Consider a monochorionic–monoamniotic gestation if no membrane is seen.
4 *Postpartum.* Confirm chorionicity by examining the placenta after delivery, including gross and histological examination.
  Among same-sex dichorionic gestations, genetic studies are required to definitively determine zygosity.

Management

Antepartum

Early ultrasonography
Ultrasonography should be performed early in gestation to confirm pregnancy dating and to assess chorionicity. If a fetal size discrepancy is noted, use biometry of the larger fetus for dating purposes.

Medications and nutritional requirements
Women carrying multiples should be counseled regarding the additional caloric and nutritional requirements. The American College of Obstetricians and Gynecologists recommends daily intake of 300 kcal more than with a singleton gestation, and a total weight gain of 35–45 pounds for women with a normal prepregnancy body mass index. Daily folic acid (1 mg) and elemental iron (60 mg) is recommended in addition to a daily prenatal vitamin.

Prenatal diagnosis

Aneuploidy screening. In dizygotic twin pregnancies, each fetus has its own independent risk of aneuploidy and, therefore, the chance of at least one abnormal fetus is increased. Both first and second trimester serum markers are approximately twice as high in twin pregnancies as in singleton pregnancies. Interpretation of abnormal serum screening results is difficult because it is not possible to determine which of the fetuses is responsible for the abnormal analyte concentration. Nuchal translucency measurement, which assesses each fetus independently, is a reasonable alternative to serum testing for aneuploidy screening in multiple gestations. Although cell-free fetal DNA testing can be used as a tool for aneuploidy screening among high-risk women with singleton gestations, there is currently insufficient data to recommend its use in multiple gestations.

Maternal serum alpha-fetoprotein screening to determine neural tube defect (NTD) risk. Maternal serum alpha-fetoprotein levels are approximately double in twins compared to singletons. A level greater than 4.0 MoM in twins is associated with an increased risk of neural tube and ventral wall defects and should be addressed with a detailed sonographic survey of these structures. Amniocentesis is offered if an open defect is suspected or ultrasound examination is inadequate.

Prenatal diagnosis. All women, regardless of age, should be counseled about the option for either screening or diagnostic testing for fetal aneuploidy. Amniocentesis may be performed on one sac only if monozygosity is certain. Otherwise, amniocentesis for karyotype should be done on all sacs. Genetic amniocentesis in multiples is usually performed using an ultrasound-guided multiple-needle approach. Indigo carmine dye may be used to confirm proper needle placement. Although pregnancy loss rates after genetic amniocentesis in twins has been considered similar to singletons, recent literature suggests an increased risk of loss after amniocentesis of twin gestations. Chorionic villus sampling offers the advantage of earlier diagnosis, and can be performed between 10 and 13 weeks with a loss rate similar to amniocentesis.

Congenital anomalies. Careful sonographic assessment of fetal anatomy is indicated in multifetal pregnancies because congenital anomalies are three to five times more common in monozygotic twins compared with singletons or dizygotic twins and dizygotic pregnancies are at increased risk compared with singletons because there are two fetuses. Anomalies unique to monozygotic gestations include acardia and conjoined twins. If one fetus in a multiple gestation has a major malformation, selective termination of the affected fetus may be offered with the technique varying with chorionicity.

Preterm birth prevention

Preterm birth occurs in more than 40% of twin and 75% of triplet gestations. Ultrasound surveillance of cervical length and fetal fibronectin testing can identify those multiple gestations at increased risk of preterm delivery. A transvaginal measurement of cervical length of less than 2.5 cm at 24 weeks is associated with an increased risk of preterm delivery before 32 weeks (odds ratio, 6.9). Similarly, a positive FFN at 28 weeks is associated with an increased risk of preterm delivery before 32 weeks (odds ratio, 9.4).

There is no evidence that prophylactic cervical cerclage, bed rest, outpatient uterine monitoring, or long-term use of prophylactic tocolytic agents are effective in preventing preterm labor or prolonging pregnancy in multiple gestations. Similarly, prophylactic progesterone has not been shown to decrease the rate of preterm birth among twin gestations.

Patient education regarding the early signs of preterm labor in multiple gestations is important. Cervical length should be measured every 2 weeks from 16 to 24 weeks in multiple gestations thought to be at highest risk for preterm delivery. Tocolysis should be reserved for women with documented preterm labor, and may be administered to allow administration of antenatal steroids. Antenatal steroids should be administered if preterm delivery is expected within 7 days and the gestational age is between 24 and 34 weeks. Magnesium sulfate is also recommended for neuroprotection before anticipated delivery before 32 weeks of gestation.

Diabetes screening

Unless individual risk factors warrant earlier screening, a glucose challenge test is recommended at 24 to 28 weeks to screen for gestational diabetes. If positive, a 3-hour glucose tolerance test should be performed to establish diagnosis of gestational diabetes.

Fetal growth assessment

Serial ultrasonography is the most accurate method to assess fetal growth in multiple gestations. Serial ultrasonographic examinations should be performed every 3–4 weeks beginning at approximately 20 weeks of gestation. Singleton growth charts may be used. Discordance should be expressed as a percentage of the larger fetal weight.

Antepartum testing

Routine antepartum testing of multiple gestations has not been shown to have benefit. However, surveillance with nonstress testing or biophysical profile is recommended for multiple gestations complicated by discordant.

Doppler velocimetry may also be used to evaluate fetal well-being in multiple gestations complicated by significant growth restriction or discordance.

Delivery
Timing of delivery
Perinatal mortality rates among dichorionic twin pregnancies nadir at approximately 38 weeks, and at approximately 35 weeks for triplet gestations. Elective delivery of dichorionic twins at 38 weeks and of uncomplicated triplet gestations at 36 weeks is therefore warranted. There is increasing evidence that, even in the setting of intensive fetal surveillance, there is a significant risk of fetal death at each gestational age in monochorionic twin gestations. Accordingly, elective delivery of uncomplicated monochorionic twins can be considered after 34 weeks and should be completed by 37 weeks of gestation. In all cases of elective preterm delivery, providers should offer a detailed discussion of the associated risks and benefits.

Mode of delivery
Several factors must be evaluated to determine the route of delivery for a patient with multiple gestations including gestational age, estimated fetal weight (EFW), fetal presentation and availability of an obstetric provider skilled in assisted breech deliveries and total breech extractions (Table 55.1).

Vertex/vertex. It is reasonable to plan for vaginal delivery for all EFWs.

Vertex/nonvertex. Route of delivery should be determined by EFWs and provider experience. In our practice, trial of labor with possible external cephalic version or breech extraction is offered if the EFW of both fetuses is greater than 1500 g and there is less than 20% discordance. If the EFW of either fetus is less than 1500 g or if there is more than 20% discordance (with B greater than A), external cephalic version can be attempted

Table 55.1   Frequency of presentation

Vertex/vertex	40%
Vertex/breech	26%
Breech/vertex	10%
Breech/breech	10%
Vertex/transverse	8%
Miscellaneous	6%

Source: Creasy *et al.*, 1994. Reproduced with permission of Elsevier.

of the second twin, but – if version is unsuccessful – cesarean delivery is performed.

Nonvertex/vertex or nonvertex/nonvertex. Cesarean delivery is indicated for all fetal weights if the presenting twin is nonvertex.

Triplets and beyond. The optimal mode of delivery is not clear; while elective caesarean is often performed, trial of labor may be considered by experienced providers.

Other considerations

Continuous electronic fetal monitoring should be used throughout labor.

The use of prostaglandins for induction and oxytocin for induction or augmentation of labor is acceptable in twin gestations.

If a trial of labor is elected, epidural anesthesia should be recommended to allow a full range of obstetric interventions to be performed if needed.

If vaginal delivery is attempted, an operating room should be available at all times, given the potential need for emergent cesarean delivery of one or both twins.

If vaginal delivery is attempted, ultrasonography should be available to evaluate position of twin B after delivery of twin A.

Twin gestation is not a contraindication to VBAC (vaginal birth after cesarean delivery).

Complications

Maternal and fetal complications of multifetal pregnancies are listed in Tables 55.2 and 55.3.

Specific complications
Monoamniotic pregnancies

Monoamniotic gestations are associated with increased perinatal mortality secondary to cord entanglement. Consider administering steroids and delivery by cesarean delivery at 32–34 weeks of gestation. Delivery should be considered earlier if there is any evidence of IUGR or significant discordance accompanied by abnormal nonstress test, biophysical profile, or Doppler studies.

Twin–twin transfusion

Occurs only in monochorionic pregnancies as a result of arteriovenous communications. Ultrasound diagnosis requires presence of a single placenta, gender concordance, and amniotic fluid discordance (polyhydramniotic recipient/oligohydramniotic donor); may be accompanied by abnormal umbilical artery Dopplers and hydrops or cardiac dysfunction. Perinatal

Table 55.2 Maternal complications in multifetal pregnancies

Hyperemesis

Urinary tract infection

Anemia

Cholestasis

Gestational diabetes*

Preeclampsia

HELLP syndrome

Acute fatty liver of pregnancy

Placental abruption

Placenta previa

Vasa previa

Preterm labor

Preterm premature rupture of membranes

Cesarean delivery

Postpartum hemorrhage

*There are conflicting reports as to whether or not twin and triplet gestations are associated with a higher rate of gestational diabetes.

Table 55.3 Fetal complications in multifetal pregnancies

Vanishing twin

Congenital anomalies

Intrauterine growth restriction

Discordant growth

Umbilical cord entanglement (monoamniotic gestations)

Twin transfusion syndrome (monochorionic gestations)

Prematurity

Perinatal mortality

Locking twins (nonvertex/vertex presentation)

mortality occurs in up to 70% of cases. Treatment includes selective laser photocoagulation of communicating vessels, septostomy, or serial amnioreduction. Intensive fetal surveillance should be performed when viability is reached.

Single fetal demise
Incidence of fetal death of one twin after 20 weeks ranges from 2.6% to 6.8% and may be as high as 17% in triplets and higher-order multiples. The

concept of an increased risk of clinically significant maternal coagulopathy after demise of one fetus of a multiple gestation has been refuted and generally is not accepted. It is reasonable to obtain baseline platelet count, prothrombin time, activated partial thromboplastin time and fibrinogen level; if normal, no further surveillance is necessary. The main risk to the surviving fetus is prematurity. Due to the common occurrence of vascular anastomoses in monochorionic pregnancies, acute hemodynamic changes associated with the demise of one fetus renders an approximately 20% risk of multicystic encephalomalacia in the viable twin. Delivery after single fetal demise does not improve outcome. Continue antenatal surveillance including nonstress testing and serial ultrasonographic examination for assessment of fetal growth and cervical length. MRI of fetal brain approximately 2 weeks after single fetal demise may help to determine the presence of cerebral injury in the surviving twin.

Prevention

Over the last several decades, the twin birth rate in the United States has increased every year, to a rate of over 30 per 1000 total births. The number of triplet, quadruplet and higher-order multiple births increased over 400% before peaking in recent years. The two major factors accounting for these increases are the widespread availability of assisted reproductive technologies and increasing maternal age at childbirth.

Multifetal pregnancy reduction

The goal of multifetal pregnancy reduction is to reduce the number of live fetuses present in the uterus and thereby decrease the risk of preterm delivery in multiple gestations. The procedure is usually performed transabdominally by injecting potassium chloride into the fetal thorax. Multifetal pregnancy reduction is usually performed between 9 weeks and 13 weeks of gestation. Although the benefit of the procedure for triplet gestation remains controversial, the majority of multifetal pregnancy reduction procedures are performed to reduce triplets to twins. A large series of 1000 cases demonstrated that the pregnancy loss rate before 24 weeks remained constant at about 5.4% in the hands of an experienced operator with the starting number of fetuses ranging from 2 to 5. Those pregnancies finishing with two or three fetuses delivered at similar gestational ages as nonreduced twins and triplets.

Selective termination

The management options available in the event of discovering an abnormality of one fetus is often an important consideration in the decision-making process involved in formulating a screening and/or diagnostic strategy. These options are expectant management (do nothing), termination of the pregnancy (both abnormal and normal fetuses), or selective termination of the abnormal fetus or fetuses. Among dichorionic gestations, selective termination is usually performed by transabdominal fetal intracardiac injection of potassium chloride. Among monochorionic gestations, selective termination can be performed using radiofrequency ablation of the cord of the anomalous twin or using other methods of cord ligation. Results of a large series of 200 cases demonstrated an overall pregnancy loss rate of 4%. Factors affecting pregnancy loss included a greater number of starting fetuses and reduction of more than one fetus.

Conclusion

Twin gestations and higher-order multifetal pregnancies comprise a significant proportion of births in the United States. Given the risk of both maternal and fetal complications, close surveillance of maternal and fetal status throughout gestation is warranted. Early confirmation of pregnancy dating and sonographic diagnosis of chorionicity are important to assess risk of specific complications. Timing of delivery should be determined based on chorionicity, and mode of delivery should be determined by gestational age, fetal weight, intertwin discordance and fetal presentation.

Suggested reading

American College of Obstetricians and Gynecologists. Screening for fetal chromosomal abnormalities. ACOG Practice Bulletin No. 77. *Obstet Gynecol* 2007;109:217–27.

American College of Obstetricians and Gynecologists. Noninvasive prenatal testing for fetal aneuploidy. Committee Opinion No. 545. *Obstet Gynecol* 2012;120:1532–4.

American College of Obstetricians and Gynecologists. Multifetal gestations: twin, triplet, and higher-order multifetal pregnancies. Practice Bulletin No. 144. *Obstet Gynecol* 2014;123:1118–32.

Barrett JF, Hannah ME, Hutton EK, Willan AR, Allen AC, Armson BA, Gafni A, Joseph KS, Mason D, Ohlsson A, *et al.* A randomized trial of planned cesarean or vaginal delivery for twin pregnancy. *N Engl J Med* 2013 Oct 3;369(14):1295–305.

D'Alton ME, Dudley DK. The ultrasonographic prediction of chorionicity in twin gestation. *Am J Obstet Gynecol* 1989;160:557.

D'Alton ME. Delivery of the second twin: revisiting the age-old dilemma. *Obstet Gynecol* 2010 Feb;115(2 Pt 1):221–2.

Fox NS, Silverstein M, Bender S, Klauser CK, Saltzman DH, Rebarber A. Active second-stage management in twin pregnancies undergoing planned vaginal delivery in a U.S. population. *Obstet Gynecol* 2010 Feb;115(2 Pt 1):229–33.

Goldenberg RL, Iams JD, Miodovnik M. National Institute of Child Health and Human Development Maternal-Fetal Medicine Units Network. The preterm prediction study: Risk factors in twin gestations. *Am J Obstet Gynecol* 1996;175:1047.

Kahn B, Lumey H, Zybert PA, *et al.* Prospective risk of fetal death in singleton, twin, and triplet gestations: implications for practice. *Obstet Gynecol* 2003;102:685.

Lee YM, Cleary-Goldman J, Thaker HM, *et al.* Antenatal sonographic prediction of twin chorionicity. *Am J Obstet Gynecol* 2006;195:863.

Malone FD, D'Alton ME. Multiple gestation: clinical characteristics and management. In: Creasy RK, (ed.) *Creasy and Resnik's Maternal-Fetal Medicine: Principles and Practice.* 7th ed. Philadelphia, PA: Saunders/Elsevier; 2014.

MacLennan AH. Multiple gestation: clinical characteristics and management. In: Creasy RK, Resnik R, (ed.) *Maternal-Fetal Medicine: Principles and Practice.* Philadelphia, PA: WB Saunders; 1994. p 589–601.

Robinson BK, Miller RS, D'Alton ME, Grobman WA. Effectiveness of timing strategies for delivery of monochorionic diamniotic twins. *Am J Obstet Gynecol* 2012 Jul;207(1):53.e1–7.

Senat MV, Deprest J, Boulvain M, Paupe A, Winer N, Ville Y. Endoscopic laser surgery versus serial amnioreduction for severe twin-to-twin transfusion syndrome. *N Engl J Med* 2004;351:136.

Vink J, Fuchs K, D'Alton ME. Amniocentesis in twin pregnancies: a systematic review of the literature. *Prenat Diagn* 2012 May;32(5):409–16.

PROTOCOL 56
Postpartum Hemorrhage

David S. McKenna
Maternal-Fetal Medicine, Miami Valley Hospital, Dayton, Ohio, USA

Clinical significance

Postpartum hemorrhage (PPH) is defined as blood loss greater than 500 cc at the time of vaginal delivery or greater than 1000 cc at the time of cesarean. The estimation of blood loss is often inaccurate, and an alternative definition is excessive bleeding that makes the mother symptomatic. Worldwide obstetric hemorrhage is the most common cause of maternal mortality, with approximately one women dying every 4 minutes as a result of obstetric bleeding. In the United States, hemorrhage affects 1–5% of deliveries, and is consistently the second or third most common cause of maternal mortality. In addition to mortality, obstetric hemorrhage often results in significant maternal morbidity.

Pathophysiology

There are several physiological adaptations to pregnancy that facilitate the maternal response to hemorrhage and coagulation. These changes include a 15–30% increase in red blood cell mass, a 40–60% increase in circulating plasma volume, increased fibrinogen, Factors VII, VIII, IX, X, XII and von Willebrand Factor, and decreased protein S. With excessive blood loss, hypovolemic shock develops and there is risk of hypoperfusion and end organ damage. Due to the physiological adaptations of pregnancy, the maternal response to hypovolemia may be delayed and blunted. Maternal comorbidity (e.g., cardiac disease) may accelerate the effects of hypovolemia.

Bleeding is normally controlled after vaginal or cesarean delivery by myometrial contraction and the activation of local decidual hemostatic factors. Defects in either of these mechanisms along with genital tract

Protocols for High-Risk Pregnancies: An Evidence-Based Approach, Sixth Edition.
Edited by John T. Queenan, Catherine Y. Spong and Charles J. Lockwood.
© 2015 John Wiley & Sons, Ltd. Published 2015 by John Wiley & Sons, Ltd.

Table 56.1   Risk factors for postpartum hemorrhage

Prolonged labor

Augmented labor

Rapid labor

Hypertension in pregnancy

Maternal treatment with magnesium sulfate, or other tocolytic agents

Uterine overdistension – macrosomia, multiple gestation, hydramnios

Operative vaginal delivery

Chorioamnionitis

History of postpartum hemorrhage in prior pregnancy or antepartum hemorrhage in current

Grand multiparity

Fetal demise

Maternal obesity – BMI more than 35 kg/m^2

Uterine factors – prior surgery, leiomyomas

Abnormal placentation – accretas, previa

Asian ethnic origin

Source: ACOG Practice Bulletin No. 76, 2006; Gabbe *et al.*, 2012; Green-top Guideline. Royal College of Obstetricians and Gynecologists. No. 52, 2009.

lacerations lead to PPH. PPH is categorized as either primary or early occurring within 24 hours, or secondary or late occurring later than 24 hours from delivery. Primary PPH is most commonly due to uterine atony defined as a failure of the myometrium to effectively contract following delivery. Risk factors for PPH are listed in Table 56.1. Uterine atony occurs in 4–6% of pregnancies and accounts for 80% of primary PPH. Other etiologies for primary PPH include retained placenta, lacerations, coagulation defects, and uterine inversion. Secondary PPH is most commonly due to infection (endomyometritis) or retained products of conception. Subinvolution of the placental site and inherited coagulation defects may also cause secondary PPH.

With sufficient hemorrhage, the maternal cardiac output eventually decreases along with oxygen delivery to the tissues. Compensatory mechanisms include vasoconstriction, increasing peripheral vascular resistance, and increasing the heart rate in order to maintain the cardiac output and diastolic blood pressure. With decreased tissue perfusion, there is the release of vasoactive substances including histamine, bradykinin, beta-endorphins, prostanoids, and cytokines. These affect membrane permeability and promote loss of fluid into the interstitium. In addition, hypoperfusion results in anaerobic metabolism and the production of lactic acid. The clinical effects include multi-organ dysfunction and, often, massive third spacing of fluid.

Diagnosis

It is important for providers caring for laboring and postpartum women to provide vigilant attention to maternal blood loss and vital signs. A high index of suspicion for hemorrhage and shock, and a low threshold for implementing treatment should be maintained. It is useful to classify hemorrhage by the amount of lost circulating volume and maternal vital signs as listed in Table 56.2. Once the diagnosis of PPH is established, evaluation, initiation of treatment, and a call for assistance should occur simultaneously. The provider should vigorously perform bimanual uterine massage, expel clots from the uterus, and empty the urinary bladder. The perineum, vagina, cervix, and uterus are assessed for lacerations, hematomas, and retained products of conception. The uterine decidua should be wiped clean with a sponge or bluntly curettaged with a large curette. This requires adequate anesthesia, lighting, instruments, assistance, and proper patient positioning. Ultrasound may be useful for examining the uterus. Early transfer to the operating room may facilitate establishing the diagnosis and management. Uterine atony should only be diagnosed once other etiologies have been excluded.

Treatment

Many evidence-based resources exist to assist in optimizing the outcome in obstetrical hemorrhage. There are two common underlying themes: checklist-based protocols and multidisciplinary team drills. It is believed that a systematic implementation of toolkits for obstetric hemorrhage will prevent many cases of maternal mortality. The reader is encouraged to review one, such as the California maternal quality care collaborative

Table 56.2 Classification of hemorrhage

	Class 1	Class 2	Class 3	Class 4
Blood loss volume (mL)	15%	15–30%	30–40%	40% or more
	900	1200–1500	1800–2100	2400
Pulse rate	<100	>100	>120	>140
Signs/symptoms	None	↑RR	Hypotension	Profound shock
		+/− Orthostasis	Hypoperfusion	Oliguria
		↓Pulse pressure		

Based on a circulating blood volume of 6000 mL. RR, respiratory rate.

(CMQCC) hemorrhage toolkit (https://www.cmqcc.org/ob_hemorrhage). A focused algorithm is depicted in Fig. 56.1.

Volume resuscitation, and treatment by medical, conservative surgical, and definitive (i.e., hysterectomy) surgical techniques, must be concurrent. Aggressive volume resuscitation is normally appropriate unless the mother has an underlying condition such as a cardiomyopathy, which would contradict a large volume infusion. Initially a volume of isotonic crystalloid, such as lactated Ringers, should be given in a ratio of 3:1 to the estimated blood loss. Colloid solutions such as albumin have not been demonstrated to be superior to crystalloid. If there is not an immediate cessation of the bleeding, preparation for blood product replacement should begin, and consideration given to initiating a massive transfusion protocol (MTP). MTPs are standardized protocols that transfuse preemptively with blood products using a balanced ratio of plasma and platelets to red blood cells. These protocols have effectively replaced the traditional approach of delaying replacement of plasma and platelets until deficiencies were demonstrated by laboratory analysis. It may be necessary to transfuse blood that is either type O-negative or type-specific while the transfusion protocol is being instituted.

In addition to MTPs, battlefield and trauma experience have given rise to other helpful agents that are not universally available. These include recombinant Factor VII, fibrinogen concentrate, and tranexamic acid which are given intravenously; as well as topical hemostatic agents such as topical thrombin, fibrin sealant, gelatin matrix, chitosan-covered gauze, and oxidized regenerated cellulose.

The level of intervention is based upon the classification of hemorrhage and the maternal response. Unless there is another obvious etiology, empiric treatment for uterine atony should be initiated with medical therapy (Table 56.3), oxygen, and uterine massage. If the bleeding continues, then activation of a predefined obstetric emergency response team should be initiated when PPH is diagnosed, or when there are clinical signs (i.e., Class 2). At a minimum the team should consist of sufficient nursing personnel to complete all necessary tasks, an anesthesia provider, the blood bank, the laboratory, and obstetric assistants. Baseline labs should be obtained, along with a red top tube for a clot test. If the red top tube clots within 6 minutes and does not lyse within 30 minutes, the fibrinogen level may be assumed to be greater than 150 mg/dL.

Preservation of fertility is the main advantage of conservative surgical intervention. Also, the likelihood of surgical morbidity will be less if hysterectomy can be avoided. However, fertility preservation must always come second to preservation of life. Therefore, when there is ongoing significant hemorrhage and the mother exhibits signs of hypovolemic shock (Class 2 hemorrhage or greater), it is imperative that hysterectomy

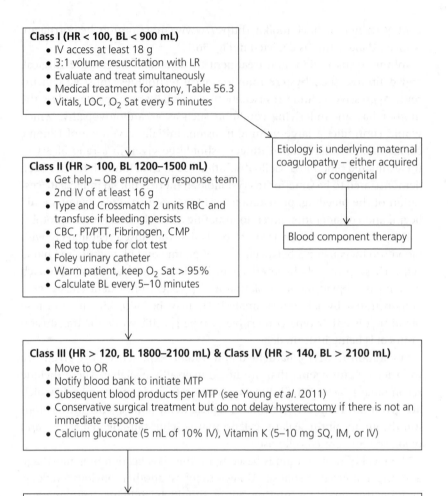

Class I (HR < 100, BL < 900 mL)
- IV access at least 18 g
- 3:1 volume resuscitation with LR
- Evaluate and treat simultaneously
- Medical treatment for atony, Table 56.3
- Vitals, LOC, O_2 Sat every 5 minutes

Etiology is underlying maternal coagulopathy – either acquired or congenital

Class II (HR > 100, BL 1200–1500 mL)
- Get help – OB emergency response team
- 2nd IV of at least 16 g
- Type and Crossmatch 2 units RBC and transfuse if bleeding persists
- CBC, PT/PTT, Fibrinogen, CMP
- Red top tube for clot test
- Foley urinary catheter
- Warm patient, keep O_2 Sat > 95%
- Calculate BL every 5–10 minutes

Blood component therapy

Class III (HR > 120, BL 1800–2100 mL) & Class IV (HR > 140, BL > 2100 mL)
- Move to OR
- Notify blood bank to initiate MTP
- Subsequent blood products per MTP (see Young *et al.* 2011)
- Conservative surgical treatment but do not delay hysterectomy if there is not an immediate response
- Calcium gluconate (5 mL of 10% IV), Vitamin K (5–10 mg SQ, IM, or IV)

Still bleeding with unrelenting coagulopathy?
- Consider risks and benefits of recombinant Factor VII
- Fibrinogen concentrate, Tranexamic acid – may consider if available
- Topical hemostatic agents
- Pre-hysterectomy – apply clamps, sponges, and pressure, then resuscitate
- Post-hysterectomy – pack the pelvis, leave incision open, complete resuscitation in the ICU, re-operate in 24 hours

Figure 56.1 Algorithm for postpartum hemorrhage. HR, heart rate; BL, blood loss; IV, intravenous; LR, lactated Ringers; LOC, level of consciousness; RBC, red blood cells; CBC, complete blood count; PT/PTT, prothrombin time and partial thromboplastin time; CMP, comprehensive metabolic panel; OR, operating room; MTP, massive transfusion protocol; SQ, subcutaneous; IM, intramuscular; ICU, intensive care unit.

Table 56.3 Medical treatment for uterine atony

Drug	Dose	Timing	Notes
Oxytocin	20–40 Units in 500–1000 mL Lactated Ringers	Usually given prophylactically after third stage	Rapid Infusion
Methylergonovine	200 µg IM	May repeat every 2–4 hours, maximum five doses	Avoid with hypertension; use caution if ephedrine has been given
Prostaglandin F2α	250 µg IM	May repeat every 20 minutes, maximum eight doses	Avoid with asthma; use caution with hypertension
Prostaglandin E1	1000 µg per rectum or sublingual	One time only	Well tolerated
Prostaglandin E2	20 mg per rectum	May repeat 2 hours	Avoid with hypotension

not be delayed. When to proceed with a hysterectomy is a judgment decision and it is generally best to err on the side of early hysterectomy.

The choice of conservative surgical procedures will depend upon the mode of delivery. After a vaginal delivery, uterine tamponade can be achieved with either an inflatable balloon (e.g., SOS Bakri Balloon™, or Foley catheter) or an intestinal bag packed with laparotomy sponges. Selective arterial embolization (SAE) by interventional radiology may be used after a vaginal delivery. This technique is best when the mother has been sufficiently resuscitated, is hemodynamically stable, any coagulopathy has been reversed, and she continues to have slow bleeding not necessitating definitive surgical intervention. There are additional conservative surgical interventions that may be attempted after cesarean delivery or after a vaginal delivery if a laparotomy is performed. These consist of uterine compression sutures (e.g., the B-Lynch compression suture), uterine, ovarian, and internal iliac artery ligation, and oversewing of the placental site in cases of invasive placentation. All conservative surgical procedures carry the risk of continued hemorrhage and worsening coagulopathy while hysterectomy is delayed. Finally, if there is an unrelenting coagulopathy, it may be lifesaving to pack the pelvis with laparotomy sponges, after completing a hysterectomy, or to apply clamps, sponges and pressure prior to a hysterectomy. This will permit catch up resuscitation. The mother may be moved to the intensive care unit, and the coagulopathy corrected there. The sponges and instruments can be removed in 24 hours, and any persistent bleeding is usually easily managed surgically or may be treated by SAE.

Complications

Women with PPH are more likely to require transfusion of blood products and the associated risks for infection and transfusion reaction, to have post-operative febrile morbidity, admission to an intensive care unit, respiratory morbidity, incidental injury to the urinary or gastrointestinal system, renal tubular or pituitary necrosis, and loss of fertility. Infants born to women with PPH, particularly those secondary to abnormal placentation are often delivered early and are at risk for complications from prematurity.

Follow up

Once the bleeding has subsided, the maternal condition must be watched closely. This involves serial assessment of vital signs, urinary output, and laboratory studies. General goals are to maintain the systolic blood pressure greater than 90 mmHg, the hematocrit at 30% or higher, and the urine output at least 30 mL per hour (or 0.5 mL/kg/hour). Attention must be paid to the respiratory and cardiovascular status, as large volume resuscitation with crystalloid will result in large shifts of fluid out and back into the intravascular space. There may be a role for vasopressors or diuretics depending on the clinical scenario. Consultation and collaboration with an intensive care specialist may help.

Prevention

In developed nations, an uterotonic medication is routinely given after delivery of the newborn or placenta to prevent PPH. Oxytocin when available is the agent of choice for prophylaxis in the third stage of labor. The practice of prophylactic uterotonics has proven to be effective in the prevention of PPH. The World Health Organization has recommended the practice be adopted in developing nations, even in deliveries attended by traditional birth attendants (www.who .int/reproductivehealth/publications/maternal_perinatal_health/ 9789241548502/en/).

In cases of placenta previa with a history of prior cesarean delivery, especially when there are sonographic findings suggestive of abnormal placental implantation, planned scheduled delivery may be beneficial. Simulation of and training for PPH will promote teamwork and may also improve outcomes.

Conclusion

PPH is best managed by a multidisciplinary team approach incorporating protocols for the evaluation and management of bleeding, and volume resuscitation and blood product replacement. All persons caring for obstetric patients should train and be equipped to respond to this obstetric emergency. Resources are available for assistance in developing a systematic response (see CMQCC OB Hemorrhage Toolkit and ACOG Patient Safety Checklist No. 10).

Suggested reading

American College of Obstetricians and Gynecologists. Postpartum hemorrhage. ACOG Practice Bulletin No. 76. *Obstet Gynecol* 2006;108:1039–47.

American College of Obstetricians and Gynecologists. Postpartum hemorrhage from vaginal delivery. Patient safety checklist No. 10. *Obstet Gynecol* 2013;121:1151–2.

California maternal quality care collaborative obstetric (OB) hemorrhage toolkit. https://www.cmqcc.org/ob_hemorrhage

Francois KE, Foley MR. Antepartum and postpartum hemorrhage. Gabbe SG, Niebyl JR, Simpson JL, *et al.*, (ed.) *Obstetrics: normal and Problem Pregnancies.* 6th Chapter 19, ed. Philadelphia: Saunders; 2012. p 415–444e5.

Rajan PV, Wing DA. Postpartum hemorrhage: evidenced-based medical interventions for prevention and treatment. *Clin Obstet Gynecol* 2010;53(1):165–181.

Royal College of Obstetricians and Gynecologists. Prevention and management of postpartum hemorrhage. Green-top Guideline. No. 52. 2009. http://www.rcog.org.uk/print/womens-health/clinical-guidance/prevention-and-management-postpartum-haemorrhage-green-top-52

World Health Organization. WHO recommendations for the prevention and treatment of postpartum hemorrhage. 2012. www.who.int/reproductivehealth/publications/maternal_perinatal_health/9789241548502/en/

Young PP, Cotton BA, Goodnough LT. Massive transfusion protocols for patients with substantial hemorrhage. *Transfus Med Rev* 2011;25(4):293–303.

APPENDIX A

Evaluation of Fetal Health and Defects

Lynn L. Simpson

Department of Obstetrics and Gynecology, Columbia University Medical Center, New York, NY, USA

Figures A.1–A.3 and Tables A.1–A.14

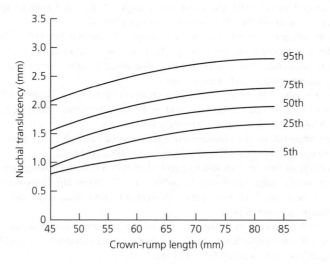

Figure A.1 Nuchal translucency measurements between 11 and 14 weeks of gestation. Nuchal translucency >95th percentile associated with risk of trisomy 21. Source: From Nicolaides KH, Sebire NJ, Snijders RJM. The 11–14 Week Scan. New York, Parthenon, 1999.

Protocols for High-Risk Pregnancies: An Evidence-Based Approach, Sixth Edition.
Edited by John T. Queenan, Catherine Y. Spong and Charles J. Lockwood.
© 2015 John Wiley & Sons, Ltd. Published 2015 by John Wiley & Sons, Ltd.

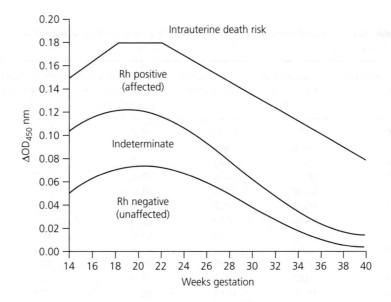

Figure A.2 Amniotic fluid ΔOD_{450} management zones. Source: From Queenan JT, Tomai TP, Ural SH, *et al*. Deviation in amniotic fluid optical density at a wavelength of 450 nm in Rh-immunized pregnancies from 14 to 40 weeks gestation: a proposal for clinical management. Am J Obstet Gynecol 1993;168:1370.

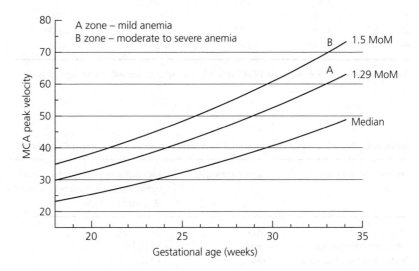

Figure A.3 Middle cerebral artery (MCA) Doppler peak velocities. Peak MCA Doppler velocity >1.5 MoM for gestational age predictive of fetal anemia. Source: From Moise KJ. Modern management of Rhesus alloimmunization in pregnancy. Obstet Gynecol 2002;100:600.

Table A.1 Estimated rates of karyotypic abnormalities related to maternal age at delivery

Maternal age (years)	Trisomy 21 at the time of live birth	At the time of amniocentesis	Any chromosomal abnormality at the time of live-birth	At the time of amniocentesis
20	1/1734	1/1231	1/526	–
25	1/1250	1/887	1/476	–
30	1/965	1/685	1/385	–
31	1/915	1/650	1/385	–
32	1/794	1/563	1/322	–
33	1/639	1/452	1/286	–
34	1/496	1/352	1/238	–
35	1/386	1/274	1/192	1/83
36	1/300	1/213	1/156	1/76
37	1/234	1/166	1/127	1/67
38	1/182	1/129	1/102	1/58
39	1/141	1/100	1/83	1/49
40	1/100	1/78	1/66	1/40
41	1/86	1/61	1/53	1/32
42	1/66	1/47	1/42	1/26
43	1/52	1/37	1/33	1/21
44	1/40	1/29	1/26	1/19
45	1/31	1/22	1/21	1/15
46	1/24	1/17	1/16	1/12
47	1/19	1/13	1/13	1/20
48	1/15	1/10	1/10	1/18
49	1/11	1/8	1/8	1/16

Source: Snijders et al. Prenat Diagn 1994;14(7): 543–52. Reproduced with permission of Wiley.

Table A.2 Significance of chromosomal microarray in fetuses with normal karyotype

Indication for prenatal diagnosis	Normal karyotype n	Pathogenic or potential for clinical significance chromosomal microarray abnormalities n (%)
Any	3822	96 (2.5%)
Advanced maternal age	1966	34 (1.7%)
Positive trisomy 21 screening	729	12 (1.6%)
Anomaly on ultrasound	755	45 (6.0%)
Other	372	5 (1.3%)

Source: Wapner et al., 2012. Adapted with permission of the Massachusetts Medical Society.

Table A.3 Frequency of chromosome aberrations in newborns.
(Modified from a summary of six surveys)

Aberration	Incidence	
Numerical		
Sex chromosomes		
47,XYY	1/1000	MB
47,XXY	1/1000	MB
Other (males)	1/1350	MB
45,X	1/10,000	FB
47,XXX	1/1000	FB
Other (female)	1/2700	FB
*Autosomal trisomies**		
No. 13 to 15 (group D)	1/20,000	LB
No. 16 to 18 (group E)	1/8000	LB
No. 21 to 22 (group G)	1/800	LB
Other	1/50,000	LB
Structural		
Balanced		
Robertsonian		
t(Dq; Dq)	1/1500	LB
t(Dq; Gq)	1/5000	LB
Reciprocal translocations and insertional inversions	1/7000	LB
Unbalanced		
Robertsonian	1/14,000	LB
Reciprocal and insertional	1/8000	LB
Inversions	1/50,000	LB
Deletions	1/10,000	LB
Supernumeraries	1/5000	LB
Other	1/8000	LB
Total	1/160	LB

FB, female births; LB, live births; MB, male births.
*Because most surveys did not use banding techniques, individual chromosomes within a group could not always be differentiated. However, group D trisomies are generally no. 13, group E no. 18, and group G no. 21.
Source: Adapted from Hook & Hamerton, 1977.

Table A.4 Available prenatal diagnosis for common disorders

Disorder	Mode of inheritance	Molecular diagnosis
α_1-Antitrypsin deficiency	AR	Determine PiZZ allele
α-Thalassemia	AR	α-Hemoglobin gene mutation
Adult polycystic kidney	AD	PKD1 and PKD2 gene mutations
β-Thalassemia	AR	β Hemoglobin gene mutation
Congenital adrenal hyperplasia	AR	CYP21A2 gene mutations and deletions
Cystic fibrosis	AR	CFTR gene mutation
Duchenne/Becker muscular dystrophy	XLR	Dystrophin gene mutation
Fragile X syndrome	XLR	CGG repeat number
Hemoglobinopathy (SS, SC)	AR	β-Chain gene mutation
Hemophilia A	XLR	Factor VIII gene inversion and mutations
Huntington disease	AD	CAG repeat number
Marfan syndrome	AD	Fibrillin (FBN-1) gene mutation
Myotonic dystrophy	AD	CTG expansion in the DMPK gene
Neurofibromatosis type 1	AD	NF1 gene mutation
Phenylketonuria	AR	Common mutations
Tay-Sachs disease	AR	Enzyme absence and gene mutation

AD, autosomal dominant; AR, autosomal recessive; XLR, X-linked recessive.
Source: Adapted from Wapner et al., 1977.

Table A.5 Relative timing and developmental pathology of certain malformations

System	Malformation	Embryology	Timing	Comment
Central nervous system	Anencephaly	Closure of anterior neural tube	26 days	Subsequent degeneration of forebrain
	Meningomyelocele	Closure in a part of posterior neural tube	28 days	80% lumbosacral
Face	Cleft lip	Closure of lip	36 days	42% with cleft palate
	Cleft maxillary palate	Fusion of maxillary palatal shelves	10 weeks	
	Branchial sinus and/or cyst	Resolution of branchial cleft	8 weeks	Preauricular; anterior to the sternocleidomastoid
Gastrointestinal	Esophageal atresia/tracheo-esophageal fistula	Lateral septation of foregut into trachea and foregut	30 days	

Table A.5 (*Continued*)

System	Malformation	Embryology	Timing	Comment
	Rectal atresia with fistula	Lateral septation of cloaca into rectum and urogenital sinus	6 weeks	
	Duodenal atresia	Recanalization of duodenum	7–8 weeks	Associated incomplete or aberrant mesenteric attachments
	Malrotation	Rotation of intestinal loop so cecum lies to the right	10 weeks	
	Omphalocele	Return of midgut from yolk sac to abdomen	10 weeks	
	Meckel diverticulum	Obliteration of vitelline duct	10 weeks	May contain gastric or pancreatic tissue
	Diaphragmatic hernia	Closure of pleuroperitoneal canal	6 weeks	Associated with lung hypoplasia
Genitourinary	Bladder exstrophy	Migration of infraumbilical mesenchyme	30 days	Associated mullerian and wolfian duct defects
	Bicornuate uterus	Fusion of lower part of mullerian ducts	10 weeks	
	Hypospadius	Fusion of urethral folds	12 weeks	
	Cryptorchidism	Descent of testes into scrotum	7–9 months	
Cardiac	Transposition of great vessels	Directional development of bulbus cordis septum	34 days	
	Ventricular septal defect	Closure of ventricular septum	6 weeks	
Limb	Aplasia of radius	Genesis of radial bone	38 days	Often accompanied by other defects of radial side of distal limb
	Syndactyly, severe	Separation of digital rays	6 weeks	

Source: Adapted from Jones, 2006. Reproduced with permission of Elsevier.

Table A.6   Prevalence of major cardiac defects by nuchal translucency thickness in chromosomally normal fetuses

Nuchal translucency	n	Major cardiac defects	Prevalence per 1000
<95th percentile	27,332	22	0.8
≥95th percentile–3.4 mm	1507	8	5.3
3.5–4.4 mm	208	6	28.9
4.–5.4 mm	66	6	90.0
≥5.5 mm	41	8	195.1
Total	29,154	50	1.7

Source: Hyatt *et al.*, 1999. Reproduced with permission of BMJ.

Table A.7   Screening for congenital heart disease: performance of current strategies

Approach	Prenatal detection rate of major congenital heart disease (%)
Four-chamber view	40–50
Four-chamber view and LVOT/RVOT	60–80
Four-chamber view and three vessels/trachea view	80
Fetal echocardiography	
Traditional risk factors alone	<20
Indication-based (risk factors and ultrasound)	50
Universal	>95

LVOT, left ventricular outflow tract; RVOT, right ventricular outflow tract.

Table A.8   Increased risk for neural tube defect (NTD)

Sibling with NTD	2%
Parent with NTD	2%
Sibling with spinal dysraphism	4%
Sibling with multiple vertebral anomalies	2%
Cousin with NTD	0.5%
Sibling with communicating hydrocephalus	1%
Elevated maternal serum alpha-fetoprotein	10%

Table A.9   Serial sonographic surveillance for twin pregnancies

Indication	Timing	Comment
Pregnancy dating	1st trimester	Optimal at 7–10 weeks using CRL
Determination of chorionicity	1st trimester	Close to 100% accuracy if done prior to second trimester
Nuchal translucency assessment	10–13 weeks	Increased with aneuploidy, malformations, TTTS
Anatomical survey	2nd trimester	Optimal at 18–22 weeks; fetal echocardiography for IVF twins and/or monochorionic twins
Placental evaluation	2nd trimester	Transvaginal imaging to exclude previa and vasa previa; color imaging for PCI
Baseline cervical length	2nd trimester	Transvaginal imaging optimal
Twin growth studies	2nd and 3rd trimester	Every 4 weeks for uncomplicated twins
Serial surveillance	2nd and 3rd trimester	Every 2 weeks for uncomplicated monochorionic twins; daily testing at viability for monoamniotic twins; frequency and type of testing of twins depends on chorionicity, risk, and complications

CRL, crown rump length; TTTS, twin–twin transfusion syndrome; IVF, in vitro fertilization; PCI, placental cord insertion.
Source: Simpson, 2013. Reproduced with permission of Elsevier.

Table A.10   Staging criteria for twin–twin transfusion syndrome

	Ultrasound parameter	Categoric criteria
Stage I	MVP of amniotic fluid	MVP <2 cm in donor sac; MVP >8 cm in recipient sac
Stage II	Fetal bladder	Nonvisualization of fetal bladder in donor twin over 60 minutes of observation
Stage III	Umbilical artery, ductus venosus, and umbilical vein Doppler waveforms	Absent or reversed umbilical artery diastolic flow, reversed ductus venosus a-wave flow, pulsatile umbilical vein flow
Stage IV	Fetal hydrops	Hydrops in one or both twins
Stage V	Absent fetal cardiac activity	Fetal demise in one or both twins

MVP, maximal vertical pocket
Source: Quintero et al., 1999. Reproduced with permission of Nature.

Table A.11   Drugs associated with congenital malformations in humans

Drug	Potential effects	Comments
ACE inhibitors	Calvarial hypoplasia, renal dysgenesis, oligohydramnios, IUGR, and neonatal renal failure	Risk increases with use in second and third trimester
Alcohol	Syndrome: prenatal and postnatalgrowth restriction, microcephaly, craniofacial dysmorphology (1–4/1000 live births); renal, cardiac, and other major malformations	Risk not limited to first trimester; late pregnancy use associated with IUGR and developmental delay; incidence of defects 4–44% among 'heavy drinkers'
Antidepressants (SSRIs)	Possible cardiac defects, NTD, omphalocele; neonatal pulmonary hypertension and withdrawal syndrome	–
Aminopterin and methotrexate	Syndrome: calvarial hypoplasia, craniofacial abnormalities, limb defects; possible developmental delay	Syndrome associated with methotrexate >10 mg/week
Androgens and norproges-terones	Masculinization of external female genitalia	Labioscrotal fusion can occur with exposure; up to 50% of those exposed are affected
Carbamazepine	NTD (1%); possible facial hypoplasia and developmental delay	–
Corticosteroids	Cleft lip/palate increased threefold to sixfold; IUGR increased with high doses	–
Diethylstilbestrol	Clear cell adenocarcinoma of the vagina, vaginal adenosis, abnormalities of the cervix and uterus, testicular abnormalities, and male/female infertility	–
Isotretinoin	Syndrome: CNS malformations, microtia/anotia, micrognathia, thymus abnormalities, cleft palate, cardiac abnormalities, eye anomalies, limb reduction defects (28%); miscarriage (22%), developmental delay (47%)	–
Lithium	Small increase in Ebstein cardiac anomaly	–
Penicillamine	Cutis laxa with chronic use	–
Phenytoin	Syndrome: IUGR, microcephaly, facial hypoplasia, hypertelorism, prominent upper lip (10%); possible developmental delay	Full syndrome in 10%; up to 30% exhibit some features
Streptomycin	Hearing loss, eighth nerve damage	–
Tetracycline	Discoloration of deciduous teeth and enamel hypoplasia	Risk only in second and third trimester

Table A.11 (*Continued*)

Drug	Potential effects	Comments
Tobacco	Oral clefts: relative risk, 1.22–1.34; IUGR, IUFD, abruption	–
Trimethadione	Syndrome: oral clefts, craniofacial abnormalities, developmental delay (80%)	–
Valproic acid	NTD (1–2%); facial hypoplasia, possible developmental delay	–
Warfarin	Syndrome: nasal hypoplasia, stippled epiphyses, growth restriction (6%); also increased microcephaly, Dandy-Walker syndrome, IUGR, preterm birth, mental retardation	Greatest risk at 6–9 weeks

ACE, angiotensin-converting enzyme; CNS, central nervous system; IUFD, intrauterine fetal demise; IUGR, intrauterine growth restriction; NTD, neural tube defect; SAB, spontaneous abortion, SSRIs, selective serotonin reuptake inhibitors.
Source: Chambers & Weiner, 2009. Reproduced with permission of Elsevier.

Table A.12 Food and Drug Administration categories for drug labeling

Category A	Well-controlled human studies have not disclosed any fetal risk. Possibility of fetal harm appears to be remote
Category B	Animal studies have not disclosed any fetal risk, or have suggested some risk not confirmed in controlled studies in women, or there are not adequate studies in women
Category C	Animal studies have revealed adverse fetal effects; there are no adequate controlled studies in women. Drugs should be given only if the potential benefit justifies the potential risk to the fetus
Category D	Evidence of human fetal risk, but benefits may outweigh risk (e.g., life-threatening illness, no safer effective drug). Patient should be warned of risk
Category X	Fetal abnormalities in animal and human studies; risk of the drug not outweighed by benefit. *Contraindicated in pregnancy*

The Food and Drug Administration has established five categories of drugs based on their potential for causing birth defects in infants born to women who use the drugs during pregnancy. By law, the label must set forth all available information on teratogenicity.

Table A.13 Hemolytic disease resulting from irregular antibodies

Blood group system	Antigen	Severity of hemolytic disease	Blood group system	Antigen	Severity of hemolytic disease
Rh subtype	C	+ to +++	Lutheran	Lua	+
	Cw	+ to +++		Lub	+
	c	+ to +++	Diego	Dia	+ to +++
	E	+ to +++		Dib	+ to +++
	e	+ to +++	P	P	
					+ to +++
Lewis	Lea	−		PPIPk (Tja)	+ to +++
	Leb	−			
I	I	−	Xg	Xga	+
Kell	K	+ to +++	Public antigens	Yta	+ to ++
	k	+		Ytb	+
	Ko	+		Lap	+
	Kpa	+		Ena	+ to +++
	Kpb	+		Ge	+
	Jsa	+		Jra	+
	Jsb	+		Coa	+ to +++
Duffy	Fya	+ to +++		Coab	+
	Fyb	−	Private antigens	Batty	+
	Fy3	+		Becker	+
Kidd	Jka	+ to +++		Berrens	+
	Jkb	+ to +++		Biles	+ to ++
	Jk3	+		Evans	+
MNSs	M	+ to +++		Gonzales	+
	N	−		Good	+ to +++
	S	+ to +++		Heibel	+ to ++
	s	+ to +++		Hunt	+
	U	+ to +++		Jobbins	+
	Mia	++		Radin	+ to ++
	Mta	++		Rm	+
	Vw	+		Ven	+
	Mur	+		Wrighta	+ to +++
	Hil	+		Wrightb	+
	Hut	+		Zd	+ to ++

−, not a proven cause of hemolytic disease of the newborn, no change in management.

+, mild, expectant management with no further diagnostic testing or intervention until delivery.

++, moderate, serial evaluations with middle cerebral Dopplers or amniotic fluid ΔOD_{450}.

+++, severe, serial evaluations with middle cerebral Dopplers or amniotic fluid ΔOD_{450}.

Source: Chambers & Weiner, 2009. Reproduced with permission of Lippincott Williams & Wilkins.

Table A.14   Fetal blood sampling

Test	Tube type	Minimum amount (mL)
Complete blood count, differential, reticulocyte count	Purple	0.3
Type and cross	Dry Bullet (Salmon)	0.5
Direct/indirect Coombs'	Dry Bullet (Salmon)	0.5
Total immunoglobulin M (IgM)	Red	0.5
Toxoplasma and cytomegalovirus CMV IgM	Red	0.5
Rubella IgM	Red	0.5
Parvovirus IgG and IgM	Red	1.0
CMV blood culture	Red	1.0
Bilirubin (total and direct)	Red	0.5
Total protein and albumin	Red	0.5
Chem-7	Red	0.5
Chem-20	Red	1.0
Kleihauer-Betke stain	Purple	0.5
Prothrombin time/partial thromboplastin time	Blue	1.8
Clotting factor level	Blue (on ice)	1.8
Venous blood gas	Heparinized TB	0.3
Arterial blood gas	Heparinized TB	0.3
Chromosomes	Green	1.0
FISH	Green	1.0
Cystic fibrosis DNA testing	Green	3–4
Polymerase chain reaction	Purple/Green	0.5

CMV, cytomegalovirus; FISH, fluorescence in situ hybridization; Ig, immunoglobulin; TB, tuberculin syringe.

Index

Page numbers in *italics* refer to Figures; those in **bold** to Tables